Ending Fibromyalgia & Auto-Immune Disease: A Comprehensive Holistic Protocol

By Tony Xhudo M.S., H.N., B.C.

Ending Fibromyalgia & Auto-Immune Disease: A Comprehensive Holistic Protocol

By Tony Xhudo M.S., H.N., B.C.
Published by Dawn Xhudo
Copyright 2013 Dawn Xhudo

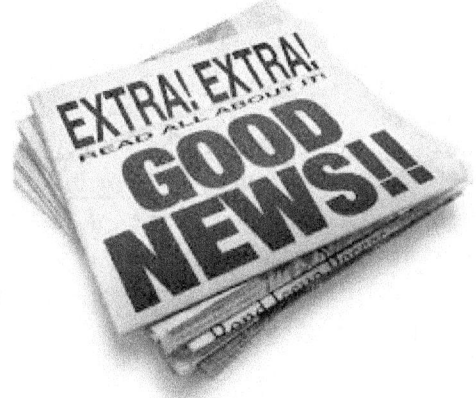

<u>Finally - No-More Pain!</u>

Disclaimer:

The information presented in this book was written for ***informational purposes only and is not by no means intended to treat, diagnose, or cure your conditio***n. This book is intended to open your mind and eyes so you can explore all potential options to help you make informed decisions for your health and wellness. The author and the publisher expressly disclaim all liability for any injury or harm that may arise from the use of the information contained in this book.

The treatments, herbs, vitamins, and supplements recommended in this book are meant to increase your knowledge of the latest developments in the use of dietary supplements, herbs, etc., and should not be taken without consulting your physician to be sure they are right for you with your particular medical condition. In the event you choose to use this information without your doctors approval, you are then prescribing for yourself, which is your constitutional right, but the author and publisher assume no responsibility.

DISCLOSURE:

DEDICATION

This Book is dedicated to the countless of millions of people who have suffered from the debilitating effects of Fibromyalgia and Auto-Immune Disease, in hopes that everyone that reads this book will bring the balance of good health back that they once lost. And to the many clients of mine that have come to me for help and guidance, in trying to cope with an illness that has had no diagnosis or specific treatment, that have suffered needlessly because of the lack of understanding by the majority of the present profession of medical practitioners.

I also, want to thank those for sharing their insights, stories, and struggles for having the confidence in me to help them with finding a remedy and cure, but have been told by many doctors that, "it's all in your head," which has inspired me to write this book. My hopes with this book is to overcome a stigma and the negative myths about this dreaded disease and help those sort through the maze of conflicting information concerning this illness.

Table of Contents

Preface

> *"The doctor of the future will give no medicine, but will involve the patient in the proper use of food, fresh air and exercise."* *Thomas Edison*

This book was carefully written to include natural healing treatment protocols that have been carefully selected and backed by scientific research from around the world that may offer hope to those that have been suffering from debilitating illnesses, FM/CFS syndrome. In this book you are about to read natural therapies that have been verified and discovered by solid scientific research. You will most definitely not run out of treatment options to chose from. Natural remedies that have improved the lives of those inflicted with FM, CFS, and Auto-Immune disease. This book also, offers complete and updated information that includes everything that you need to know to cure yourself from FM, CFS, and Auto-Immune System disorders.

You will explore for once and for all an illness that has escaped medical science from finding a possible cure or treatment that works, since doctors have been describing what we now know as Fibromylagia, since the early 1800's. And yes, it goes back that far. In 1884, a Scottish physician described tender points, <u>the hallmark of Fibromyalgia</u>. In 1904, Dr. William Gowers coined the phrase "fibrositis", which implies a disorder related to inflammation, and it wasn't until the late 1970's and 1980's that the medical researchers began to identify Fibromylagia and focused on diagnosing and treating it. In 1987, the American Medical Association (AMA), recognized FMS as a true illness and a major cause of disability. Now, unfortunately more than 20 years later most physicians still lack the training to diagnose and treat it!

<u>But unfortunately</u>, that is all they have been doing since then, just "<u>treating</u>" (Key word here), an illness that lingers on forever, that has now escalated to over <u>20 million people world wide</u>. For years medical science has been <u>treating the symptoms of Fibromyalgia and not the root cause of the disease</u>. <u>Example being, no one with a headache suffers, because of a deficiency of aspirin. And no one with depression has a deficiency of Prozac.</u>

Our medical system has been subduing symptoms with drugs but does not deal with the underlying causes of the disease itself. At the root of most ailments today in America, is poor nutrition. The good news is that a well nourished body can better manage and beat this disease. The bad news is that we have lost the war on Auto-Immune related illnesses, after spending billions of dollars in therapies chasing an illness that had no known diagnosis or treatment for over a century now.

Yet, it has also been known since as far back as 400BC when the "Father of Medicine" Hippocrates, who once said "Let Thy Food Be Thy medicine", meaning that optimal nutrition feeds the body and mind. It was Hippocrates who first developed the concept of – diet, exercise and happiness as the cornerstones of Health. Your diet being the host defense mechanism while empowering the mind of the diseased inflicted with the awareness that - "I Can Do Something About My Condition."

Naturopathic Medicine in practice considers the fundamental components of health – biochemistry, biomechanics, and the emotional predisposition – in order to help a person restore balance that we describe as good health. Many studies in the past of medical science and research have been supporting this concept all along with the use of optimal nutrition as a part of a comprehensive nutritional protocol. In fact, many years ago it was common for many doctors to prescribe natural medicine as a remedy for many of those who were stricken with disease and illness. For centuries natural remedies were keeping people alive, easing their pain, and preventing reocurring symptoms. Our medicines of the early 1800's were mostly herbal. Diseases such as Scurvy (vitamin C), Goiter (Iodine/Kelp) were cured with nutrition, not by medicine.

Today if you have arthritis, drugs treats the pain, but the arthritis doesn't go away. If you have high blood pressure, drugs are given to lower your blood pressure, but the problem does not go away, and if you go off your blood pressure medication, your blood pressure shoots up again. Treating these symptoms allopathically is different from treating them holistically. Recently, the World Health Organization estimated that 80% of the people worldwide rely on herbal medicine for some part of their primary health care. In Germany, 70% of the German physicians prescribe about 600-700 plant based medicines to their patients.

Fibromylagia is a disease that includes just about every symptom of pain you can imagine, but since there is known cause, and no known cure, there is just endless and profitable treatment for continuing pain. Those inflicted with this wretched disorder are very motivated to pay for treatment. The doctors have no incentive to cure, but rather suggest "treatments" that will prolong or even worse increase their symptoms with adding cocktails of additional drug therapy. Therefore, its the perfect disease!

As you read further on in this book you will see the proof of this proposition and description of Fibromylagia, and you will know with certainty that you have had it, or have it, or will get it, unless you are very lucky. You will also know that this disease covers any and every pain you could have, with only a slight stretch of fact. This has become the disease of choice for doctors and many drug producing companies looking for a profitable venture.

The value of nutritional dietary means cannot be over simplified, but yet modern science refuses to acknowledge this simple basic down to earth concept. But still yet, we as people are faced with "Life & Death" diseases that fall on the hands of big pharmaceutical companies to brew-up powerful drugs to line there pockets on exotic drugs that make billionaires out of them and the state representatives and politicians that support them.

An interesting article from the book - "Why Animals Don't Get Heart Attacks....But People Do!" by Dr. Matthias Rath's book, in which I urgently encourage you to read, expresses the pharmaceutical industry main primary function and existence. Which he strongly states that -

(1) Their purpose and driving force is to increase sales of pharmaceutical drugs for ongoing diseases and to find new diseases to market existing drugs.

(2) By their very nature, the pharmaceutical industry has no interest in curing diseases. Therefore, their eradication of any disease inevitably destroys a multi-billion dollar market of prescription drugs. Their cause and primary concern is only to develop drugs to relieve symptoms, but not to cure them.

(3) If eradication therapies for diseases are discovered and developed, the industry has a basic interest to suppress, discredit and obstruct these medical breakthroughs in order to make sure that diseases continue as the very basis for a lucrative prescription drug market.

(4) The economic interest of the pharmaceutical industry is the main reason why no medical breakthrough has been made for the control of most common diseases such as cardiovascular disease, high blood pressure, heart failure, diabetes, cancer, and osteoporosis, and why these diseases continue like epidemics on a worldwide scale.

(5) For the same economic reasons, the pharmaceutical industry has now formed an international cartel bt the code name "Codex Alimentarius" with aim to outlaw any health information in connection with vitamins and to limit free access to natural therapies on a worldwide scale.

(6) At the same time, the pharmaceutical companies withhold public information about the effects and risks of prescription drugs and life-threatening side effects are omitted or openly denied.

(7) In order to assure the status quo of this deceptive scheme, a legion of pharmaceutical lobbyists is employed to influence legislation, control regulatory agencies (e, g., FDA), and manipulate medical research and education. Expensive advertising campaigns to deceive the public.

(8) Millions of people and patients around the world are defrauded twice: A major portion of their income is used to finance the exploding profits of the pharmaceutical industry. In return, they are offered a medicine that does not even cure. And so with that I might add that "The money as they say, is not in the cure, but in the medicine!

Keep in mind that the above was written by a medical doctor. A doctor that honestly endeavors to heal and cure, and who is passionate about his beliefs in healing. There are many passionate doctors that take their profession serious and there are those that do not, but merely dispense medications as if they were candy. This conspiracy of the pharmaceutical industry is nothing new, it has been going on for quite some time now. There have been many doctors and scientists whom have been working together to find cures for diseases, that when they do, they get harassed by the *authorities and are told to keep quite or else!*

Many of them have also found cures to cancers, tumors, diabetes, etc., but instead of making it public are given ultimatums. The internet and libraries are full of conspiracy factors concerning nutrition and drugs, and many doctors and scientists that have also gone into exile because of it.
Today, Dr. Rath and others have joined in a struggle in Europe to fight for our rights in the freedom of use of vitamins, minerals, and herbs. The new "Codex Law" which chooses to take away our rights, if in affect, will take away our given right to purchase supplements as you wish for your own beneficial health and well being. For information on this subject that concerns every American's right for the use of supplements, please visit (www.mnwelldir.org).

There is a solution to this problem, contact your state representative and vote against the new "Codex Almentarius Law." Don't let the FDA & the FTC take away your rights for nutritional freedom. This new law wants to set new regulations that aim to outlaw any health information in connection with vitamins and limit your free access to natural therapies on a world wide scale. Their purpose is to regulate dietary supplements worldwide and set international safety standards for the purpose of increased trade. Pharmaceutical interests stepped in and began exerting their influence for their own personal greed, because supplements work and do benefit health to fight disease.

Their objective is to outlaw health products and any information on vitamins and dietary supplements, except those under direct control. If in affect, it would supersede the United States domestic laws without the American people's voice or vote in the matter. It is urgent that we as people do not let this happen and let this sort new type of dictation take affect on your God given freedom and own personal right to purchase dietary supplements. What will be next? Taking away our right to purchase health books, or any books for that matter. This could very well happen!

Please see – www.natural-health-information-centre.com/codex-alimentarius.html for further information.

People in general have to become passionate about their health and re-educate themselves on nutritional wellness & disease manifestations. Your health depends on your freedom to choose what you feel is right for you. It is within the scope of this book that not only covers about Fibromyalgia and Auto-Immune Disease, but also how disease manifestation occurs, and whole body detoxification techniques and methods you can employ to rid yourself of pathogens and create a healthy body and state of mind!

Know that diseases do have known causes and well understood mechanisms for producing symptoms. That is why most of the Naturopathic Physicians have cured and remedied nature's most debilitating disease, where modern medicine looks to treat and profit from diseases they say that there is no known cure for. Ask yourself why, that in some other parts of the world diseases like diabetes and cancers either don't exist or are cured. But in America where profits in medicine, medical doctors, hospitals and pharmaceutical drugs are very large, they just seem to never go away only to re-introduce newer type of drugs to deal with the symptoms.

They are the biggest business in America period, Two Trillion Dollars a year, and yet, <u>still haven't found the cure for the common cold?</u> Treatments for it? Yes, there by the hundreds from pharmaceutical over-the-counter medicine, to the more powerful prescription versions. The point that I'm trying to state here, is that "You can Heal Yourself" of any illness or any disease, if you just stop doing what's making you sick in the first place, and start doing what will create a healthy lifestyle or a healthy way of living that will cause your body to cure disease and heal itself. Know that your healing results are a direct response or reflection of the dedication and effort that you put in creating your healthy and healing lifestyle!

The human body was designed to heal itself of disease or illness, by eating foods that nourish your body that contain the highest concentration of nutrition and life force. Not by eating junk foods devoid of nutrition that are loaded with substances, and chemicals that block and congest your body's life force. <u>You have of whats in this book a plethora of informational wealth of potent supplement resources made available to you to basically live a clean, healthy, and disease free lifestyle!</u> And ward off disease and sickness.

<u>*This book was written for those who are ready to take responsibility for their health and well-being and do what ever it takes to heal themselves.*</u>

<u>*To Your Health & Awareness of Living Life Fruitfully,*</u>

The Author..Tony Xhudo, M.Sc./H.N.
March 19th, 2013

INTRODUCTION

FM & CFS: WHY ME?

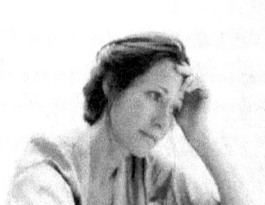

As a Holistic Health Practitioner I frequently get to hear whats on the hearts and minds of each client, listening as they reveal their lives and pains, their anxieties and fears. Each client's story is unique, and I'm perpetually astonished with some of the profound courage, pain, and endurance that each client of mine displays concerning their specific health problem. As a concerned Holistic Health Practitioner, I'm committed to treating the whole person, and not simply their disease, but what caused their illness and any other specific tale that may lead to any other underlying factors that may have contributed to their illness.

Through the years of consulting and helping each individual client make a complete recovery, I've discovered that Fibromyalgia has destroyed and wrecked the lives of many who are trying to cope with this debilitating illness. That is one of the main reasons why I chose to write this book. Fibromylagia has undermined and wrecked havoc on millions of people, an illness that resists typical medical treatment that only manifests additional symptoms. Let's clear the air right away and state that many of these poor souls that have been enduring Fibromyalgia/CFS have been basically experiencing the consequences of a susceptibility of past accumulative stress responses that have been built over time. Their symptoms, which I believe are the result of a three prong attack consisting of:

- *Stress. The main contributor to sickness and disease.*
- *A shortage of brain chemicals (neurotransmitters), specifically Serotonin, the master brain controller. Responsible for regulating pain, sleep, and emotional moods and behavior.*
- *A disrupting of unbalanced and/or inadequate hormone levels (estrogens, testosterone) – Adrenal (cortisol, dhea, pregnenolone), Thyroid (T4/T3), and Growth Hormone.*

And that is why I decided to write this book. The six finest words that any health care practitioner can ever hear are "I Feel So Much Better Now." This is what my clients tell me when they have applied the methods in this book. Nothing is more gratifying than helping those who have suffered from illnesses a good part of their lives when they walk in my office stating that they got their lives back.

With the aid of this book you will be able to resolve the many symptoms this illness has brought upon you. Your situation is far from hopeless. In fact, with a few lifestyle changes, nutritional supplements, and some safe, gentle alternative therapies, you can turn things around and get your life back as well!

With Fibromyalgia/CFS, the truth is the more you hear about it, the more you find out that many people have it. It just seems to be everywhere! Even the name of it seems horrifying! **F-i-b-r-o-m-y-a-l-g-i-a**, *which means – "a generalized musculoskeletal pain, stiffness, chronic aching, chronic fatigue, no energy, headaches, migraines, irritable bowls, depression, mood swings"*, etc.

But here's what it really means – *I can't sleep, I'm stressed out, I just want to lay in bed all day, I hurt all over, what hell is wrong with me?, and 'please' - "will somebody just shoot me!"*

But hey!, the good news is that you can feel good again, because what you have in your hands is a wealth of enormous scientific information to help speed you on your way towards recovery! My goal is to provide you with the most updated information you need; what causes your symptoms, how you got this dreaded disorder, and how you are going to feel great again. By applying the most effective holistic health therapies, that will help you get back on your feet, so you can kick the butt of this dreaded disease once and for all!

Having Fibromyalgia **(FMS)** and Chronic Fatigue **(CFS)** is like saying - *"which came first the chicken or the egg?"* Because of all the horrible symptoms of just about every bodily function that this disease affects, it makes one wonder, *"**how the hell did I wind up with this odd combination of mental and physical problems", was it caused by a physical thing or was it an emotional one?*** The sad thing is, you're not alone. Fibromyalgia affects over 20 million of people around the world, young, old, and the numbers just keep on growing. It got so bad that in 1990, the World Health Organization accepted Fibromyalgia as a disease. And so, it became official that all the symptoms were not in your head, they were for real! (as most doctors back then would say).

According to modern medicine fibromyalgia and chronic fatigue still have no known cause and no known cure. This is another reason why I chose to write this book, to tell you and the rest of the world that there is a remedy and a cure, but that depends on you! With all the information presented in this book about FMS and CFS, you can pretty much be rest assured that help is finally here, in getting rid of this disease, and starting a whole new healthy life.

This book is about learning how and why you got into this condition, and what you need to know to finally end this God forsaken illness. It isn't going to be easy, but the results and the relief of being miserable will be well worth it!

Chapter 1

UNDERSTANDING FIBROMYALGIA & CHRONIC FATIGUE SYNDROME

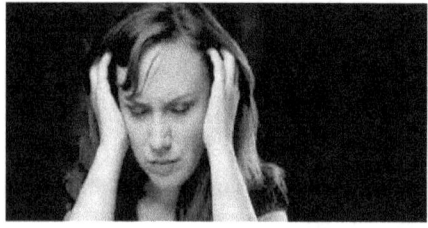

For most people who have had, or has FM /CFS, know that it can be a very complicated condition affecting you mentally and physically. Because of its complexity, Fibromyalgia can have an impact on virtually every part of your body. At the beginning of onset, you may have been told by your physician that, *"it's all in your head."* Unfortunately, this is one of the main reasons why Fibromyalgia is so misunderstood, misdiagnosed, and not properly treated.

Sort of an invisible illness that many find it so hard to believe that some one can hurt so much all of the time. Medical practitioners are quick to run tests to no avail, prescribing various medications from A to Z which may include: *anti-inflammatorys, anti-depressants, anti-convulsants, muscle relaxants, sleeping pills, and anxiety drugs, the list goes on,* thinking that maybe one or the other will do the trick. But not realizing they are only masking the symptoms and worsening their illness by not curing the problem. The end result of all this ***"prescription cocktail,"*** is that they wind up being more confused, more symptoms, and disoriented than ever, concluding, ***"Maybe I'm crazy, after all."***

But take heart, cause you're on your way to freedom! Freedom from feeling so miserable and no longer on the end of your rope thinking that impending doom is on the way, but that's not going to be the case here. The solutions to your debilitating dilemma is at it's end. Because by the time you finish reading this book, you will know how to solve this <u>mystery illness,</u> so labeled. My goal is to get you, to get to the root of the problem, and to help you to get your body's healing ability to return back to normal.

About Fibromyalgia & CFS

Fibromyalgia syndrome (FMS) and CFS is an 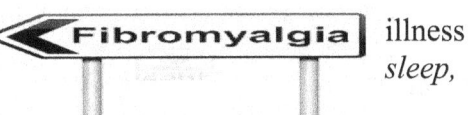 illness characterized by *diffuse muscle pain, poor* sleep, *and un-relenting fatigue,* being the most common, but there are a host of other symptoms that tag along as well. Over 10 million Americans suffer with FMS & CFS; ninety percent of them are women between 25 to 50 years old. At the moment diagnostic tests are currently unavailable to confirm or pinpoint these illnesses.

The diagnosis is usually reached after ruling out other conditions that include *neurological, auto-immune, endocrine, musculoskeletal, immunological, and mental disorders.* Hence, most of those who are stricken with this illness for at least 7 years and have been seen by a dozen of different doctors before they're diagnosed with fibromyalgia.

Fibromyalgia **(FM)** and Chronic Fatigue**(CFS)** are very similar, and actually in my belief and study, <u>Fibromyalgia is what you often end up with as a result of having Chronic Fatigue syndrome for a lengthy period of time</u>. That is why they are often called cousins. They both share the same set of symptoms and both being the result of a <u>self generated auto-immune disorder.</u> The research on **FM and CFS** both grew out of the field of immunology. The diagnosis of CFS was based on fatigue and at least 3 of the following symptoms that you have had for at least 6 months which include:

1. **Short-term memory loss(brain-fog)**
2. **Variations of symptoms in relation to activity, stress, and weather changes.**
3. **Muscle and joint pain**
4. **Headaches and increased thirst**
5. **Disordered and unrefreshed sleep**
6. **Recurrent or persistent infections and poor immunity**
7. **Tiredness after exertion that lasts for more than 24 hours**
8. **Yeast overgrowth, bowl infections, among others**
9. **Hormone deficiencies**
10. **Nutritional deficiencies**

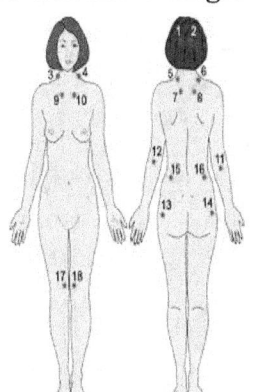

While a diagnosis of Fibromyalgia requires testing for a certain number of tender points on wide spread pain in all four quadrants of the body with a sensitivity in 11 of the 18 tender point sites of the body with a minimum of 3 months duration. The symptoms of Fibromyalgia primarily focus on pain, with the same similarities of CFS which includes – *severe fatigue, disordered sleeping patterns, tension headaches, tiredness, frequent infections, cold intolerance, and depression (McCain, 1998).*

One of the more devastating symptoms of Fibromyalgia is **sleep disorder.** But in those Fibromyalgia, the pain in the muscles and tissues make it impossible to lie in one position for an extended period of time. 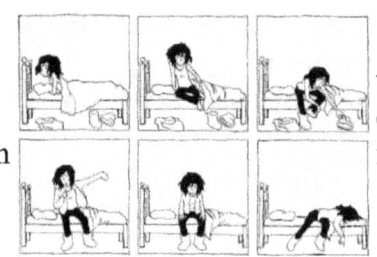 with connective

As a result of that the patient is continuously woken up into light sleep. Fibro' patients do not get the normal deep stages of sleep that allow for complete rest and recuperation. This situation creates a disturbance in growth hormone secretion which almost abolishes growth hormone production. This is also one of the "Key" points in Fibromyalgia regarding the muscle pain that Fibromyalgia patients often suffer from.

It has also been known for 25 years that FM patients have an abnormal sleeping pattern involving stages 3 and 4 of non REM sleep. As GH is secreted predominantly during stages 3 and 4 of non-REM sleep *(From Bennett et al, J. Rheumatol. 24:1384-1389, 1997)*

These low levels of growth hormone has also been associated with low energy, muscle weakness, sensitivity to cold, weakened ability to remember and think, and other problems that are seen in many people with Fibrobmyalgia. According to Dr. Alfonso Leal-Cerro, MD, professor of Endocrinology at the Hospital Universitario Virgen del Rocio in Seville, Spain, states that FM definitely has a hormone component that is attributed to this chronic condition.

What is Happening To My Body?

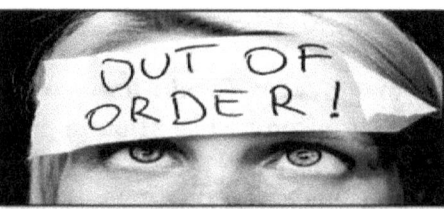

In 1843, a physician named Robert described the condition now known "Fibromyalgia" as rheumatism with places" that could be felt in many the body. Froriep first by the name of painful hard locations on

If you're suffering from this chronic condition that never seems to get better but only results in new symptoms you never had or felt before, then welcome to the world of **auto-immune disorder.** And I'm sure the most important piece of information that you want to hear if you have Fibromyalgia is that relief is possible. Your pain level will drop from a ten to a one and your fatigue will melt away as if it was never there, and finally sleep through the night to awaken refreshed. But first let's go ahead and explain to you of how you could of been so lucky (no-pun intended), to have acquired such a dreadful annoying syndrome that causes you to have this wide spread-pain from head to toe.

Fibromyalgia (FM) and Chronic Fatigue Syndrome (CFS) are considered separate but related disorders, a "phantom" chronic pain and fatigue that affects 5% (20 million), of the American population, with women being (75% - 90%) the most likely victims **(Pellgrino, 1989)**. People suffering from Fibromyalgia
experience a variety of painful and debilitating symptoms, including:

Symptoms

- **Chronic fatigue**
- **Wide spread chronic musculo skeletal pain from head to toe**
- **Disrupted and un-refreshed sleep**
- **Tenderness on palpation of specific anatomical sites generally referred to as tender points on the body.**
- **Chronic achy feeling**
- **Subjective soft tissue swelling**
- **Gastrointestinal disturbances**
- **Stiffness of the soft tissues of the body – muscles, ligaments, and tendons**
- **Anxiety, brain-fog, and cognitive difficulties**
- **Depression and mood swings**
- **Chronic bladder and vaginal infections**
- **Insomnia**

The symptoms of Fibromyalgia may also be worsened by *physical exercise, mental stress, poor sleeping habits, daily activity around the household, or exposure to the cold*. There are three variations of Fibromyalgia: primary, secondary, and localized. Primary fibroblast is the most common type of Fibromyalgia and is much more prevalent in women than men (7 times). And the primary symptoms are usually accompanied by other symptoms, including – *poor sleep, anxiety, depression, fatigue, and irritable bowl syndrome.*

Secondary Fibromyalgia occurs in people in which the symptoms of Fibromyalgia are the result of an underlying condition, such as hypothyroidism and adrenal fatigue. Secondary symptoms of Fibromyalgia is also wide-spread in the body. Localized Fibromyalgia is more common in men and the symptoms come on more rapidly than in primary or secondary Fibromyalgia. The symptoms of localized Fibromyalgia are usually the result of an occupation or sports, and are generally localized in a particular area of the body.

Meeting The Criteria of Fibromyalgia & Chronic Fatigue

Despite much research and more speculation on the subject, much of Fibromyalgia remains poorly understood. It is a complex and

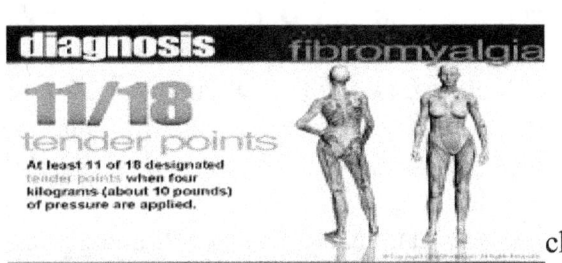

chronic

disease that causes wide spread pain and profound fatigue. The many associated symptoms of Fibromyalgia affect a wide variety of disparate parts of the body which often makes it difficult for doctors to grasp the connections among a *foggy brain, pains throughout the body, frequent bladder infections, brittle nails,* and poor hair quality, and try to understand them as relevant symptoms of the same disease.

That is the problem often found with Fibromyalgia, the symptoms are common with other diseases as well, and can mimic a variety of other medical problems. Like auto-immune diseases such as multiple sclerosis, under active thyroid, anemia, lyme disease, irritable syndrome, TMJ syndrome, lupus, allergies, CFS, heavy metal toxicity, and clinical depression.

To patients as well as doctors, Fibromyalgia can be quite frustrating as it is confounding. Test results given often show negative, as there are no validating laboratory X-rays, or scanning techniques to provide sound footing for physicians to confirm that something is wrong. Instead, doctors make their diagnoses based on a pattern of symptoms that consists of diffuse pain present for 3 months or more and 11 areas that are tender or painful to deep touch.

To see if you meet the criteria, a doctor applies firm pressure to 18 different areas on the body to see which areas elicit pain. If 11 of those areas are painful, the pain has been present for 3 months or more and other medical conditions are ruled out, the diagnosis of fibromyalgia can be made. For these reasons, Fibromyalgia is often described as an **"invisible disability."** Because of this, Fibromyalgia was considered a **"psychogenic"** (mental rather than physical condition), which many people have gone for years without a correct diagnosis, with only sporadic, but largely ineffective treatments.

However, it is now been firmly established as a real disease **(Arthritis & Rheumatism 1997;40(4):752-60).** It is associated with disability of a magnitude comparable to that of other chronic pain conditions. And as of today, fibromyalgia has become increasingly common, to that it was - recognized as a disease by the **"World Health Organization in 1990."** Studies have confirmed that Fibromyalgia is a **real disease**, described as the most common cause of wide spread chronic muscle pain. It's range of symptoms makes everyday tasks daunting, difficult, and often impossible. and that the altered responses to pain and exercise are physiologically based source **(Arthritis & Rheumatism 2002;461136-1138, 1333-1350).**

Although, Fibromyalgia is not a terminal illness, it is a demoralizing and debilitating one. The symptoms for some people can be very unbearable – so much so that the famous so-called **"Suicide Doctor", Jack Kevorkian, in 1997,** helped a few patients of his end their suffering. One of these Fibromyalgics, was a forty-year old Janis Murphy. Doctors now know that pain interferes with recovery; it can bring direct consequences, such as increased blood pressure, heart attack, seizure, brain hemorrhage and stroke. This is the truth about chronic pain to suicide.

Research shows that nearly every FMS patient considers suicide at one point or another, and the suicide rate among FMS patients is high. From this as well as as it's current wide spread popularity for those unfortunate one's stricken with this disease, Fibromyalgia cases have reached epidemic proportions in the form of US Social security disability claims, workers' compensation, and accident litigation. There are over 25% of American Fibromyalgia patients that have received some form of disability or injury compensation.

The name Fibromyalgia, a Greek word meaning **"pain" in the muscles and fibers,** has now largely replaced the previously popular term *"fibrositis",* which was once used to describe this disorder. The *"itis" meaning inflammation of a bodily process that can result in - pain, swelling, stiffness, and redness.*

But Fibromyalgia is part of a *wider syndrome encompassing headaches, irritability, irritable bladder, dysmenorrhea, cold sensitivity, exercise intolerance, complain of weakness, restless legs, atypical patterns of numbness and tingling.* Earlier research has also described this dreadful condition as a chronic inflammation in the muscles, tendons, and ligaments, but recent information and research has proved that the inflammation of Fibromyalgia is *really a form of a muscular and soft tissue rheumatism, rather than arthritis of the joints.* It typically presents itself in young or middle aged women (25 to 50 yrs. old), and it can also occur in men as well.

CFS/Fibromyalgia Checklist - Diagnostic Criteria

This basic checklist will help those determine if you have CFS or FMS? If you have had severe fatigue or widespread pain persisting over 3 months without any obvious cause, and have had insomnia, and disturbed sleeping patterns, and headaches. Then you might have CFS and/or FMS. The checklist below can help you access the possibility of this. This criteria has been established by the ACR(American College of Rheumatology).

CFS -Checklist

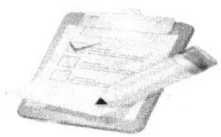

1. Do you frequently experience unusually long periods of fatigue?
2. Is your fatigue the result of some ongoing physical exertion that you are not aware of?
3. Does you fatigue go away after you have rested normally?
4. As a result of your ongoing fatigue, have you substantially reduced your previous levels of occupational, educational, social, or personality activities?
5. **Check off each of the following symptoms below** that began at the same time as your fatigue, and that has persisted for at least 6 months.
- Impairment in short term memory or concentration, severe enough to cause substantial reduction in previous levels of personal activity?
- Sore throat?
- Tender neck or axillary(armpit) lymph nodes?
- Muscle pain?
- Multi-joint pain without swelling or redness?
- Headaches of a new type, pattern, or severity?

- Unrefreshed sleep?
- Post-exertion fatigue lasting more than 24 hours?

FMS Checklist

Check off each area you've had pain over the last week.
- Left shoulder girdle
- Right shoulder girdle
- Upper left arm
- Upper right arm
- lower left arm
- Lower right arm
- Hip buttock, trochanter, right side
- Hip buttock, trochanter, left side
- Upper left leg
- Upper right leg
- Lower left leg
- Lower right leg
- Jaw left side of face
- Jaw right side of face
- Chest
- abdomen
- Upper back
- Lower back
- Neck

Rate the severity of your fatigue during the past week
- No problem
- Slight or mild problems, generally mild or intermittent.
- Moderate, considerate problems, often present and/or at a moderate level.
- Severe: pervasive, continuous, life-disturbing problems.

Rate the severity of your having felt unrefreshed sleep after you've woken up each morning
- No problem
- Slight or mild problems, generally mild or intermittent.
- Moderate, considerate problems, often present and/or at a moderate level.
- Severe: pervasive, continuous, life-disturbing problems.

Rate the severity of your cognitive dysfunction (i.e., feelings of "Brain Fog") during the past 6 months.
- No problem
- Slight or mild problems, generally mild or intermittent.
- Moderate, considerate problems, often present and/or at a moderate level.
- Severe: pervasive, continuous, life-disturbing problems.

Check each of the following symptoms that you have experienced during the past 6 months.

- Headaches
- Pain or cramps in lower abdomen
- Depression

Possible Causes of FMS & CFS

While the underlying cause still remaining a mystery, new research findings continue to bringing us closer to closing the gap of understanding the basic mechanisms of fibromyalgia and chronic fatigue. Most researchers tend to agree that (FM) is a disorder of endocrine/neurotransmitter deregulation brought on by chronic and unrelenting stress. The links between Fibro and Chronic Fatigue and stress have now been established. Research has made it clear that these two diseases have been influenced by stress in a number of ways.

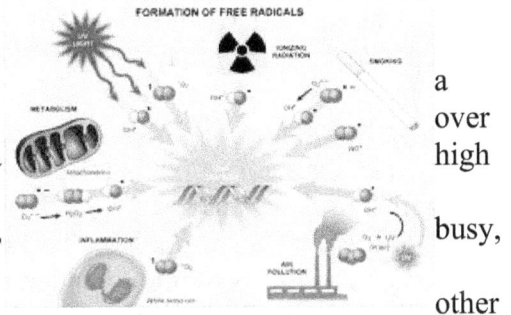

Stress plays a key role in many people that suffer from these diseases, they all tend to have a history of chronic stress, often due to stress over load taking on too many responsibilities. With a high number of them being young women who have "Type A" personalities and who lead ambitious, busy, stressful lives, suffer the most of from the consequences of stress over-load. Men on the other hand with Fibro' often have worked in jobs that have resulted in physical job related stress.

The onset of Fibromyalgia is triggered by an extremely stressful experiences. This onset of this crippling disease results in 50% of auto-immune disorders that were triggered by stress. Physical and psychological stress has been implicated in the development of auto-immune disease, since numerous animal and human studies demonstrated the effect of sundry stressor on immune function. Moreover, many retrospective studies found that a high proportion (up to 80%) of patients reported uncommon emotional stress before disease onset. Unfortunately, not only does stress cause disease, but the disease itself also causes significant stress in people, creating a vicious cycle.

It also presumed that the stress-triggered neuroendocrine hormones lead to immune deregulation, which ultimately results in auto-immune disease, by altering or amplifying cytokine production. Therefore, the treatment of auto-immune disease should include stress management and behavioral intervention to present stress-related immune system imbalance.

Stress Response and Auto-Immune Disease: The Cause and The Effect

According to Dr. Esther M. Sternberg, Chief of the Section on Neuroendocrine Immunology and Behavior at the National Institute of Mental Health, speaks of how stress can worsen disease, and how understanding the cross-talk between brain and the immune system can help us structure our lives to help us heal. He states, that a blunting of the brain hormonal stress response is also an important contributor to the development of auto-immune disease. The reasons for this is that cortisol, the potent anti-inflammatory hormone that is released from the adrenal glands in response to stress, is also released after exposure to inflammatory triggers.

In normal circumstances cortisol keeps the immune system in check, preventing inflammation from going out of control. In many patients with auto-immune disease, this cortisol response and the cascade of brain hormones that stimulate its release are impaired, so there is no shut off valve to end inflammation when it is no longer needed.

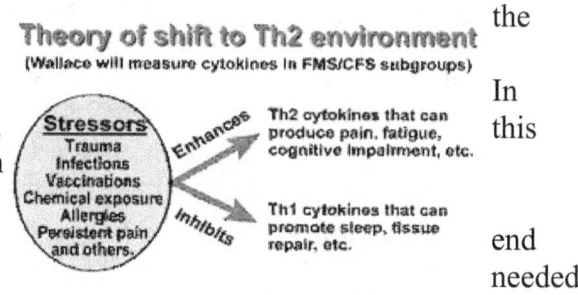

Cortisol is also one of the main stress hormones that is released by the adrenal glands when we are under stress. And not just the normal "flight or fight" response type of stress, but also the everyday, chronic levels of stress that we are under these days.

 When you are under a lot of stress your body produces high levels of cortisol and Fibromyalgia is a condition that is mainly known for it's high pain levels. Interestingly enough, cortisol does have a very positive job in all this and that is as an inflammatory agent. This is also very important, because cortisol is the main way our body tries to counter act the effects of inflammation and reduce inflammation as well. The problem however, happens when the inflammation becomes chronic, because this chronic inflammation is a physical stress on our body and it continually triggers the release of cortisol.

The more and more, our lives are filled with stress and sometimes seem to spin out of control, the more cortisol we tend to produce. This excess cortisol triggers the breakdown of other bodily functions that interfere with normal everyday functions. Left unresolved, it can create a host of health problems. When this goes on for too long of a time period, many different ill-health conditions arise, contributing to symptoms of pain and inflammation, affecting a cascade of endocrine related manifestations.

Chronic stress is one of the main triggers for auto-immune disorders. Your immune system is a complex network of organs, glands, and special cells that encompasses your entire body, designed to protect and guard you against foreign invaders that can harm you or compromise your body's ability to function in a healthy way. One reason why stress is believed to play an important role in auto-immune disorders is because of its effects on hormonal and cellular changes in the body. Stress can also have effects on other hormones, brain neurotransmitters, prostaglandins, crucial enzymatic systems, and metabolic activities that are still unknown. Understanding these concepts are very important in understanding the diseases caused by stress and to create a plan of action for the management of stress and stress induced diseases. Besides being a trigger for auto-immune disorder, there are many other stress induced diseases that include:
- High Blood Pressure
- Acid Peptic Disease

- Tension or Migraine Headaches
- Insomnia
- IBS
- Psychoneurosis
- Sexual Dysfunction
- Skin Diseases – Psoriasis, Urticaria, Pruritus, Neurodermatitis, Lichen planus, etc.
- Asthma
- High Cholesterol
- Heart Disease
- Alcoholism
- And many others!

It has become fairly obvious now that stress is the number one killer in the US that leads to many chronic health issues. But what most people don't know or realize is how damaging chronic stress can actually be for you!

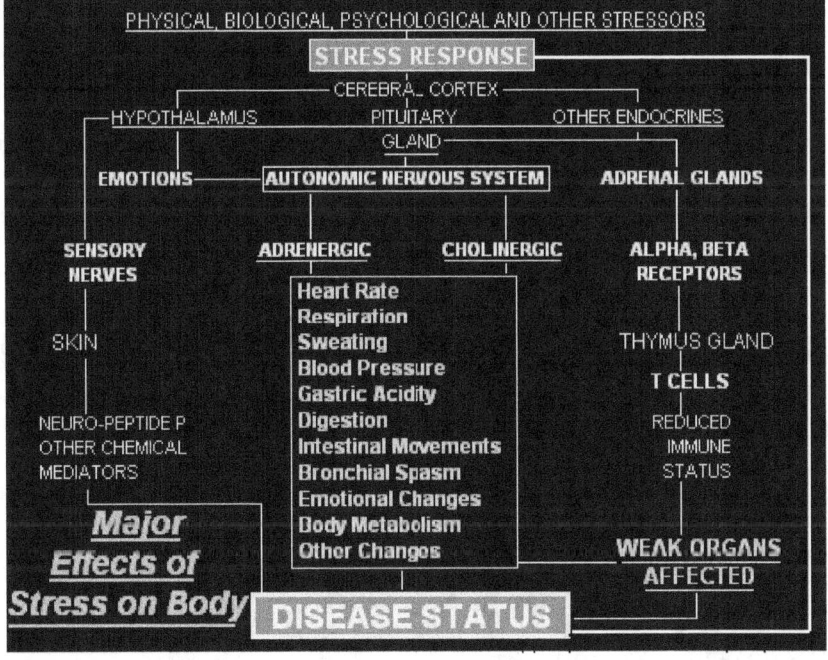

For instance, many people do not realize that when the body is highly stressed it will not heal itself. And when left in this chronic stressful situation, it begins to inhibit the immune system causing a malfunction in its ability to self regulate. This puts a tremendous strain on the body, and can cause severe damage if its left "on" too frequently. The digestive system begins to shut down affecting every part of the digestive system. It can increase the acid in your stomach causing indigestion. It can also cause your esophagus to go into spasms. Make you feel nauseous, constipated, and cause diarrhea. And worse, it can lead to malabsorption problems, Leaky Gut syndrome, IBS, Crohn's disease, etc.

Remember, the stomach is also believed by many to be the *"seat of all human* _emotions.__"_ How many times have you come to a thought or difficult situation or decision, and have said _"I've got a bad feeling about this",_ well the reason being is our digestion is controlled by the enteric nervous system, a system composed of hundreds of millions of nerves that communicate with the central nervous system.

Your body is a marvelous, complex, and miraculous system. And as with any system, the ability of the whole to function smoothly and efficiently depends upon each small part remaining intact and in optimum working order. Your digestion in all its detail is the foundation of good health. Chronic stress if left unresolved can assault the immune barrier between the digestive system and the nervous system as they interact in the case of auto-immune diseases. Hopefully you've gained a little bit of understanding and insight of how stress can impact the start of a debilitating illness such as auto-immune disorder.

Although, all stress in life is unavoidable. We all have some form of daily stress to daily with, some may have more than others and some may not. Stress management becomes crucial in dealing with any stressful situations that may occur in the future. Learn to apply some of the stress techniques listed in this book, and add some of the herbal adaptogens that will help you manage stress in a much more more healthful and beneficial way.

Chapter 2

Auto-Immune Disorders & FM/CFS

The most common cause of all disease in the world today is auto-immune disease. Auto-immune disease is a real terror that threatens the entire body. There are more than 80 different types of auto-immune disorders. And a person can generally have more than one auto-immune disorder at the same time. It is also estimated that 75% of auto-immune related disorders occur in women, and most frequently during their child bearing years. Why? It seems that higher estrogen levels seem to stimulate the immune system, which may explain why men are less affected. Some examples of auto-immune or auto-immune-related disorders include:

- Addison's disease _(adrenal insufficiency, hypocortisolism))_
- Celiac disease _(gluten sensitivity)_
- Dermatomyositis _(skin disorder)_
- Graves disease _(enlargement of the thyroid gland gland, overactivity)_
- Hashimoto's Thyroiditis _(hypothyroidism, chronic thyroid damage)_
- Multiple Sclerosis _(an inflammatory disease, leading to damage of the myelin sheaths)_
- Myasthenia Gravis _(auto-immune neuromuscular disease)_
- Pernicious anemia _(red blood cell disorder, lack of)_
- Reactive Arthritis _(a chronic, systemic rheumatic disease)_
- Rheumatoid Arthritis _(chronic systemic inflammatory disorder affecting many tissues & organs)_
- Sjogern Syndrome _(destruction of the exocrine glands, tears & saliva)_
- Systemic Lupus Erythematosus _(a systemic auto-immune disease affecting any_

part of the body)

- Type I Diabetes (*destruction of insulin producing beta cells of the pancreas*)
- Fibromylagia/CFS (*a chronic widespread painful inflammatory disorder & severe fatigue*)
- Chronic Lyme Disease (*an infection caused by a bacterium "Borreelia burgdoferi, causing pain and fatigue conditions*)
- And many others!

Fibromyalgia and chronic fatigue, also share a common link with Auto-Immune disease, they can all be defined as an idiopathic disease being labeled as <u>one that develops without any apparent or unknown cause.</u> One widely accepted estimate of FM/CFS syndrome sufferers world wide are at a staggering 90 million people, and that was nearly 20 years ago! With over 300,000 people in the U.K. that have been diagnosed with CFS and Fibromyalgia. Today the official figure probably represents the tip of the iceberg with more and more people being diagnosed with these dreaded diseases.

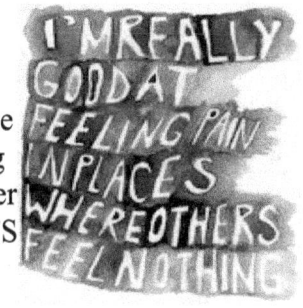

Researchers are beginning to believe that there is a strong auto-immune relationship with Fibromyalgia and Chronic Fatigue sufferers, as well as other idiopathic diseases. These diseases may in fact be found to be varying manifestations of the same underlying autoimmune problems.

What Is Auto-Immune Disorder

Auto-Immune disorder is when our body produces an inappropriate immune response against its own organs. In other words, the body actually begins to attack its own cells. When our body encounters something foreign in its own environment it needs to be able to build an immune response against these foreign substances to protect itself from harm. When this happens the body will start to produce anti-bodies that attack its own cells, tissues, and other organs which may be restricted to certain organs (e.g. in thyroiditis), or involve a particular tissue in different places (e.g. the kidneys/adrenals), overall affecting over 23 million Americans. This is what causes the inflammation and damage that leads to auto-immune disorder.

Your Body's Main Components of The Immune System
"Information You Need To Know"

<u>**Thymus gland**</u>- This is the master gland of the immune network. Located above the heart, it secrets various hormones that are responsible for regulating the immune system functions. It also produces T-cells, which are another major player in the immune system functioning. The thymus gland is extremely susceptible to damage from stress, environmental toxins, infections, and chronic

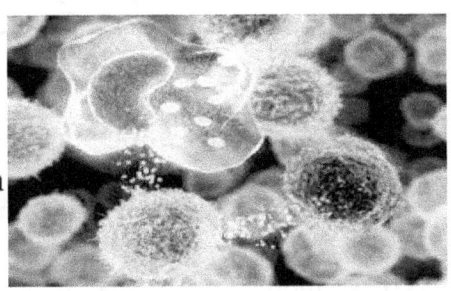

illness.

Skin and Mucous Membranes – The skin is your body's largest organ which is also its first line of defense against foreign intruders. The mucus membranes of the gastrointestinal tract, lungs, vagina, nose, mouth, and so on, are the body's "internal skin", and are also a line of defense against invaders.

Bone marrow – The center portion of the bone is an area rich in blood vessels and other substances. It is here that many types of immune cells are manufactured.

Spleen – The dark red organ, located on the left side of the upper abdominal area, manufactures lymphocytes, attacks bacteria, and recycles damaged blood.

Lymph Nodes – These tiny, gland like structures are found throughout the body, including the under arms, in the groin, and behind the ears. If you've ever had "swollen glands", what you had were inflamed lymph nodes. And the reason being that they were inflamed or swollen is because the lymph node as act as an inspection station for foreign substances, which they remove from the body's tissues.

The Lymphatic System – This network consists of lymph vessels, lymph nodes, and lymph, a thick fluid that is made up of fat and white blood cells. While the circulatory system is the transportation system for the blood, the lymphatic system carries immune cells to parts of the body where they are needed.

Lymphocytes – Types of white blood cells, produced in the bone marrow and are found in the blood and in the spleen, lymph nodes, thymus, and other tissues. Lymphocytes perform perform four primary functions, all of which must work properly for a healthy immune system. They recognize invaders, they prepare a line of defense, and communicate with other essential immune system cells by producing cytokines and deploying them to act against the invaders; and stop the action of the immune cells once their job is done. If anyone of these steps goes awry, disease, including auto immune conditions, can be the result.

When your immune system is functioning normally - when all its components are operating optimally it can alert you and effectively fight off many of the different types of enemies, such as bacteria, viruses, parasites, and fungi, and the harmful effects of stress. Unfortunately, people with unhealthy immune systems that are the result of nutritional deficiencies, unhealthy lifestyles, chronic stress are burdened with chronic life altering symptoms that eventually wind up with some type of auto-immune disorder. When this happens, instead of fighting foreign invaders with anti-bodies-substances, the immune system components start to attack the body's own healthy cells, the bones, glands, joints, blood, brain, nerves, or other parts as if it was the enemy. This is known as an auto-immune disorder.

Possible Causes of Auto-immune Disease

There are more than 80 separate medical conditions that

have been recognized as being the result of an auto-immune response, with fibromyalgia being one of them. Some of these like rheumatoid arthritis, lupus, multiple sclerosis, hypothyroidism (Hashimoto's thyroiditis), hyperthyroidism (Grave's disorder), Chrohn's disease, ulcerative colitis, type 1 diabetes, autism, **chronic fatigue syndrome**, ankylosing spondylitis, auto-immune hepatitis, auto-immune kidney disease, polymyostis, scleroderma, Sjogren's syndrome, and vascultis. With evidence proving that these diseases all share a common source, here are some additional factors that weigh into this theory -

- Family or personal history of auto-immune disease.(possible risk factor)

- **Gender or hormone status** – 75% of auto-immune disease occurs in women, and in most frequencies of child bearing years. Higher estrogen levels seem to stimulate the immune system, which may explain why men are less affected.

- **Bacterial and viral infections and illness** - are all implicated in auto-immune disease. Often a battle of Epstein- Barr virus triggers the onset of auto-immune disease.

- **Toxic metal exposure** – 25% of the public has some form of toxic metal exposure.

- **Toxic chemical exposure** – toxins such as pesticides, solvents, industrial chemicals, household cleaners and hair dyes have all been implicated in auto-immune disease.

- **Vaccinations/Immunizations** – scientists have found a connection between auto-immune disease and vaccinations.

- **Stress and Trauma** – Many studies have shown a direct link between a major stressful lifestyle event and the development of an auto-immune disease within 6 to 12 months later. Unmanaged stress is a risk factor for the development of all major diseases, including heart disease and cancer. Our thoughts and feelings have a direct effect and impact on our immune system. Loneliness is now recognized as the number one predictor of disease due to its immune suppressing action. Laughter and feelings of happiness, on the other hand, increase and enhance the action of our immune cells.

- **Smoking** – Smoking increases the risk of several auto-immune diseases, primarily because of the chemicals found in cigarettes.**Nutritional deficiencies** – Poor diets are an important factor in auto-immunity because poor nutrition compromises the immune system. Processed foods are loaded with chemicals, hormones, steroids, trans fats, and sugars, which promote the creation of free radicals in the body, which in turn damages the cells.**Associated Factors In The Development of Auto-Immune Disorder?**According to scientific research and study, the cause of autoimmune disorder is still unknown, but it appears to be an inherited predisposition, or a relentless state of chronic stress in many of the cases. Auto-Immune disease can affect anyone. Yet certain people are at a greater risk, including:

- **People with a family history of auto-immune diseases** that run in families, such as lupus, and multiple sclerosis. Inherited certain genes that can make it more likely to get an auto-immune disease.

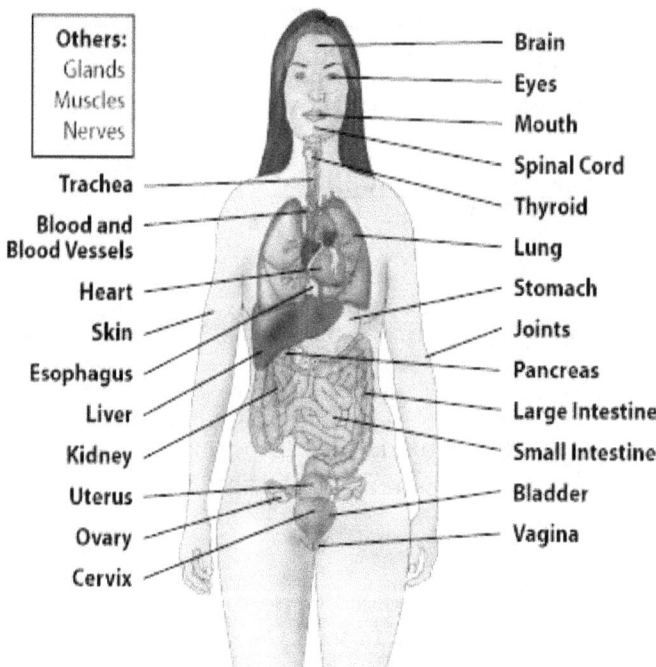

Body Parts That Can Be Affected by Autoimmune Diseases

- **People who are around certain environmental exposures** including, chemical solvents, chemical factories, and viral and bacterial infections are also linked to many auto-immune diseases.

- **People of certain races and ethnic backgrounds** that can affect certain groups of people more so than others. Example, type I diabetes are more common in white people than in other ethnic groups. With Lupus being more prevalent in African and Hispanic people.

- **Chronic Stress & Trauma sufferers**. Stress, the number one cause of all related disease manifestations can be the main contributor and the direct link to the start of all disease related conditions. Stressful emotions can unleash a torrent of cortisol and free radicals that can affect many organs and tissues of the body, and can act as a trigger for many auto-immune diseases. Unmanaged stressful events can be a severe development of all major diseases having a direct impact on the immune system. Even loneliness is now recognized as the number one predictor of disease due to its immune suppressing actions on the body.

- **Gender or Hormonal status** – more than 75% of auto-immune disorders occur in women, possibly due to higher estrogen levels, caused by dietary factors and environmental.

- **Bacterial and Viral infections and Illnesses**, a virus such as Epstein-Barr virus, which can trigger the onset of auto-immune disease.

- **Toxic Metal Exposure**. It has been estimated that over 25% of of people have some form of heavy metal poisoning such as, mercury, lead, cadmium, arsenic, aluminum, nickle, and other heavy metals that can be linked to the auto-immune process. Heavy metals induce auto-antibodies which can create auto-immune illness.

- **Vaccines/Immunizations** – it has been found by science linking some auto-immune diseases with vaccinations. The February issue of Auto-Immunity, with 10 research articles evaluated the link between vaccinations. Example, the controversial Anthrax vaccine has been linked to the development of auto-immune related diseases.

- **Smoking** – also increases the risk for the development of several auto-immune diseases, primarily due to the chemicals and additives that have been found in cigarettes.

- **Nutritional Deficiencies** – poor diets will compromise the immune system. Processed foods are loaded with chemicals, additives, synthetic hormones, steroids, sugars, trans-fats which can promote the creation of free radicals in the body, which in turn damage the cells and tissues of the body.

The incidence of these diseases also continues to rise by 8% on a yearly basis, and between 10 to 30% of all doctor office visits are due to symptoms that resemble those of Fibromyalgia and chronic fatigue.

Researchers reported in the Journal of Clinical Investigations that there is a clear indication of autoimmune components in FM and CFS, and that approximately 52% of CFS and FM syndrome patients developed auto-antibodies indicative of autoimmune reactions.

German researchers also acknowledged this relationship between these debilitating syndromes and autoimmune disease. **(See - 1994 article published in the German Medical Journal) -** *Wein Med Wochenschr,* **[link url=http://www.ncbi.nlm.nih.gov./htbin-post/Entrez/query?]**

Common Signs & Symptoms of Auto-Immune Disease

Extreme Fatigue – a severe persistent fatigue not alleviated by rest. This also experienced by almost all universal auto-immune disease sufferers.

Muscle & Joint Pain – also found in almost every auto-immune disease. A general pain, burning, aching, and soreness in muscles or joint pain and aches.

Swollen Glands – Can be all over the body, but generally in the throat area, under arms, groin area, and top of the legs.

Inflammation - early warning sign of pain, especially when chronic, is a sign that something needs immediate attention. This is also a part of every auto-immune disease disorder.

Susceptibility to Infections - frequent colds, bladder infections, ear infections, sore throat, sinus problems, yeast infections, that all have a slow recovery time.

Sleep Disturbances – disturbed rest from sleeping 7 to 8 hours of normal sleep periods.

Weight Loss or Gain - changes of weight, typically in the 10 to 15 pound range, which may be unexplainable.

Low Blood Sugar – A sign of adrenal gland failure.

Blood Pressure Changes – most auto-immune sufferers have low blood pressure, but also not uncommon to have high blood pressure as well. Signs of feeling dizziness or vertigo, fainting spells, palpitations, and fluctuations in heart rate.

Candida Yeast Infections - Common in virtually all auto-immune sufferers. Can manifest as a digestive disturbance, sinus infection, vaginal yeast infections or thrush.

Allergies - having numerous food allergies, chemical and environmental sensitivities.

Digestive Disturbances – Abdominal pain, bloating, tenderness, heartburn, cramps, constipation, diarrhea, excessive gas, all can reflect a condition known as "leaky gut syndrome", very common with all auto-immune disorders.

Anxiety & Depression – mood and emotional changes, panic attacks, excessive irritability, common in all auto-immune disorders.

Memory Problems – Known as "Brain fog", common also in auto-immune disorders.

Thyroid Problems – Many are known to have hypothyroidism, although hyperthyroidism is also common. It may also not show up in normal thyroid tests. Can also manifest as low body temperature and excessive hair loss.

Re-Currant Headaches – Excessive periods of severe headaches or migraines in some people with auto-immune disease.

Low Grade Fevers – very common and might be experienced on a daily basis.

Re-Currant Miscarriage – Very common symptom in many auto-immune diseases.

As you can see by the above list that these symptoms are quite extensive and may be hard to believe that they may be connected, but usually they are the prelude to the manifestation of auto-immune disorder. If you are experiencing these symptoms it is important to follow up with further tests and consult with an auto-immune specialist to further diagnose a possible connection with auto-immune disease.

Testing For Auto-Immune Related Problems

Testing for auto-immune disease can start with your primary care physician that will proceed with a physical exam depending on the typical signs and type of the disease, and/or which he or she may refer you to an auto-immune specialist to diagnose an auto-immune disorder which may include:

- **Antinuclear antibody tests**
- **Auto-antibody tests**
- **CBC**
- **C-reactive Erythrocyte sedimentation rate (ESR)**

Getting a diagnosis may be also be a long and stressful process, as each auto-immune disease is unique, and may share some of the same symptoms. Which make it hard for doctors to find out if you really have auto-immune disease, or which one it may be. It is important to also help yourself with the process by writing down a complete family health history that includes an extended family history to share with your doctor. You can take these additional steps to help with a quick and positive diagnosis to find out the cause of your symptoms by:

- **Writing down an extended family health history.**
- **Record all possible symptoms your having, even if they seem unrelated.**
- **See a specialist who has experience in dealing with your most major symptoms.**
- **List your dietary regimen that you currently are following.**
- **Work related history.**
- **Any stressful and traumatic experiences.**
- **And if your doctor does not take your symptoms seriously or tells you that your symptoms are stress related or in your head (*which has been done many times before)*, if so, always get a second, third, or fourth opinion.**

Doctors that treat auto-immune disease are;

- **Nephrologists** – **treats kidney related problems.**
- **Rheumatologistologist** – **treats arthritis, and other rheumatic diseases.**
- **Neurologist** – **treats nerve related problems.**
- **Hematologist** – **treats blood related problems.**
- **Gastroenterologist** – **treats digestive related problems.**

- **Dermatologist** – treats skin related problems.
- **Physical Therapist** – treats speech related problems associated with multiple sclerosis.

Conventional Medical Treatment For Auto-Immune Disorder

The goals of conventional medical treatments are to reduce symptoms of the disorder, control the auto-immune process, and maintain the body's ability to fight the disease. Drugs normally used in the treatment of auto-immune disorder are:

- **Hormone replacement therapy – for damaged hormone producing glands.**
- **Enzyme replacement therapy – for damaged enzyme producing glands.**
- **Corticosteroids – Prednisone.**
- **NSAIDs – non-steroidal anti-inflammatory drugs used to treat inflammatiion.**
- **Immuno-suppresants – (a general class of immune suppressing drugs) Cytoxan, Neoral, and Sandimmune.**

NOTE: Side effects of immuno-suppresant drugs can have very serious effects leaving you vulnerable to a variety of opportunistic infections that would normally be prevented by the immune system. Which could make for the risk of serious and numerous complications.

Another approach that is often suggested in this book, is to get a complete "Hair Tissue Mineral Analysis" done to find out if there are any loads of toxicity concerning heavy metals that may contributed to an auto-immune illness. This test can provide you with a much needed information about mineral ratios that can be toxic and causing an imbalances in your body, especially if you are suffering from symptoms of auto-immune disease.

It has also been found that in a large number of cases, the cause of auto-immune disease can be traced to an over abundance of toxicity that the body had to deal with over many years, particularly heavy metals. It would be to your benefit in completing a hair analysis tests to determine your vulnerabilities. Contact a health care practitioner in your area and check to see if they offer this service for you, or you can check on the back of this book for laboratory's that can instruct you in obtaining a comprehensive hair analysis test for further information.

The Solution To Beating Auto-immune Disease

The solution to beating auto-immune disease lies in addressing the "root cause of auto-immunity", and in regulating the immune system response. Ideally this can happen without the side effects associated with pharmaceutical drugs such as interferon, predninsone, or methotrexate.

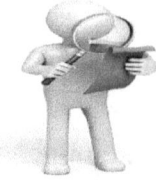

In a large number of cases, the cause of auto-immune disease can be traced to the overload of toxicity the body has had to deal with over so many years, particularly chronic stress and heavy metals. I suggest you consider having a hair tissue mineral analysis test done to determine which heavy metals the body is high in and which essential minerals the body is deficient in. This test can provide you with valuable information about mineral ratio's that can be toxic and that may be causing an imbalances in your body, especially if you are suffering from auto-immune disease.

The other solution is learning to manage your stressors and decide in having a lifestyle change in certain measures that can be of help in reducing the stress-related effects from every day issue's, with a nutrient dense dietary plan. A hair tissue mineral analysis can also help determine the severity of your internal organs such as your adrenal glands, your thyroid, thymus, liver, and kidney irregularities.

 I have found this test to be a very important factor for cases that I have been confronted with to help determine the exact cause of specific allergies towards foods, heavy metals, nutritional deficiencies, glandular problems, and imbalances. Also, in helping one know of any probability factors of health related diseases. A hair tissue analysis can be a great tool in establishing a proper health protocol in determining what your nutritional needs may be. I highly recommend it.

Hair tissue mineral analysis usually needs to be obtained through a health care practitioner. However, there are services that can be found through the internet from a federally licensed laboratory. Bare in mind also, that some states do not allow hair analysis tests to be submitted. Each hair analysis contains a detailed 10 to 15 page report from the laboratory itself, which shows you a bar graph readings indicating high, low and reference range levels for toxic metals, essential minerals, and significant mineral ratios. It also includes a metabolic profile, recommended for diet and supplement based on individuals.

Natural Treatment For Auto-Immune Disease

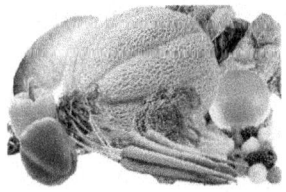

Your immune system is the most sensitive system of our whole entire body. It is easily subjected to the excessive demands of emotional and physical stressors, and it can begin to function erratically in a short period of time. Sometimes, it can even begin to attack your own body. So, the goal of a comprehensive healing program is to bring the body back into balance by using as many natural interventions as possible. The most useful interventions include some or all of the following:

- **Eliminate** all junk foods, processed and refined foods, all sugar by products.
- Include a **whole Body cleanse** to eliminate toxins, chemicals, parasites, yeast over growths, etc.

- **Add specific** herbs, amino acids, and phytonutrients during preparation for detox. (see section on body cleansing & detoxification)
- **Include a sound dietary plan** with some natural *therapeutic foods* and begin to adhere to a quality food diet, *juicing fresh vegetables & fruits* several times a week is also a great source of getting fresh live enzymes, vitamins, and minerals for super glandular health. (see section on body cleansing and dietary plan for detox).
- **Add an exercise program plan**, very important in health and well being.
- **Reduce your stressors** and include a stress management plan of course to follow which include yoga, tai-chi, and meditation. (see section on stress and diet, and *adaptogenic herbs*)
- **Induce an emotional and spiritual growth attitude.**
- **Take a hormone balancing supplement** to balance your hormones & neurotransmitters.
- **Include micronutrient supplements and super foods** that include *Colostrum,*** Royal Jelly, and Velvet Deer Antler.* They have done wonders in healing auto-immune disorders.
- Adding *Pancreatic Enzyme*s to your supplement program is one of the major healing protocols in reversing auto-immune disease.

Your goal here is to gradually diminish the use of potentially harmful *junk foods, chemicals, and medications* over time. Eventually, your body will return back to it's healthy state of good health and most of your medications can be slowly stopped. Healing will occur if the original imbalances and unhealthy lifestyle are corrected. Remember, the symptoms you have developed are your own body's way to communicate with you that it has become unhealthy and out of balance. Heed its messages, because relapses are possible if you revert back to your old ways. Good Health to You! Let the healing begin!

If you are living with auto-immune disease, there are many alternative things you can do each day to feel better and eventually eliminate the disease altogether. The list above are the basic guide lines to help you determine the proper course of action. There are also many alternative methods/supplements that are very effective in reversing this condition as you will soon begin to see, as I list them in their important perspective categories. The first main objective in healing auto-immune disease, is going to be, to come up with a healthy dietary plan, as always is the case when dealing with illnesses. That is the first important guideline, *"Let Thy food Be Thy Medicine & Thy Medicine Be Thy Food.",* Hippocrates 400 BC.

Dietary Plan & Healing Auto-Immune Disease

Throughout the ages human beings have been the product of their environmental conditions. Basically, we are what we eat. If we eat like crap, we become like crap, setting the stage for disease manifestation to begin. Of course, we as humans always tend to eat what tastes good to our pallets. Usually sweets, salty, and spicy combinations of foods. And generally what can be prepared in a fast and tasty way, junk foods, fast food restaurants, hot dogs, hamburgers, tacos, etc., etc. The list goes on!

Dietary changes as a holistic health practitioner has always been the number one difficult thing for me to employ concerning my past clientele of individuals. People, in generally when they have been accustomed to eating certain dietary foods consisting of processed, fatty, and hormonal active based foods, devoid of any nutritional means are one of the most contributing factors in their health. However, those that do recognize the importance of good and healthy nutrition do often make the change, why? Because they actually are tired of feeling sick, and want to get better.

It can not be stressed enough just how important diet is to health and disease, and I'm sure that a lot of health care physicians agree with me on this. But before I begin listing the basic requirements to this dietary change that you must employ, I would like to also add the **importance of regular exercise,** which helps the immune system function most responsively. An aggressive dietary nutritional approach to auto-immune illness should always be tried first when the disease is in its infancy. And logically of course the more advanced the disease is, the more damage that has been done by the disease you will respond. But that does not mean to its end also. It just would require an additionally strong and aggressive course of action. Remember, all diseases are curable! Never let anyone tell you differently!

The first requirement would be to cleanse the body of any impurities and toxins to begin adding your nutritional requirements. This has to to be done, if your seeking complete recovery from your illness. I mean would you move into a house that's filthy and dirty contaminated with germs and pathogens? Of course not! Its the same thing with detoxing your body. When you begin, follow the section on whole body detoxification on **chapter 16** for a complete guide line. *For specific dietary guidelines and procedures please see chapters 21, 22, 23, 25, and 26 for a complete breakdown on a dietary protocol of action.*

Dietary Plan

Because people with auto-immune diseases appear to have a predisposed weakness in their immune systems, it is strongly recommended that you adhere to a diet of foods in the *"super foods" category in chapter 18.* Also, avoiding contact with chlorinated water is of the utmost importance. As the chlorinated water kills bacteria, friendly and unfreindly, in the intestines. It can just as well be absorbed through the skin when bathing or taking a shower. So, it is recommended to install a shower filter to remove the chlorine for an uninterrupted healing response.

Therapeutic Healing Foods For Auto-Immune Disease

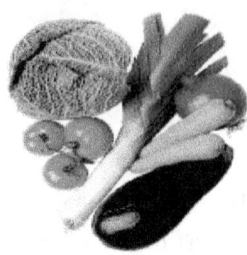

Making a change to therapeutic foods can make a big difference in your healing response and can contribute greatly to the health of your immune system and digestive tract. Remember, virtually all diseases manifest in the stomach! A healthy stomach (digestive system) makes for a healthy body and mind. Taking care of your gastrointestinal health is "Key" to your overall health ----- whether your battling cancer, heart disease, auto-immune disease, diabetes, or any other ill health related condition.

Individuals that have followed these specific healing protocols have dramatically improved their assimilation and absorption of foods and nutrients. And specifically have healed their long standing symptoms and have remained disease free by following these healing protocols. These specific foods should be consumed as often as possible.

Mushrooms – *Shiitake and Chag*a mushrooms contain more immunity building properties than most of the mushroom varieties. Incorporating these beneficial immune enhancing mushrooms can greatly help you to establish a proper functioning immune system.

Fresh Vegetable Juice (Juicing Machine) – consume vegetable juices that are low in carbohydrates, such as celery and green juices mixed with a small amount of higher carbohydrate veggies such as carrots or beets. Mix in some sort of healthy fat with each glass of juice. One to three tablespoons of cultured Goat's milk, extra virgin coconut oil, canned or fresh coconut milk and cream, or flax seed oil enhances absorption of minerals and prevents spikes in blood sugar. *(see the "Juicing Bible" by Pat Crocker, for excellent juicing recipes)*

Cultured Goat's Milk – consume 8 to 32 ounces of the highest quality goat's milk (See Probiogurt). Do not purchase any yogurt that contains the organism "Strepoccus thermophilus," it contains a bacterial microbe that has been known to make the immune system disorders worse.

Omega – 3 Eggs – consume as many as three eggs high in omega-3 fatty acids each day. These eggs contain DHA, vitamin E and B12, and anti-oxidants including lutein.

Extra Virgin Coconut Oil – perhaps the healthiest of available oils. It contains large amounts of Lauric Acid, a potent anti-microbial and one of the chief fatty acids found in breast milk. It is recommended to try and cook almost exclusively with this oil. Consume as much as two to four tablespoons per day of the oil in cooking, smoothies, or right off the spoon.

Ocean Caught Fish – The healthiest of all protein sources. Salmon, sardines, mackerel, herring, and albacore tuna are high in the omega 3 fatty acids (EPA) and (DHA). Ocean fish can be consumed every day if you choose to do so, it enhances the digestive system and the immune system.

Cod Liver Oil – Take one to three teaspoons of Olde World Icelandic Cod liver oil each day. The amount consumed is based on the amount of sunlight you receive each day. People in colder climates generally need to consume larger amounts. Cod liver oil is a fantastic source of omega 3 fatty acids, vitamin A and D.

Fermented Vegetables - A great source to aid in digestion, a naturally occurring source of probiotics and enzymes. Consume a few table spoons of fermented vegetable such as sauerkraut, fermented cabbage, pickles, and green tomato's with each meal.

Stocks/Broths – made from the bones of chicken, lamb, beef, and fish contain minerals, gelatin, cartilage, collagen, and electrolytes from the vegetables. Stocks are an excellent source of proteins, especially collagen which can help heal the gut lining and reduce inflammation.

Grass Fed Meats - A great source of protein from grass fed cattle, buffalo, and lamb, rich in minerals, iron, B12, vitamins, A, D, and omega 3 fatty acids. Can be eaten a few times per week.

Supplements For Healing & Reversing
Auto-Immune Disease

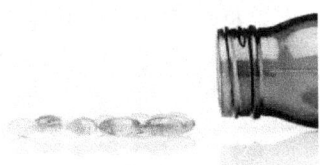

Goatein – **(100% Natural Goat's Milk Protein/ Garden of Life)** The only protein powder on the market made from organically produced goat's milk. This protein powder is partially pre-digested, and is usually well tolerated by those with food allergies and digestive problems. Take one to four tablespoons per day mixed in water, juice, smoothies, yogurt or can be used in baking. Many people that can not drink cow's milk can take Goatein.

Goatein contains all the essential amino acids for optimal health. Goatein also, contains 14 different strains of probiotics and is abundant in digestive enzymes.

FYI (*For Your Inflammation*) by the makers of ***Garden of Life (Goatein)*** is a specific formula of natural occurring compounds that contains enzymes, collagen extract, and phytonutrients specifically designed to reduce inflammation and support joint function and mobility. FYI also supports anti-oxidant function in the body. Dosage recommended is 6 tablets first thing in the morning and six before bed for three to six months or until health has greatly improved, and then reduce down to a maintenance level of three to six tablets per day.

Perfect Food – *by Garden of Life*, contains a super green formula powder consisting of 8000mg of greens per serving. It consists of *46 phytonutrient-dense foods, 13 sprouted ingredients, fermented whole food ingredients, made from young cereal grass juices*.

Perfect Food also contains *10 probiotic strains,* delivering one billion live cell count per daily serving to support digestive health, and *spirulina* to support healthy immune system activity. An excellent source of *vitamin A in the form of beta-carotene and natural vitamin C*. This formula is a perfect choice for those who are unable to eat enough green foods. Take one to two table spoons daily with 8 ounces of water or fresh vegetable juice. It is best taken on an empty stomach away from food.

Omega-Zyme – Is a highly effective enzyme product that helps the body digest proteins, carbohydrates, fats and dairy. Omega-Zyme contains 20 different digestive enzymes, making it effective for digesting difficult known foods such as *nuts, seeds, broccoli and beans*. Omega-Zyme also has 20 times more lipase for the digestion of fats than other leading brands. Another effective and powerful product by Garden of Life manufacturers. Omega-Zyme comes in powder and in capsule form. Take one to three capsules with each meal or snack.

Bovine Colostrum - One of the primary functions of the immune system is the production of anti-bodies in response to the presence of invading organisms like viruses or bacteria. And nature has provided us a miracle substance called **Colostrum**, a special substance that looks sort of like milk, but has a yellowish to orange tint, secreted by all female animals in the last few days of pregnancy and during the first few days of an infants life. Colostrum is the most incredible life supporting substance on the planet! Why? Because Colostrum is life's first food produced by the mother's mammary glands to support and sustain the infants life force for adulthood.

Our life support system (immune system) depends on the special growth and immune factors depend on colostrum to protect us as infants from contaminants, bacteria, and viruses during the very early stages of infancy to insure a progressive and healthy survival rate as we grow up into manhood. Colostrum has also been shown to be the only substance that can replace the vital components of life, and only bovine colostrum, from cows, has been shown to be safe and very biologically active and transferable to humans.

That is why, it is very important for pregnant mothers to breast feed their newborns upon birth. It has been noted that newborns that have been breast fed have endured a much stronger immune system growing up into adulthood than non-breast fed infants. And are much less likely to contract sicknesses and diseases during their stages of life.

Why? Because colostrum is loaded with life enhancing ingredients that contain, vitamins, minerals, enzymes, essential fatty acids, proteins, immunoglobins, lactoferrin, growth factors, and antibodies, and much more. Bovine colostrum is also 4 times richer than human colostrum and is found to be virtually identical to human colostrum.

Colostrum also has a long history in the treatment of auto-immune diseases, and bovine colostrum offers a proven means of effectively alleviating disease symptoms and treating the underlying conditions associated with disease progression over time. The component in colostrum that is most beneficial in regulating the immune system in patients with auto-immune disorder is Proline-Rich polypeptide (PRP).

Discovered in 1983, PRP is a small protein chain present in colostrum that has the ability to regulate the immune system as the hormones of the Thymus Gland. PRP from colostrum has been demonstrated to improve or eliminate symptomatology of both allergies and auto-immune diseases by inhibiting the over production of lymphocytes and T-cells reducing the major symptoms of allergies, that include pain, swelling and inflammation. *(The American Journal of Natural Medicine, March 1998)*

Colostrum's healing affects do not stop there either, its growth factors, lactoferrin, and immunoglobin components further go on and aid in the healing of the intestines (leaky gut syndrome), repairing of the myelin sheaths (multiple sclerosis), nerve tissues, connective tissues (arthritis), reducing inflammation and swellings (FM/CFS/Lupus, Etc.), and proved also to be remarkable in lowering insulin needs of diabetics, balancing blood sugar levels, which makes colostrum a very important healing aid in not only all auto-immune related diseases, but also in general sickness of any kind.

Colostrum, in medical treatment, with some cultures have used colostrum to treat the sick, theorizing that the high nutritional value and useful beneficial factor can be a potential new technique for immunization which could use colostrum, rather than vaccines. Now that would be an ideal method for preventing and treating the many associated illnesses associated with auto-immune disease. But unfortunately, the money hungry grubbers of the world (Pharmaceutical Industries) would obviously prevent or eliminate it altogether. <u>Because the money is in the medicine and not in the cure!</u> Hence the conspiracy factor, that is for another book to be explained in a later time.

Colostrum's many beneficial effects include: *rebuilds the immune system, destroys bacteria, viruses, fungi, accelerates healing of all body tissues, burns fat, used as a weight loss product, increases bone density, builds muscle, increases growth hormone and IGF-1 production, and reverses aging.* There have been many clinical studies and trials that have demonstrated the healing and rejuvenating effects of colostrum. Pharmaceutical companies have also synthesized the components of colostrum, such as *interferon, protease inhibitors, gamma globulin, growth hormone (GH), and insulin growth factor (IGF-1)*, which has been used in many anti-aging clinics for the past 10-15 years.

Colostrum's significant effects with healing allergies, CFS, FM, compromised digestive disturbances, osteoporosis, auto-immune disease, yeast infections, and basically anything to do with affecting the immune system can help you restore balance back to a non-disease state. It's profound natural healing capabilities can be used in virtually all disease states of the human body. It is also important to recognize that the best high quality colostrum should come from the first 6 hours after calving, where high quality colostrum with natural Immunoglobulins and lactoferrin are found. Look for reputable companies that recognize this important fact.

Conclusion: There are many studies that indicate that colostrum can provide significant support for individuals with auto-immune disease. Colostrum may potentially slow or stop the progression of the auto-immune disease, by healing injury in the gastrointestinal tract and by eliminating the leaky gut connection associated with the disease. Scientific studies and evidence have shown the powerful immune enhancing effects and its growth components in colostrum which can regulate the overactive immune response as well as heal tissues damaged by auto-immune disease.

Below is a list of some recommended companies that sell high quality colostrum. Colostrum is very safe and is basically listed as a food. With a rich source of natural proteins, carbohydrates, essential fats, vitamins, minerals, and biologically active growth factors, lactoferrins, and immunoglobulins. Note that all colostrum is not the same. Reputable and high quality colostrum can be bought from "Symbiotics Colostrum", "Immune tree Colostrum", New Zealand Colostrum", all can be found on line through the internet.

Dosages for Colostrum: 1,000mg to 2,000mg twice a day taken on an empty stomach. Colostrum can be found in capsules and in powder, which can also be mixed with a high quality biologically active, 100% hydrolyzed protein powder (see Proto-Whey protein powder by BioNutritional research group), a 100% micro peptide formula, which is also high in Glutathione, giving you a powerful synergistic effect.

NOTE: dosage can be increased or decreased till the desired results are obtained. For additional and much more in depth information on Colostrum please read Chapter 23: targeted natural therapies for FM/CFS.

Recommended reading: *The Colostrum Miracle by* The Editors of The Doctors' Prescription for Healthy Living Magazine & *Colostrum Life's First Food* by Daniel G. Clark, MD and Kaye Wyatt.

Pancreatic Enzymes – can be used as a powerful anti-inflammatory and immune support supplement for auto-immune disease and additional digestive support. They are also one of the most useful dietary nutritional supplements available. Enzymes in general help to speed up chemical reactions that take place within the digestive system to build new molecules or split the bonds that join them together to break them into smaller units. They are derived from the pancreas of hogs (pancreatin), fungal, or by plant sources. They function similar to the way the digestive enzymes secreted by the human pancreas and is required for digestion and break down of fats, proteins, and carbohydrates for the absorption of food.

The pancreas is the primary human organ in the abdomen situated just below the stomach. The enzymes include lipase that digests fats, proteases which digest proteins, and amylases which digest starch. A normally functioning pancrease secretes about 8 cups of fluid juice, daily into the duodenum, the portion of the small intestine that connects with the stomach. This fluid contains pancreatic enzymes which helps to neutralize stomach acid as it enters the small intestine.

Pancreatic Insufficiency

Pancreatic enzymes are need when an insufficiency arises and the absorption of food is generally impaired. Having an insufficient amount of pancreatic enzymes is also very common in people who have pancreatic cancer. Some other conditions that may cause pancreatic insufficiency are:

- *Cystic fibrosis*
- *Chronic Pancreatitis*
- *Blockage or duodenal tumors*
- *Pancreatectomy*
- *Stomach ulcers*
- *Celiac disease*
- *Crohons disease*
- *Auto-Immune Disease*

When pancreatic insufficiency occurs, malabsorption (impaired absorption of nutrients) by the intestines may result, leading to deficiencies of essential nutrients will occur. Mild forms of pancreatic insufficiency are often difficult to diagnose, and there is controversy among researchers regarding whether milder forms of pancreatic insufficiency need treatment. However, the normal signs of pancreatic insufficiency are – excess oil in their stools (steatorrhea), which is associated with symptoms of pale, foul-smelling, bulky stools to the side of the toilet bowl or are difficult to flush, oil droplets floating in the toilet bowl after bowl movements, and abdominal discomfort, constipation, gas, and bloating. People with pancreatic insufficiency may also have bone pain, muscle cramps, night blindness, and easy bruising. Another indicator of pancreatic insufficiency is the intestinal over growth of yeast Candida Albicans. As well as being necessary for protein absorption, the protease serve other important functions.

For example, the protease, as well as other digestive secreti0ons, are largely responsible for keeping the small intestines free from parasites (including bacteria, yeast, protozoa, and intestinal worms. Alcoholism is also one of the main causes of pancreatic insufficiency and pancreatis, and total abstinence from alcohol is strongly recommended. Cigarette smoking decreases pancreatic secretion and increases the risk for chronic pancreatic also. Providing you with yet another reason to quit smoking!

In a large international study, the major risk factors for early death in groups of patients with chronic alcoholic and nonalcoholic pancreatic included smoking and drinking alcohol.

Enzyme preparations have been shown to be useful in the following situations:

- Cancer
- Digestive support
- Hepatitis C
- Hepes zoster
- Multiple sclerosis
- Auto-Immune disease
- Food allergies
- Rheumatoid arthritis
- Sports injuries and trauma (inflammation)
- Pancreatic insufficiency

The Importance of Pancreatic Enzymes In Auto-Immune Disorder

After about the age of 27 to 28, the body declines in its ability to produce its own enzymes. In response to age and poor diet, chronic degenerative disease develops. This has much to do with the diet. When a diet consisting of overcooked and processed foods that are heavy in sugar and depleted of any mineral value, the body begins to suffer from a lack of fresh, viable enzymes. Slowly as enzyme depletion takes effect, symptoms from poor digestion soon start to manifest. Biological processes necessary for your body to build raw material, begin to show weakness in some of your normal activities resulting in a reduction of:

- Energy production
- Absorption of oxygen
- Fighting infections
- Reducing inflammation
- Lack of nutrients to your cells
- Carrying away waste toxic products
- Breaking down fats in your blood, regulation of cholesterol & triglycerides
- Dissolving blood clots
- Hormone regulation
- Slowing down the aging cycle

A lack of enzymes can affect profound changes within the body. They are the catalyst of life's evolving cycle and are essential for biochemical reactions to take place, sort of like the spark that ignites the fire to a mind boggling several million reactions per second! Hence the importance of enzymes.

Enzymes also rely on other elements to accomplish their tasks, such as vitamins, and minerals. These elements are called c that you're probably familiar with is – *co-enzyme Q10*. *CoQ10* is found in the mitochondria of your cells where it is involved in making ATP, every cell's principle source. Another example is *Magnesium*, which participates in over 300 enzymatic reactions.

One of the most knowledgeable men in the world on enzymes, is Dr. Edward Howell, who has spent his entire life studying enzymes, credited with catalyzing enzyme research. Dr. Howell believed you were born with a limited enzyme producing capacity, and that your life expectancy depending on how well you preserved your enzyme potential. His theory was that if you do not get enough enzymes from the foods you eat, a great strain will be placed on your digestive system to "pick up the slack," i.e., produce enough enzymes to accomplish the task.

A deficiency in digestive enzymes then reduces availability of your metabolic enzymes. Howell believed this metabolic enzyme deficit was the ***root cause most chronic diseases.***

A sad fact is that 90% of Americans in the US buy processed foods. Diets heavy in cooked, processed, and sugary foods, combined with the overuse of pharmaceutical drugs such as anti-biotics, deplete your body's ability to make enzymes. Enzymes are also heat sensitive, heating your food above 116 degrees F renders most enzymes inactive. This is one of the mo to eat raw foods as much as possible, especially in your later years. Raw foods are exceptional rich in natural live enzymes. Consuming them will decrease your body's burden to produce its own enzymes.

You should be getting 75% of your digestive enzyme intake from raw foods, and the more you can eat, the healthier you will be. Chronic malabsorption can lead to a variety of illnesses. Not having sufficient enzymes can impair your ability to recover from illness, can also be the start of an ongoing illness, and can basically compromise your immune system making you vulnerable to disease and infections. Research has shown that every 10 years, your body's production of enzymes decrease by 13%. So by the age production could be 25% lower than it was when you were a young child. And by the time your 70 years of age, you could be producing one-third of the enzymes you need. And to make matters worse, your stomach also produces less hydrochloric acid as you age as well. Hydrochloric acid is crucial in activating your stomach's digestive enzymes.

Now that you know the importance of digestive enzymes and their ability to catalyze energy production. You will learn how pancreatic enzymes play an important role in healing auto-immune disorder.

Systemic Enzymes & Pancreatic Enzyme
Healing Auto-Immune Disease

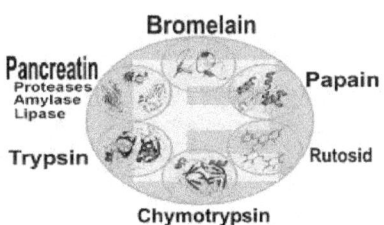

Systemic enzymes, or proteolytic systemic oral enzymes are those that operate not just for digestion but <u>throughout the body in every system and organ</u>. The word "Systemic" means body-wide. And are involved in almost every metabolic process in the human body, especially helping the human body to maintain healthy inflammation and immune activity levels. When taken on an empty stomach, proteolytic enzymes will pass through the stomach or intestinal lining and enter the circulatory system. This is why they are called "Systemic" - once they enter the circulatory system, they circulate throughout the body.

The Importance Of Systemic Enzymes

The most important thing that they do is to break down excess fibrin in your circulatory system and in other connective tissue, such as your muscles. These enzymes help to bring vital nutrients and oxygen rich blood that help to remove waste produced by inflammation and excess fibrin. Enzymes are the first line of defense against inflammation. When the immune system senses any irritation in the body it creates a protein chain called *"circulating immune complex"* (CIC), specifically for that particular area of inflammation. In 1999, the Noble prize was awarded to a scientist who discovered this tagging mechanism called (CIC).

Aspirin, Ibuprofen, Celebrix, Vioxx and the rest of the NSAIDs all work by keeping the body from making all CIC's. This ignores the fact that some CICs are vital to life, like those that maintain the lining of the intestine and those that keep the kidneys functioning! Not to mention the fact that the NSAIDs, along with Acetamophen, are highly toxic to the liver and kidneys. It is estimated that 20,000 Americans die every year from these over the counter drugs, and another 100,000 will wind up in the hospital with liver and kidney damage, or bleeding in the intestines from the side effects of these drugs.

Systemic enzymes on the other hand are perfectly safe and are free of any dangerous side effects, and have no toxic dose level. And best of all systemic enzymes can tell the difference between the good CICs and the bad ones because hydrolytic enzymes are a lock and key mechanism and their *"teeth"* will only fit over bad CICs. So instead of preventing the creation of all CICs, systemic enzymes just *"eat"* the bad ones and in doing so lower inflammation and pain anywhere in the body.

Systemic enzymes have been used successfully in the treatment of the following conditions:

- Arthritis
- Atherosclerosis
- Back pain
- Chronic Fatigue Syndrome
- Fibromyalgia
- Fibrocystic breast disease
- Sciatica
- Spinal Stenosis
- Strains and Sprains
- Post -operative scar tissue
- High Blood Pressure
- Cancer

- Tumors
- Traumatic Inflamation
- Uterine Fibroids
- Endometreosis
- Osteoarthritis
- Pulmonary Fibrosis
- High Cholesterol
- Clogged Arteries
- Wrinkles
- Joint & muscle Inflammation
- Allergies
- Circulatory Disorders
- and many others!

Their powerful anti-inflammatory action has out performed aspirin, ibubrophen, celebrex, vioxx and all other NSAIDs! Systemic enzymes also function as an Immune modelator, restoring a steady state back to the body. They break down and digest the coating that protects and houses viruses to render them inert and harmless. Digests spider veins, and helps to create tremendous energy and a feeling of well being.

Systemic Enzymes That Help Modulate The Immune System

Enzymes are adaptogenic, they seek to restore a steady state back to the body. When the immune system is running to low, it becomes susceptible to infectious diseases. When it's amp up too high, then the immune system creates anti-bodies that attack it's own tissues, as seen in auto-immune diseases of MS, Lupus, Rheumatoid Arthritis, and Graves Disease. Here systemic enzymes will help to tone down immune function and eat away at the anti-bodies the immune system is making to attack its own tissue.

When the immune system is running too low, the enzymes increase immune response, producing more natural killer cells, and improve the efficiency of the white blood cells, all leading to improved immunity.

List of Proteolytic/Systemic Enzymes

- Protease – derived from fruits such as pineapples and papaya.
- Chymotrypsin – a pancreatic enzyme
- Bromelain – a natural enzyme found in pineapples
- Papain – a proteolytic enzyme derived from papayas.
- Serratiapeptidase – a proteolytic enzyme derived from silk worms.
- Pancreatic enzymes – derived from pancreas of hogs.

Tips to obtain the best results from taking pancreatic enzymes:

- *Take enzymes with every meal or snack*
- *Start with the smallest dose and adjust accordingly*

- *Purchase enzymes with an <u>enteric coating</u> to prevent breakdown in the stomach.*
- *Pancreatic enzymes may also have reduce effectiveness if taken at the same time with calcium-or magnesium containing anti-acids, such as maalox, mylanta, tums, rolaids, and others.*

<u>**NOTE:**</u> *<u>Enzymes are generally not recommended two days before any scheduled surgeries.</u>*

Pancreatic enzymes are generally well tolerated and are not associated with any significant side-effects. Even in people with presumably normal pancreatic function, taking pancreatic enzymes produced no unwanted side effects.

<u>**Recommended Brands:**</u> *Twin Lab "Pancreatin"* one capsule will digest 50 grams of protein (3/4lb steak), 50 gms of starch (3lbs. White potatoes), and 67 gms of fat 1 ¾ oz. Italian salad dressing). *<u>Dosage</u>* – one capsule after each meal. *<u>Other good brands are</u> – Pancreatin Quadruple strength by Solgar, Michael's Health Products – W-Zymes Xtra-10x pancreatin, and Country Life Pancreatin.*

<u>**Goatein**</u> – **(100% Natural Goat's Milk Protein/ Garden of Life)** The only protein powder on the market made from organically produced goat's milk. This protein powder is partially pre-digested, and is usually well tolerated by those with food allergies and digestive problems. Take one to four tablespoons per day mixed in water, juice, smoothies, yogurt or can be used in baking. Many people that can not drink cow's milk can take Goatein.

Goatein contains all the essential amino acids for optimal health. <u>Goatein also, contains 14 different strains of probiotics and is abundant in digestive enzymes.</u>

<u>**FYI**</u> (*For Your Inflammation*) by the makers of *Garden of Life (Goatein)* is a specific formula of natural occurring compounds that contains enzymes, collagen extract, and phytonutrients specifically designed to reduce inflammation and support joint function and mobility. FYI also supports anti-oxidant function in the body. Dosage recommended is 6 tablets first thing in the morning and six before bed for three to six months or until health has greatly improved, and then reduce down to a maintenance level of three to six tablets per day.

<u>**Perfect Food**</u> – *by Garden of Life*, contains a super green formula powder consisting of 8000mg of greens per serving. It consists of *46 phytonutrient-dense foods, 13 sprouted ingredients, fermented whole food ingredients, made from young cereal grass juices*. Perfect Food also contains *10 probiotic strains,* delivering one billion live cell count per daily serving to support digestive health, and *spirulina* to support healthy immune system activity. An excellent source of *vitamin A in the form of beta-carotene and natural vitamin C*. This formula is a perfect choice for those who are unable to eat enough green foods. <u>Take one to two table spoons daily with 8 ounces of water or fresh vegetable juice. It is best taken on an empty stomach away from food.</u>

<u>**Omega-Zyme**</u> – Is a highly effective enzyme product that helps the body digest

proteins, carbohydrates, fats and dairy. Omega-Zyme contains 20 different digestive enzymes, making it effective for digesting difficult known foods such as *nuts, seeds, broccoli and beans*. Omega-Zyme also has 20 times more lipase for the digestion of fats than other leading brands. Another effective and powerful product by Garden of Life manufacturers. Omega-Zyme comes in powder and in capsule form. Take one to three capsules with each meal or snack.

References & Resources

Drs. Staroscik et al., Molecular Immunology; Bovine Colostrum's PRPs ability to regulate activity of the immune system, and hormones of the thymus gland; Allergies & Auto-Immune disease.

Playford RJ. (1999) Bovine colostrum is a health food supplement which prevents NSAIDs induced gut damage. Gut 44(5): 653-8.

Henderson D. (2000) Colostrum: Nature's Healing Miracle, CNR publications, Sedona, AZ.

"Colostrum: Life's First Food – The Ultimate Anti-aging Weight-Loss and Immune Supplement": Daniel G. Clark, MD., Kaye Wyatt.

"The Colostrum Miracle: The Anti-aging S Immunity & prevent Premature Aging": The Editors of The Doctors' prescription for Healthy Living magazine.

Goronzy JJ, Weyand CM. The innate and adaptive immune systems. In: Goldman L, Ausiello D, eds. Cecil Medicine. 23Rd ed. Philadelphia, Pa: Saunders Elsevier; 2007: chap 42.

Ghosh S, Vestrgaard, M, Pedersen, O, Serjrsen, K. (2007) Biological activity of bovine milk on proliferation of human intestinal cells. Journal of Dairy research 74(1):58-65. Bovine milk contains a number of biological that affect growth development of human intestinal tissue. The degree of activity depended on the stage of lactation.

Drs. Tortora, Funke & Cast; Microbiology "Clinical studies show that IgE (Immunoglobulin), found in bovine colostrum, may be responsible for regulating allergic response."

Ebina, T., et al., "Treatment of multiple sclerosis with anti-measles cow colostrum. "Med Microbiol Immunol (Berl), 1984; 173(2):87-93.

Lamoureux, G. et al., Transfer Factor of Proline-rich Polypeptides from Bovine Colostrum: A clinical and immunological study of the effects of transfer factor on multiple sclerosis. Clin Exp Immunol. 1981 March; 43(3): 667-564.

Important: For more information on Auto-Immune Disease, a must read, is the book titled *"Auto-Immune – The Cause & The Cure"* by **Anness Brockley and Kristin**

Urdiales. This book covers the causes of auto-immune disease with a collective of evidence that offers valid proof, not only of the cause of auto-immune disease, but also the possible ways to cure it. This book identifies the cause and the cure for: CFS, FM, Lupus, Rheumatoid Arthritis, Type II Diabetes, etc., etc. This book also shares many of the recommended remedies listed in this book as well.

Also please read for further interesting information concerning diet and auto-immune diseases the book by Dr. Fuhrman titled "Eat To Live."

Ransberger K: Enzyme treatment in comparison with immune complex diseases. Arthritis Rheuma 1986; 8: 16-9.

Ransberger K., Van Scaik W: Enzyme therapy in multiple sclerosis. Der Kassenarzt 1986;41: 42-5

Murray, MT, Pizzorno J: Encyclopedia of Natural Medicine 2nd ed. Prime Publishing, Rocklin, CA; 1998.

Biochemistry, Mary Campell, Ph.D., and Shawn Farrel, Ph.D.; Jan 23, 2011 National institute of Health: Proteolytic Enzymes

"Enzymes – A Drug of The Future", Prof. Heinrich Wrba MD and Otto Pecher MD.

"Enzyme Nutrition: The Food Enzyme Concept" by Dr. Edward Howell

Chapter 3

FMS/CFS – Auto-Immune Link
Vitamin B12 Connection

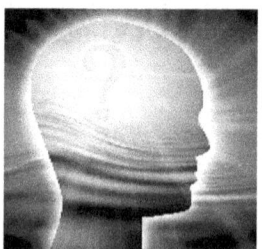

<u>**Auto-Immune disorder**</u> is when our body produces an inappropriate immune response against its own tissues and organs. In other words, the body basically attacks its own cells. When our body encounters something foreign in its own environment it needs to be able to build an immune response against these foreign substances to protect itself from harm. When this happens the body will start to produce antibodies that attack its own cells, tissues, and other organs. This is what causes the inflammation and damage that leads to an autoimmune disorder. <u>Antibodies</u> also destroy your vitally important <u>acid</u>-secreting cells lining the stomach through auto-immune inflammation, and so less stomach acid is secreted and **vitamin B12 (cobalamin)** deficiency is often the result. How important is B12?

<u>B12 is one of the most biologically active substances known</u>. It is involved in the metabolism of every cell in the human body, DNA replication, formation of red blood cells, and helps form the fatty substance, called "myelin," around your nerve cells for protection.

If stomach acid is not secreted due to auto-immune inflammation of parietal cells lining the stomach, breakdown and solubilization of food is prevented. As a result, vitamin B12 is trapped within its food-bound protein matrix, unable to freely bind and be absorbed. And secondly, if auto-antibodies are formed against **"intrinsic factor"**, they will bind intrinsic factor, preventing formation of the IF-B12 complex. It is important that the binding of vitamin B12 to intrinsic factor within the intestines is absolutely essential before absorption can occur. The IF-B12 complex induces proper configuration of the intestinal receptor for binding and absorption.

To ameliorate B12 deficiency, a direct injection of a B12 shot into the body, by passing the dysfunctional digestive tract or administration of a high dose of oral B12 supplementation are the general treatment options for this important form of vitamin B12 deficiency. Also, any form of pancreatic insufficiency such as a lack of pancreatic enzymes, calcium, etc., inhibits absorption at the intestinal wall. If these conditions persist, a vitamin B12 deficiency will eventually develop.*[References, Andres E, Goichot B, Schlienger JL. Food cobalamin malabsorption: a usual cause of vit-B12 deficiency. Arch Intern Med. 2000;160:2061-2.]*

Strict vegetarians (vegans) that consume a strict vegetarian diet will eventually become deficient in vitamin B12, if they do not supplement their diet with sufficient amounts of B12. Plant-based diets do not contain vitamin B12 in their tissues. A strict plant-based diet (vegan) will therefore eventually cause a B12 deficiency. However, your body is extremely efficient in conserving vitamin B12 and unlike any other water-soluble vitamins, vitamin B12 is actually stored in the liver. In sharp contrast, people with absorption malfunctions like atrophic gastritis, auto-immune inflammation or pancreatic insufficiency may develop vitamin B12 deficiency symptoms within 2 to 3 years. **Chronic alcoholics**, are also at risk of a vitamin B12 deficiency, as alcohol reduces vitamin B12 absorption and at the same time increases clearance of the vitamin B12 in the urine.

Vitamin B12 Deficiency & FMS/CFS

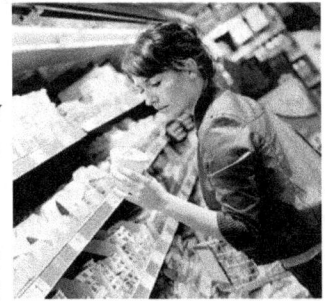

Any one can actually be low in B12, severe alcoholics and especially if your a vegetarian, and have been for several years and don't take supplemental B12. It could also be low if you don't make intrinsic factor, which is made in the stomach and is needed to absorb B12. Lack of intrinsic factor is usually an auto-immune disorder. The impact vitamin B12 has in your life is far reaching. This important vitamin is intimately involved with protein metabolism and DNA synthesis, two major biochemical processes controlling everything from heredity to metabolism, and plays a vital role in the formation of red blood cells, nerve system functioning, DNA &

RNA production, certain hormones, and fats. Consequently, the results of a B12 deficiency are very serious.

Consequences of B12 Deficiency

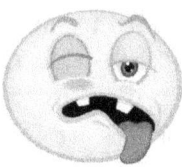

Vitamin B12 deficiency puts the brakes on DNA synthesis and protein metabolism, which creates a wide spectrum of dysfunction. And is the only vitamin that contains essential mineral elements. Deficiencies for example can cause:

• **Deficiency causes - "Megaloblastic Anemia" - is a debilitating condition characterized by fatigue, lack of energy, diarrhea, nausea, decreased appetite, weak muscles, headaches, tingling sensations and sore tongue. (sound familiar? FMS/CFS)**

• **Irreversible Degenerative neuropathy is a hallmark of B12 deficiency. This causes serious deterioration of the peripheral and Central Nervous system, including brain occurs if B12 deficiency is not resolved.**

• **Deficiency of B12 also increases levels of "Homocysteine" - a toxic amino acid associated with significant cardiovascular risk.**

• **Lack of B12 – will also trap another important B vitamin called Folate in a metabolically useless form. Both B12 and Folate (Folic acid) are highly interrelated and deficiencies of either vitamin are grave threats to your good health.**

• **Vitamin B12 also participates in the regeneration of a form of folate called "Folic Acid" - Folic acid is the required form of folate for re-entry into the cycle of a single carbon metabolism and continuous flow of carbon. If vitamin B12 is deficient, folic acid can not be regenerated and becomes trapped in a metabolically useless form, unable to re-enter the cycle of single carbon metabolism.**

<u>Symptoms associated with vitamin B12 deficiency include</u> **– anemia, fatigue, weakness, constipation, decreased appetite, decreased sensory perception and weight-loss. In addition, neurological symptoms may also be present and include numbness and tingling of the hands, and feet, balance, depression, confusion, dementia and memory loss, and sore mouth and tongue.**

Vitamin B12 has long been thought by many researchers to aid in several nerve related disorders, including multiple sclerosis and Alzheimer's disease. The typical CFS and FMS patients also suffers from symptoms that are distinctly neurological, such as numbness and tingling in extremities, memory loss and balance disorders. Some doctors who specialize in the treatment of CFS and FMS are choosing to augment oral supplementation of B12 with injected doses comparable to or higher than those typically prescribed for patients suffering from B12 deficiency (pernicious anemia).

Studies reported in the New England Medical Journal of Medicine, revealed that high doses of B12 therapy had either cured or greatly improved the symptoms of patients suffering from CFS and fibromyalgia-like neurological symptoms. Which including numbness and tingling in the extremities, memory loss, weakness of limbs, changes in moods and personality, and even fatigue.

Also interesting, a writing in the **Scandinavian Journal of Rheumatology in 1997, Swedish scientists** described their study of 12 patients who fulfilled their diagnostic criteria for both FMS and CFS. Although all the patients had normal levels of B12 in their blood, they had extremely low or non-detectable levels of B12 in their spinal fluid, and by inference, in their brains. The low levels of B12 in the spinal fluid correlated with the degree of fatigue experienced by the patient. The findings suggested that at least some of CFS and fibromyalgia patients fail to metabolize B12 properly.

One year later, these same researchers reported that not only did CFS and FMS patients lack B12 in their nervous systems, they also had abnormal high levels off "Homocysteine", an amino acid like substance that is normally regulated in the cells by B12. Among other things, high levels of homocysteine have been linked with heart disease.
The Swedish scientists also discovered that the higher the homocysteine levels in CFS and fibromyalgia patients were three times higher than in healthy people --- the greater the severity of fatigue. They also concluded that the absence of B12 in the nervous system and high homocysteine levels among CFS and fibromyalgia suffers constitute "an underlying factor" in both diseases.

The B12 deficiency in CFS and fibromyalgia patients occurs because of a defect in the patient's ability to transport the nutrient into cells. It was also discovered that the same patients in the study also appeared to have a similar problem transporting magnesium and potassium into cells. Why this defect occurs remains to be explained, but they point out, that large doses of B12 markedly improve cognitive ability, mood, irritability, and numbness and weakness in a majority of patients.

Doctors who practice at the Hunter-Hopkins Center in Charlotte, North Carolina, recommend a subcutaneous dose of 3,000mcgs every 2 to 3 days of B12 for a "continuous and satisfactory level of improvement." Worries of toxicity are generally unwarranted, as B12 is water-soluble, and any excess is simply excreted through the urine. It is also strongly advised for those that suffer from FMS and CFS to take oral supplements of other vitamins, particularly **B6** and **folate**, since excess B12 can potentially compete with other B vitamins in cells and hinder absorption. Scientists aren't exactly sure what causes FMS, but they have noted some correlations between vitamin B12 deficiency and FM/CFS that provide some important clues towards understanding the pattern of these dreaded diseases.

Conclusion

Vitamin B12 therapy should definitely be listed in your treatment protocol for fibromyalgia and chronic fatigue. Dr. Keith Berndtson of American Whole Health in Chicago suggests that patients who are either shy of injecting themselves with vitamin B12 shots who are functioning and not fully disabled by their illness – should try taking one to two milligrams of B12 under the tongue each day. It would definitely benefit those who especially suffer from the neuro-cognitive problems of FMS and CFS. Based on studies and reports which suggest that there is oxidative neuro-stress going on in FMS and CFS patients that the vitamin B12 deficiency may be a hallmark of the fibromyalgia and chronic fatigue *[source - Dr. Keith Berndtson, American WholeHealth – Chicago, Illinois, Pub. 9/13/2000].*

Note: **There several kinds of vitamin B12 that are called vitamin B12, but there is only one form of vitamin B12 that should be used in the majority of cases, which is "Methylcobalamin".**
B12 is more scientifically called "cobalamin" and there are three forms of cobalamin's generally used as dietary supplements, namely– Hydroxocobalamin, Cyanocobalamin, and Methylcobalamin.

All three types are considered vitamin B12, but they are not all the same and using the right one can be a critical decision. Cyanocobalamin is probably the most commonly used in the medical world and is given as "B12-shots" in the doctors office for certain medical conditions. But cyanocobalamin is actually the worst one to use despite the fact that doctors all over the US prescribe it over any other form.

Not only does cyanocobalamin require higher dosages for the same effectiveness as hydroxocobalamin, but it is entirely ineffective for several different conditions related to a B12 deficiency.

It has been suggested by many researchers in the field that cyanocobalamin should be removed from the market (*Dr. AG Freeman, 1970, cyanocobalamin – a case for withdrawal: discussion paper*) While hydroxocobalamin is preferred over cyanocobalamin, another formulation called methylcobalamin is actually the BEST CHOICE.

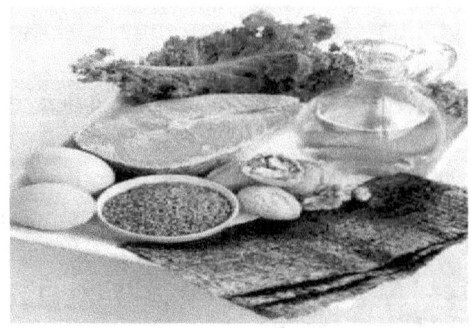

Natural Dietary Sources of Vitamin B12

Methylcobalamin is is the preferred form found in food and has a much higher bio-availability than the other two forms widely made available in supplements today. For deficiency purposes, Methylcobalamin has been shown to work in neurological diseases, which also helps in the elimination of toxic substances in the body. Choosing correctly, could very well mean the difference between good health and disease.

<u>Guidelines for use</u> – Vitamin B12 is frequently used in a combination with B vitamins, such as a B complex that includes B1, B2, B3, B5, B6, and folic acid. B12 should also be combined with calcium during absorption to benefit the body properly. The preferred form of B12 should be lozenges or sublingual containing 1,000mcgs of B12 Methylcobalamin.

<u>Cautions</u> – Be sure to take a folic acid supplement along with B12, as a high intake of one can mask a deficiency in the other. Because B12 contains cobalt, people who are allergic to cobalamin and cobalt should avoid taking vitamin B12. (see book on "The Ultimate Healing System: The Illustrated Guide To Muscle-Testing & Nutrition," by Dr. Donald J. Lepore)

<u>General Interactions</u> – Potassium supplements and numerous drugs interfere with the absorption of B12, in particular chloramphenicol (antibiotic), interferes with red blood cell formation.

<u>Natural Dietary Sources</u> – Milk, eggs, liver (desiccated liver is an excellent source), fortified brewer's yeast, peanuts, bananas, sunflower seeds, concord grapes, raw wheat germ, and bee pollen.

Health Benefits of Vitamin B12 You Can Experience

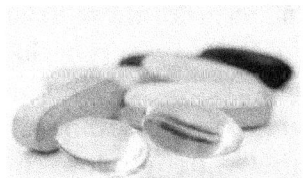

1.   Regenerates another important vitamin folic acid.

2.   Vitamin B12 & Folic Acid support synthesis and metabolism of proteins and DNA bio-synthesis.

3.   Supports healthy red blood cell formation and depends on synthesis of DNA. Without B12, DNA shuts down causing Megaloblastic anemia. Symptoms include – fatigue, no energy, diarrhea, nausea, decreased appetite, weak muscles, headaches, tingling sensations and sore tongue.

4.   B12 supports the synthesis of another important amino acid methionine, a

crucial building block of proteins.

5.   B12 promotes the activity of hormones and neurotransmitters affecting your moods, these include dopamine, serotonin, and melatonin.

6.   Promotes the synthesis of another important amino acid Sam-e, which is required for 100 enzymatic reactions required for normal activity within your body.

7.   B12 helps you reduce dangerous levels of Homocysteine, a dangerous toxic amino acid associated with cardiovascular disease.

8.   B12 helps prevent irreversible neurological impairment. Peripheral and central nervous system deterioration due to B12 deficiency which has been linked to the onset of Alzheimer's Disease and Dementia.

9.   B12 supports the maintenance of the Insulative Mylin Sheath surrounding your nerves.

10.   B12 benefits your nervous system – depression, memory, moods and behavior.

<u>Conclusion</u> – The benefits of vitamin B12 are far-reaching – ranging from the formation of healthy red blood cells, generation of energy levels, control of mood, focus, concentration, memory, and protection from degenerative nerve damage that may lead to Alzheimer's and even potential protection from atherosclerosis and cancer.

Sometimes, certain factors interfere with your ability to absorb cobalamin from foods you eat. Fibromyalgia is an auto-immune disorder, and so often is vitamin b12 deficiency. And having one auto-immune disorder also raises your risk for having others, according to the latest research. So it is not that uncommon for somebody with Fibromyalgia to also suffer from auto-immune vitamin B12 deficiency. It is also not uncommon for a vitamin B12 deficiency to be misdiagnosed as arthritis, diabetes, depression, chronic fatigue and Fibromyalgia.

Also, gastrointestinal ailments associated with fibroblast often will lead to a B12 deficiency from the inability to produce intrinsic factor, a necessary enzyme needed to absorb B12.

For those of you interested in further information of this vital and important vitamin, I urge you to read the book - <u>"Could it Be B12?: An Epidemic of Misdiagnoses"</u> by Sally M. Pacholok, R.N., B.S.N. and Jeffrey J. Stuart, D.O.

Knowing Your Hormones & FMS / CFS

"Your Hormones Define Who You Are, They Are a Reflection of Your Personality"
'As Your Hormones Go, So Do You'

Your hormones basically influence the health of every cell in your body, *your moods, drive, motivation, intellectual capacity, lean body mass, visceral fat, blood sugar, libido, sexual function, orgasmic satiety and social interactions* are just a few functions that can be affected by *testosterone, estradiol, progesterone, DHEA, adrenal hormones, cortisol, thyroid hormones, insulin, growth hormone, leptin, prolactin, melatonin*, or any of more than 50 hormones that are produced by your body on a daily basis, 24 hours a day and every day of your life. Basically your hormones rule your life and define who you are, how you feel, act, do, and say.

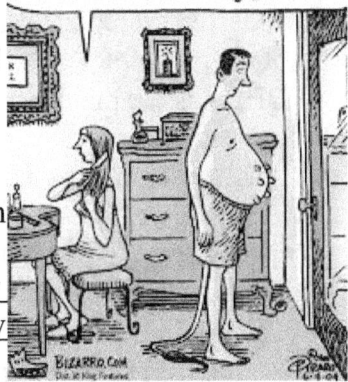

Knowing a bit about some of these vital and necessary hormones that play a significant part on Fibromyalgia and Chronic fatigue will help you understand a little bit more of how it relates to your current condition of FMS and CFS. Your hormones also have a significant effect on all of your neurotransmitters, estrogen effects serotonin, testosterone effects dopamine and progesterone effects GABA. Simply put, your hormones are really, really very important. The conductor that orchestrates your hormonal balance is nothing bigger than the size of a pea and situated in the brain. The pituitary gland in conjunction with the hypothalamus gland controls vital bodily functions by excreting the following hormones:

- The **Antidiuretic hormone (ADH)** controls the absorption of water by the kidneys.
- **Oxytocin** is the "cuddle" hormone responsible for the release of mother's milk and uterus contraction after child birth.
- **Prolactin** stimulates female breast milk production.
- **Growth hormone (GH)** regulates body and bone growth, improves muscle strength and increases protein synthesis, fat usage and carbohydrate storage.
- **Adrenocorticotropic hormone (ACTH)** stimulates the adrenal glands to release the stress hormones **cortisol**.
- Follicle Stimulating hormone (FSH) stimulates female or male organs.
-In the Female: stimulates growth of eggs and produces estrogen
-In the Male: stimulates growth of sperm.
- Luteinizing hormone (LH) stimulates female or male organs.
-In females: stimulates the release of eggs and produces progesterone.
-In Males: stimulates the release of testosterone.
- Thyroid Stimulating hormone (TSH) regulates the thyroid gland.
- Endorphins are the body's natural pain killers.

Note: All of these hormones stimulate the relevant glands and organs to secrete specific hormones that are essential for functioning namely:

Adrenal Glands:

- Adrenalin causes the heart rate, blood sugar, and blood pressure to increase.
- Noradrenalin raises the blood pressure.
- Cortisol mobilizes our stress response.
- Aldosterone regulates sodium and mineral balance through kidney s to control blood pressure.
- DHEA is the main building block for the manufacture of of estrogen and testosterone.
- Small amounts of estrogen, progesterone and testosterone.

Thyroid & Parathyroid gland:
- Thyroxin regulates our metabolism.
- Calcitonin lowers our blood calcium levels and builds bone strength.
- Parathyroid Hormone (PTH) increases the calcium and phosphate in the blood & bones.

The Thymus Gland:
- Thymosins promotes the development of t-lymphocytes for the immune system.

The Kidneys:
- Renin regulates the blood pressure.

The Pancreas:
- Insulin enables cells to take up glucose.
- Glucagon stimulates the body to convert stored energy (glycogen) to glucose.

The Uterus:
- Produces the hormones estrogen and progesterone.

The Testes:
- Produces testosterone.

This is by no means a complete list but is limited to the more well known glands and organs. And, as you can see the inner workings of our bodies hormones are very complex and there is a lot than can go wrong, especially when illness manifests, as such when dealing with FMS and CFS.

All these hormones work automatically when everything works as designed you don't even notice about them. However, when something does go wrong you will know and feel the effects, because hormonal imbalance has all kinds of nasty effects and symptoms. Such as in FMS and CFS.

Balancing Hormones Naturally

Since your hormones effect every aspect of your bodily function, it is essential to keep them in balance for your health and well being. The most common hormonal imbalance with women is estrogen and progesterone. The reason being is that progesterone is the "mother" hormone used to manufacture all the other hormones. Thus when there is insufficient progesterone it causes an excess estrogen build up that results in unpleasant side effects such as PMS, hot flashes, mood swings, depression and other menopausal symptoms.

Estrogen that is not balanced with progesterone is role of estrogen is to make cells grow it has been implicated in breast cancer, fibroids, ovarian cysts, endometriosis, osteoporosis, etc. High estrogen levels is also implicated in men as well because some testosterone is converted into estrogen and DHT, which stimulates the prostate to grow. When there is too much estrogen it also interferes with your thyroid hormone thyroxine. And if Thyroxine can't work properly your metabolism slows down and you gain unnecessary weight. You also typically will retain water.

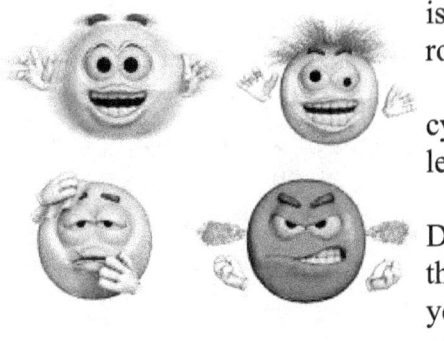

Since the stress hormone cortisol is also made from progesterone there is a big drain on progesterone when you are stressed. Cortisol is needed to allow Thyroxine, which regulates your metabolism, and insulin, which manages your energy utilization, to function properly. However, too much cortisol and your metabolism slows down and you become insulin resistant. Although stress is inevitable it is chronic stress that is extremely detrimental for your health since cortisol is the main hormonal disruptor and the main reason for hormonal imbalance.*(Holford, P.2004. Optimum Nutrition Bible. Piatkus: London)*

Disruptors of Hormonal Balance

Excess cortisol (stress) is the single biggest cause of hormonal imbalance, however, it is not the only reason. Synthetic compounds are the other cause that are estrogen mimics, which we are exposed to on daily levels. These compounds mimic the role of natural estrogen disrupting the body's biochemistry and changing sexual and reproductive functioning. It is also increases the risk of cancer rates. What are synthetic estrogens? These are compounds such as bisphenol A and phathalates present in soft plastic bottles, plastic bags, cling wraps, and pesticides, industrial compounds and estrogen hormone replacement therapy (HRT).

These hormones and synthetic compounds are finding their way into the food chain as well as in our drinking water supply. The estrogen in HRT end up in our drinking water while most of the beef we eat comes from feedlots where cattle are injected with estrogens to make them grow faster and fatter increasing the farmer's yield of meat and such to charge more money by the pound during market sales.

This brief explanation on hormones was to give you a basic understanding of how your hormones work and function, and how they can affect your health when they go unbalanced, and on top of that show you how it can correlate, and/or affect your primary health problem FM and CFS.

How To Avoid Exposure To These Hormone Disruptors?

- When purchasing your groceries of *meat, poultry, vegetables and fruits*, make sure their of an *organic supplier* and thoroughly wash your vegetables & fruits to reduce exposure to pesticides. A good idea when washing your produce is to add a cap full of hydrogen peroxide to your water bath and submerge and wash off any residue from prior handling during shipping and manufacturing. Another common and clean, healthy way is to add one cap full of bleach to one to two gallons of water to disinfect any pollutants.
- Drink distilled or filtered water to remove any potential hormone disruptors.
- Remove soft plastics as soon as possible especially cling wraps. Do not heat food in plastics, the chemicals that keep plastics flexible get absorbed by fats in the food.
- Avoid HRT thereby reducing your exposure to synthetic estrogens.
- Periodic Whole body cleanses are a great idea to rid your body of any past or current harmful synthetics, toxins, parasites, and heavy metals.

Balancing Your Hormones Naturally

Balancing your hormone levels naturally requires you to make some lifestyle changes that are reasonably easy to do. It's importance concerning FM and CFS can go a long way in making you feel healthy and well. That is if you want to restore some normality to your life and recover your health it is vital that you take the effort to make some changes and enhance your hormonal balance. Starting with the following list below:

1. **Stress Less** - Stress is the biggest disruptor of every hormone function in your body. Anything that triggers your flight or fight reaction, emotional or physical can be defined as stress, such as: **Physical stresses** like working too hard and too many hours, less sleep and rest, too hot or too cold temperatures, too much exercise, etc.

2. **Emotional stresses** – such as anger, guilt, traumatic experiences, unresolved conflict or perceived dangers causing anxieties and worries that activate your flight or fight response. These types of emotions are exceptionally stressful as they can usually last over a long periods of time.

3. **Eating Habits** – Reduce your consumption of sugar, refined carbohydrates and stimulants (caffeine) as it results in the release of stress hormone cortisol.

4. **Balance your blood sugar** with supplemental aids like - Chromium Picolinate, Alpha Lipoic Acid, or a specific formula such as "Enzymedica Reduce" by Premier Research.

5. **Decrease your intake of red meats and dairy products** that are not of an organic nature and hormone free, as they can contain synthetic estrogen, especially in the fat.

6. **Consume more fish or omega 3** to help the body cope with stress better and subsequently balance your hormones levels.

7.   **Supplement** your body with hormone balancing herbs, that include **Maca, or Macafem (Lepidium Meyenii)** is a non-estrogenic herb that stimulates the endocrine system in a safe and natural way to produce the necessary hormones naturally. This specific formula is formulated as "Maca' being the main ingredient added with additional supporting nutrients. Can be found online at "www.macafem.com." It can also be used by men as well.

The most important thing to remember is, STRESS is the single biggest reason why your hormones can become unbalanced, and unfortunately, it is virtually impossible to eliminate it completely from our lives, so take the time to relax and be happy, apply some of the stress techniques mentioned in this book to allow you to be better manage stress.

Resources - *"Is It Me or My Hormones?" Marcelle Pick*
"The Hormone Solution" Thierry Hertoghe

Stress – The Fibromyalgia Trigger

The links between stress and Fibromyalgia have now been well established. The research has made clear that stress does influence Fibromyalgia and chronic fatigue in a number of different ways. Many Fibromyalgia patients have a history of chronic stress, often due to personal problems, family matters, work relations, environment, financial matters, friendships, marriages, relationships, etc., etc. Which can all be an overload on the stress glands of the body, eventually building up over time creating a viscous cycle for an extended period of time. This causes certain neurotransmitters to release chemicals that tend to shock the body and weaken the immune system, thus making the Fibromyalgia symptoms and circumstances worse and increasing the risk of creating other diseases.

Some researchers also believe that the onset of of Fibromyalgia is triggered by an extremely stressful experience. While this stress may be associated with an emotional or physical trauma, such as an automobile accident, a divorce, relationship break ups, financial difficulties, and physical abuse, there is now sufficient evidence to suggest that both CFS and FMS and post traumatic stress disorder may be the significant factors in the onset of of Fibromyalgia. The correlation between health and stress is obvious. In fact, the majority of Fibromyalgia victims I have worked with have all experienced a traumatic experience of some kind which caused a long period of undue chronic stress in their lives.

Health Conditions Associated with Stress Response

- **Stress intolerance**
- **Depression**
- **Insomnia**

- **Allergies**
- **Osteoporosis**
- **Hypothyroidism**
- **Hypo-Adrenia**
- **PMS**
- **Accelerated Aging**
- **Anxiety**
- **Poor Immune Functioning**
- **Obesity**
- **Fibromyalgia/Chronic Fatigue Syndrome**
- **Glucose intolerance**
- **Yeast Over Growth**

How Stress Can Aggravate The Symptoms of FMS & CFS

For CFS and FM patients, stress can also make the condition worse and can trigger particular physical symptoms. People who suffer from FM and CFS often have trouble knowing their personal limitations, which can make it hard for them to know when they are in danger of over exerting themselves. When 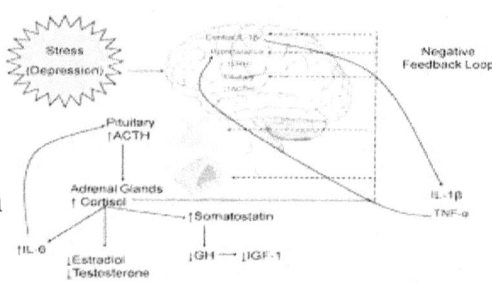 Fibromyalgia patients physically over exert themselves, this can often lead to increased stress, which results in increased pain. A vicious cycle can easily develop, because the pain can lead to more stress, which in turn, can lead to more pain. For this reason, stress management can also help greatly with fibroblast pain management.

Defining Stress

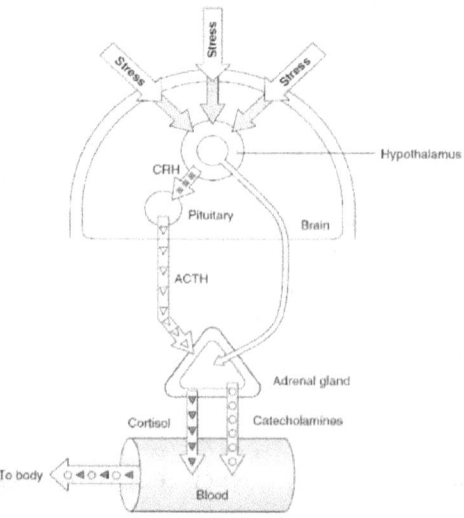

Schematic diagram of how stress affects the body.

Recent studies show that over 43% of Fibromyalgia patients have low thyroid function (hypothyroid) with symptoms of mental fatigue, depression, and poor memory.

Chronic stress on the other hand can be a factor here in regards to the disruption of the hypothalamus gland. And understanding the biochemical interactions that constitute the stress response requires a definition of stress. In the realm of biology, stress refers to what happens when an organism fails to respond appropriately to threats. While the "threats" humans face today often take more benign forms compared to those our hunter-gathered ancestors faced, they can be equally taxing on our bodies.

Some stress, of course, can be beneficial. The pressure it can exert can be incentive enough to accomplish necessary goals. Often, however, stress reaches chronic, harmful levels, and deleterious consequences follow, from compromised immune function to weight gain to development impairment. The intensity of stress is governed largely by glucocorticoids, the primary molecules involved in the stress response. Proper stress management takes on a great importance given the wide range of bodily systems impacted by stress hormones. During periods of increased stress, the immune system is compromised due to the effects of excess levels of cortisol *(Leproult et al.)*

Stress signals activate the hypothalamus-pituitary-adrenal (HPA) axis and the sympathetic nervous system. The elements derived from those systems (eg., cortisol, catecholamines and neuropeptides) can impact the immune system and create possible disease states, hence auto-immune disease *(Psychological Bulletin, 133, 25-45)*.

Since people with Fibromyalgia are often diagnosed with auto-immune disease such as rheumatoid arthritis and lupus, it has been theorized that Fibro' has an immune system basis too. One study indicated an increased number positive antinuclear anti-body blood tests among people with fibroblast. This finding may be coincidental though since it is known that a small percentage of healthy people are also positive for anti-nuclear anti-bodies (ANA). The high prevalence of Fibro' in the general population may suggest that its occurrence in people with auto-immune disease is purely coincidental. I on the other hand tend to disagree with this, as most of those afflicted with Fibromyalgia and CFS all reported chronic stress had played a part to their affliction of this disease.

Cortisol Levels & Fibromyalgia

A team of researchers from Massachusetts found that cortisol levels are low in people with Fibromyalgia. Produced by the adrenal glands it affects many bodily systems. Low levels of cortisol are ever present in the body but we produce more during times of stress. When the body is deficient in cortisol, the symptoms of Fibro are mirrored, such as:

- **Fatigue**
- **Weakness**
- **Muscle pain**
- **Abdominal distress**
- **Thinking problems**
- **Mood swings**
- **Sleep disturbances**

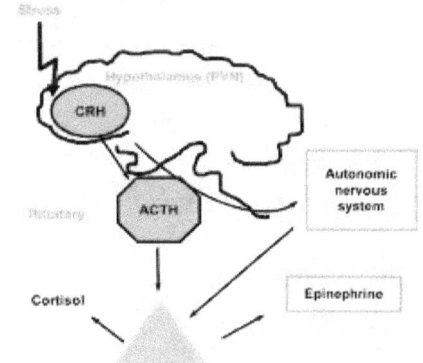

The researchers from Massachusetts found that Fibromyalgia patients produce less cortisol in response to stress than do healthy people, possibly having to do with a defect in the hypothalamus-pituitary-adrenal axis which controls cortisol production. It is not clear how important cortisol deficiency is in the onset or course of fibroblast. Giving patients corticosteroid medications does not improve the condition.

While cortisol is an important and helpful part of the body's in response to stress, it's also important that the body's relaxation response to be activated so the body's functions can return to normal following a stressful event. But unfortunately, in our current high-stress culture, the body's stress response is activated so often that the body doesn't always have a chance to return to normal, resulting in a state of chronic stress. This is what actually starts the creation of disease and ill health conditions that excess cortisol production often creates. These high and prolonged levels of cortisol in the blood stream (like those associated with chronic stress) have been shown to have negative effects, such as:

Effects of Excess Cortisol Levels

- **Impaired Cognitive performance**
- **Suppressed Thyroid functioning**
- **Adrenal Fatigue dysfunction**
- **Blood Sugar imbalance**
- **Decreased Immune system levels**
- **Decreased Bone density**
- **High Blood pressure**
- **Increased Abdominal fat**

To keep cortisol levels healthy and under control, the body's relaxation response should be activated after the flight or fight response occurs. You can learn how to relax your body with various stress management techniques, and you can make lifestyle changes in order to keep your body from reacting to stress in the first place. The following have been helpful in relaxing the body and mind, aiding the body in maintaining healthy cortisol levels:

- **Exercise**
- **Yoga**
- **Nutritional supplementation**
- **Herbal therapy (Adaptogens for adrenal support)**
- **Meditation**
- **Breathing exercises**
- **Guided imagery**
- **Listening to music**

Cortisol secretion may also vary from person to person, and people are wired biologically different in their reaction to stress. One person may secrete higher amounts of cortisol than any other in the same situation. Studies have also shown that people who secrete higher levels of cortisol in response to stress also tend to eat more food, and the food that is higher in carbohydrates than people who secrete less cortisol. If you are sensitive to stress, it's especially important for you to learn stress management techniques and maintain a healthy lifestyle.

Adrenal Exhaustion and Fibromyalgia

Adrenal exhaustion typically happens after an extended period of time of continual stress and high cortisol levels, where the adrenal glands become over worked and fatigued. This is primarily caused by too much mental, emotional, and physical stress. The first stage of adrenal exhaustion is where cortisol levels are high and DHEA levels are usually low. The next stage is where DHEA levels drop too low, but the cortisol still remains high. The final stage is where the adrenal glands are worn out and both cortisol levels and DHEA will drop too low which results in inadequate amounts of stress hormones produced in a normal daily rhythm.

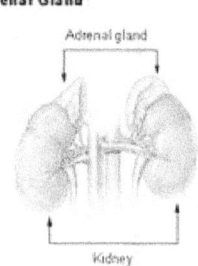

Adrenal Gland

Low levels of DHEA have been associated with:

- **Obesity**
- **Immune dysfunctional**
- **Auto-immune disease**
- **Type II Diabetes**
- **Lupus**
- **Memory loss**
- **Depression**
- **Cardiovascular disease**
- **Low libido**
- **Erectile dysfunctional**
- **Osteoporosis**

When your adrenal glands become exhausted and produce less cortisol, you will suffer from *fatigue, sugar cravings, irritability, muscle weakness, difficulty exercising, suppressed immune system, increased susceptibility to infections and viruses and much, much more*. This also encourages insulin resistance and weight gain, especially in the abdomen area. (All of these symptoms and more are symptoms of low cortisol and Fibromyalgia). When this is the case, you will find it to be very difficult coping with everyday stresses and become very irritable and over whelmed very easily. On top of that, you will also feel depressed and have feelings of helplessness and hopelessness.

The relationship between low cortisol levels, and Fibromyalgia is inflammation. Cortisol is known as a natural anti-inflammatory. When you get to the point of adrenal exhaustion, cortisol levels drop to a very low level. This in turn triggers inflammation. A normal daily pattern of cortisol levels is a peak rise in the morning, decreasing throughout the day, and low at night. In a healthy cycle cortisol levels goes down at night so you can sleep, dream, rejuvenate and rest and awaken feeling refreshed. Then at 7 to 8am it peaks, and you wake up! When the adrenal glands become dysfunctional, this pattern reverses.

Stress plays havoc with neurotransmitter function, thyroid function, and hormonal balance. Chronic stress can also raises cortisol, cholesterol, adrenalin, insulin, blood sugar, and it lowers growth hormone secretion, testosterone production, and suppresses immunity levels. It causes infertility and loss of sex drive and sleep. Stress imbalances the hormones of the endocrine system, the neurotransmitters of the nervous system, and the cytokines of the immune system.

Some people have abnormal response to stress. Their body is saying, "Now that my stress hormones are up, I had better keep them up, because another stressful thing is bound to happen." So instead of stress hormones returning to normal in twenty minutes, they are still up four hours later. And if there is more stress in the meantime, stress hormone levels are going to stay high for another four hours after that. These people find it hard to relax and are wired, but tired. Adrenalin, drugs, toxins, pesticides, metals, hypothyroidism, and infection all increase the time it takes for cortisol levels to return to normal.

The Many Consequences of Cortisol

Cortisol is catabolic, it breaks down tissues of the body. It has a devastating effect on the brain if its really high for a long period of time. Prolonged levels of excess cortisol causes impairment of brain dendrites by damaging the hippocampus, the master controller of the hypothalamus. This damage makes stress even worse by preventing access to information that is needed to decide whether or not something is really a threat or not.

In the initial stages of stress, when cortisol levels are high you may get thyroid resistance, where the cells can't let the thyroid hormone come in and do its job. Too much cortisol is responsible for weight gain (especially belly fat) blood sugar imbalance, thinning skin, muscle wasting, and aging. In the final stages of adrenal dysfunction, when cortisol levels drop due to adrenal exhaustion, there is not enough cortisol to allow the thyroid hormones to do their job of increasing energy and keeping metabolism up. This is why adrenal issues must be treated first, before the thyroid. If you treat the thyroid without treating the adrenals, you may feel worse than ever, because you are stressing an already overstressed system that can't respond to stress properly.

When you are under the effects of chronic stress, you break down more than you build up. You are accelerating the aging process. Your body will steal DHEA, resulting in lower estrogen, testosterone, and androstenedione. DHEA will get converted to make more cortisol because cortisol is more important. Pregnenolone may also be stolen to make cortisol. Pregnenolone is formed from cholesterol. Pregnenolone is used by the adrenal glands to form DHEA or used to make cortisol. Without pregnenolone, you can't make progesterone, DHEA, cortisol, or other hormones.

Testing For Cortisol & DHEA

The best way to test for cortisol and DHEA is through the saliva. The saliva test is preferred over blood and urine because saliva hormone values are more **"bio-available"** than the other biopsies. Unlike blood or urine hormone testing, saliva testing analysis assess the biologically active compounds (free fraction form) at the cellular level. It represents the patients true hormonal activity, especially with multiple samples collected over the course throughout the day. In comparison, blood analysis assess compounds as they travel through the blood serum, most of which are protein bound, preventing them from attaching to cell receptors. Saliva testing can identify the impact of chronic stress and the underlying dynamics of all your health complaints concerning your stress hormones. Here's a quick view of the importance of saliva testing benefits:

1. **Saliva testing should be performed on all patients with auto-immune disorder, FMS, CFS, and sex hormone insufficiency; evaluating progesterone, testosterone, and the estrogen.**
2. **It provides a window into each persons core state of health.**
3. **Identifies Cortisol rhythm with DHEA sulfate to determine the stage of adrenal fatigue.**
4. **Identifies Melatonin and night time cortisol levels to help with the evaluation of sleep problems.**

Always dig for the underlying cause of your health issues. Cortisol output by your adrenal glands is one of the most reliable indicators of your adrenal function and how well your body is dealing with stress.

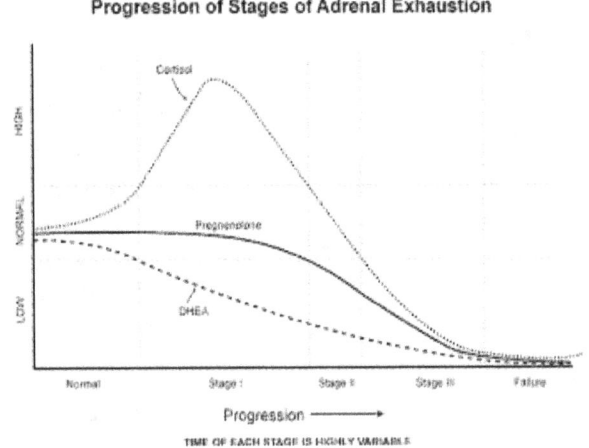

Progression of Stages of Adrenal Exhaustion

The Cortisol/DHEAS Saliva test measures the levels of the stress hormones DHEAS and cortisol in your saliva, and it provides you an evaluation of how cortisol levels differ throughout the day. Most saliva tests can uncover biochemical imbalances that can be underlying causes of such conditions as *chronic stress, adrenal fatigue, anxiety, chronic fatigue, obesity, diabetes, depression, insomnia, and many other chronic conditions.* Saliva testing is an important way to assess your DHEA, and Cortisol levels, in adrenal functioning that can profoundly affect an individual's energy levels, disease resistance, and general sense of well-being.

The synthesis of steroid hormones begins when the body uses cholesterol to make pregnenolone, the basic hormonal substance. From pregnenolone the makes DHEA and progesterone. The hormones in the progesterone pathway include cortisol and progesterone itself, are not directly derivable from DHEA. From this we can rightly intuit that although DHEA can be a remarkable help in the case of DHEA, estrogen, or testosterone deficiency, the truly balancing hormone substance is Pregnenolone. In fact, even though taking DHEA, better results can be obtained from taking Pregnenolone than DHEA.

One of the important requirements of pregnenolone is, you need to eat cholesterol containing foods to insure adequate pregnenolone production and to keep your body from manufacturing cholesterol. *These foods include butter, shellfish, avocados, eggs, and meat.* Don't deprive yourself from these important cholesterol containing foods. If you are taking Statins, then you can't make your own cholesterol and may have inadequate pregnenolone levels and steroid hormone production, if you don't eat enough cholesterol. Testing of all hormones should be performed on all patients with FMS and CFS to identify the underlying non-functioning hormones. This is a key in restoring balance back to the body.

Adrenal Symptoms Cortisol Test Questionnaire
(Men & Women)

(This questionnaire reveals the significant symptoms that indicates the need for Adrenal Saliva Testing)

<u>Adrenal Deficiency</u>
Early morning fatigue
Low blood sugar problems
Allergies
Chemical sensitivities
Stress
Heart Palpitations
Arthritis
Aches & pains
Irritability
Decreased concentration
Cold body temperature

<u>Adrenal Excess</u>

Weight gain
Sleep disturbances
Elevated triglycerides
Irritable, anxious, nervous
Depression
Headaches
Low libido
Hair loss
Stress
Memory lapse
Acne
Increased body hair (women)
Increased facial hair (women)

Check off each item that persists over time. If you have more than half of these symptoms that have persisted over time and nothing else you tried worked, then an adrenal function saliva test is indicated. At minimum an AM cortisol test is indicated. Note that for optimal adrenal gland function, they requires DHEA, Progesterone, and pregnenolone; These hormones are crucial in support of

adrenal exhaustion, stress, fatigue, and burnout.

Symptoms of Adrenal Dysfunction

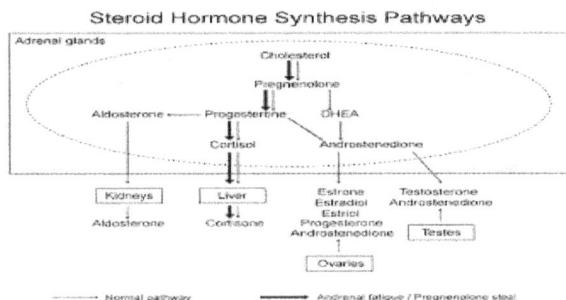

One will notice cortisol deficiency in the morning hours. With a loss of restorative sleep, you wake up exhausted and stay exhausted until bedtime. Without sleep, growth hormone (GH) and thyroid stimulating hormone (TSH) production is impaired. And without GH and thyroid stimulating hormone, and with increased cortisol and prolactin, your tissues begin to break down. Sleep deprivation interferes with nerve cell renewal causing major depression. People with more severe adrenal dysfunction will have a sudden drop in energy levels during exercise. Typically hitting the wall just after 30 minutes of exercise.

People with even more severe adrenal dysfunction often have low blood pressure. But sometimes people with clear signs of adrenal fatigue have high blood pressure. With sometimes having inflammation issues with their cardiovascular system or metabolic syndrome. But they still have low adrenal function. Low adrenal reserves is also associated with auto-immune disorders. This includes Fibromyalgia, chronic fatigue, lupus, thyroiditis, and rheumatoid arthritis. Interestingly enough, Salt cravings is a common symptom in all stages of adrenal fatigue. It's one of your body's ways of crying out for something it needs. However, the majority of people with adrenal fatigue have low blood pressure, not high. And for over seventy years, it has been known that people with Addisons disease benefited from the addition of sodium (salt) to their diet.

In adrenal fatigue it helps to raise blood pressure, in addition to restoring some of the other functions related to sodium loss within the cells. So, if you have salt cravings, use sea salt instead of regular table salt and salt your food liberally, as the trace minerals in sea salt are very beneficial to the health and functioning of your adrenal glands. If you are also concerned about your blood pressure buy a blood pressure machine and monitor your blood pressure readings those with low blood pressure, may experience a temporary rise in blood pressure toward normal when they add salt (sodium) to their diet. However, not to worry, as this does not lead to high blood pressure in most cases of adrenal fatigue patients that have low blood pressure. In most cases it benefits those who have added it to their diet.

In fact, if you happen to be one of those rare people with adrenal fatigue and high blood pressure, salt your food. Some of the symptoms of adrenal fatigue are caused by your body's need for sodium. Look for iodized sea salt in your grocery store. Also, some of the most nutrient rich sources of salt are kelp and a preparation of salt and sesame seeds called "gomasio". To improve the nutrient content of sea salt, it is a good idea to mix it half and half with kelp, this makes it exceptionally fortifying for those who suffer from severe adrenal fatigue. <u>On the other hand foods high in potassium such as fruits (especially bananas and dried figs) can make adrenal fatigue worse!</u> *Learn to avoid fruits and fruit juices in the early morning hours.* <u>The combination of sugar and potassium from fruits make it a dangerous combination for people with hypoadrenia.</u>

Yogurt with fruit for breakfast will put a lot of hypoadrenia people on the floor in a hurry, and one of the signs of hypoadrenia is increased fatigue with shakiness after a high fruit breakfast.

Symptoms of adrenal dysfunction include the following:

- **Severe fatigue**
- **Sleep difficulty (from elevated cortisol levels at night)**
- **Persistent illness (low immune function)**
- **Weight management issues**
- **Focus and concentration difficulty**
- **Anxiety, anxiousness (wired and tired)**
- **Mood swings**
- **Poor sleeping patterns with difficulty getting up in the morning hours.**
- **Salt cravings**
- **Low Libido (men & women)**
- **Impotence**
- **Low body Temperature**
- **Low or High Blood Pressure**
- **Carbohydrate Cravings**
- **Postural Dizziness**
- **Possible Ulcers**
- **Decreased Metabolism**

Testing For Adrenal Dysfunction: You Can Do At Home

Laboratory tests for adrenal fatigue typically used by doctors today are designed to detect adrenal fatigue in its varying degrees of severity as in several standard blood and urine tests to look for indications of hypoadrenia, their indications although interpret as inexact.

Their standard blood and urine tests include everything but the most severe cases of adrenal malfunction, such as ***Addison's disease (extreme low function of the adrenal glands)*** and ***Cushing's Syndrome (an extremely high functioning of the adrenal glands)***. So unless your hypoadrenia is this severe, your doctor will interpret your test results as indicating your adrenal gland function to be within normal range.

However, there are relatively new lab tests that accurately measures several hormones, especially for measuring the adrenal hormones, called **"Saliva Hormone testing"**. There are also, several different type of tests that you can do at home to help yourself to further determine if your adrenal glands are under functioning. These tests that are listed for home use, can be quite helpful, in the privacy of your own home to determine if your adrenal glands are functioning normally. The first test that was discovered in 1924 by Dr. Arroyo, is called the *"Iris Contraction Test"* and you can do this test at home yourself. The only equipment you'll need is a **chair, a small flashlight (penlight), a mirror, a watch with a second hand and a dark room.**

The Iris Contraction Test – First darken the room and sit in a chair facing a mirror. Then shine a lash light across one eye(not directly in the eye) but across from the side of your head. Keep shinning the light steadily across one eye and watch in the mirror with the other eye. You should see your pupil (the dark circle in the center of your eye) contract immediately as the light hits your eye.

This occurs because the iris, a tiny circular muscle composed of small muscle fibers, contracts and dilates the pupil in response to the light. Just like any muscle, after it has been exercised beyond normal capacity, it likes to rest. The pupil will normally remain contracted in the increased light. But if you have some form of *hypoadrenia,* the pupil will not be able to hold its contraction and will dilate despite the light shinning on it.

This dilation will take place normally within 2 minutes and will last for about 30 to 45 seconds before it recovers and contracts again. Time how long the dilation lasts with the second hand on the watch and record it along with the date.

After you do this once, let the eye rest. If you have any difficulty doing this on yourself, have a friend assist you and shine a light across your eye while both of you watch the pupil size.

Important – Retest monthly, if your eye indicates that you may be suffering from adrenal fatigue, this will serve as an indicator for recovery. As you recover from adrenal fatigue, the iris will hold its contraction and the pupil will remain small for longer. This diminished ability of the iris to remain contracted is present in moderate to server adrenal fatigue, but may not be present in mild cases.

The Low Blood pressure and Postural Low Blood pressure Test – Blood pressure is an important indicator of adrenal gland function. Although there are other causes associated with low blood pressure, low adrenal function is probably the most common and the most neglected by doctors. *Before you begin taking this test make sure that when you do that you are well hydrated with fluids (water) as this can give a false indication in measuring your blood pressure readings.*

For this test, all you need is a blood pressure gauge called a *"sphygmomanometer"* from a local drug store, or medical supply house, or the internet. Get the type that takes your blood pressure without the stethoscope. Some of them also have a convenient printed readouts. After learning how to work your blood pressure measuring device, lie down quietly for 10 minutes and then take your blood pressure while still lying down.

Next stand up and take your blood pressure again right after you stand up. Normally the blood pressure will rise 10 to 20mmHg= millimeters of mercury. If it drops when you stand up, you likely have some form of hypoadrenia or you may be dehydrated. If so try it again after you have had plenty of water. This will not work if you just drink one glass of water and trying again right away because your tissues take time to re-hydrate after drinking.

If your blood pressure still drops 10mmHg or more when you are sure you are not dehydrated, you probably have some form of *hypoadrenia*. The more severe the drop in blood pressure is, the more your *hypoadrenia* is. If you discover you are one of the many people with adrenal fatigue and low blood pressure, you should then find your blood pressure increasing to normal as you follow the program in this book.

Note: Occasionally, some one can have a normal blood pressure reading and still have *hypoadrenia,* the reason for this is due to the lack of elasticity in the arteries seen in those who have **"atherosclerosis" (hardening of the arteries).**

Also, if you are a complete vegetarian, and your blood pressure may be 95/65. If so, then your lower over all blood pressure does not necessarily mean you have *hypoadrenia*. However, a drop in blood pressure upon standing up from a lying position will still indicate *hypoadrenia*.

Sergent's White Line Test – This test was first described in 1917 by a French physician named Emile Sergent, as a simple test to check for low adrenal dysfunction that is still used to this day.

To do this test, you will need a *ball point pen*, take the dull end of the ball point pen and lightly stroke the skin of your abdomen, making a mark about 6" long. Within a few seconds a line will appear. In a normal reaction, the mark made by the penis initially white but reddens withing a few seconds.

If you have *hypoadrenia*. The line will stay white for about 2 minutes and will also widen. This test, although not always positive in people with *hypoadrenia (about 40% of cases) is a slam dunk confirmation of the presence of hypoadrenia.*

Summary: It is always best to do all 3 tests: the iris contraction test, the blood pressure lying and standing test, and Sergent's White Line test. The first two tests are reliable indicators found in nearly every moderate to severe cases of adrenal fatigue, but not in mild cases. Sergent's white line is only present in moderate to severe cases of *hypoadrenia* and in borderline cases, may only be present when the adrenals are at low ebb.

When this is the case, the "questionnaire test" of signs and symptoms, of adrenal fatigue can be your guide, especially in mild cases, because symptoms of adrenal fatigue usually precede signs.

Restoring Adrenal Health

Adrenal health can be measured with a four point cortisol saliva test, also called "cortisol test-saliva collection" (4x) or adrenal rhythm test. Using a four point measuring system, this cortisol test assesses saliva samples and is non-invasive. The test contains 4 test tubes for specimen collection, as well as the necessary lab paper work and a per-paid shipping label for quick specimen delivery. Test results include recommended treatments for addressing cortisol related issues. A reliable cortisol test is an excellent method of effectively measuring cortisol levels, assessing where they are throughout the day, and determining the best natural treatment options to ensure those levels are healthy and under control.

Treatment Methods for Adrenal Dysfunction

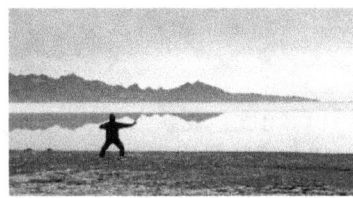

- **Apply stress reduction techniques**
- **Ensure adequate sleep patterns**
- **Use herbal adaptogens**
- **Adjust or ensure a proper lifestyle change**
- **Use and apply glandular extracts**
- **Use and apply vitamins and minerals for adrenal gland support**
- **Eliminate all processed foods**
- **Establish a corrective nutritional diet plant-based**
- **Eliminate the energy robbers(things that drain your energy) – alcohol consumption, smoking, processed foods, sugar by-products, junk and fast foods, etc.**
- **Take your dietary supplements regularly**
- **Keep a journal, jot down your experiences each day.**
- **Try having a glass of water with ½ to 1 teaspoon of sea salt stirred until dissolved. (for severe adrenal fatigue)**
- **Learn to salt your food with sea salt, eliminate regular table salt. Eat lots of colored vegetables, high quality proteins – lean cut meats, turkey, fish, and beans.**
- **Make the necessary lifestyle changes you need to make to regain your health.**
- **Take a 1,000mgs of vitamin C complex with 400mgs of magnesium and B5 500mgs every day with a small snack at 2:00pm.**

Avoid These Things

Getting over tired
Coffee, sugar, alcohol, and white flour products

Staying up late at night past 12am
Never skip breakfast
Avoid fruit in the morning hours
Never eat (starchy carbohydrates like bread, pastas) by themselves
Avoid over working and pushing yourself to the extreme
Chronic stress robs you of your brain power, shrinks and destroys the brain's region of memory.
Ending romantic or long term relationships can be devastating. It was found to be similar to the same brain changes as Post-traumatic Stress Disorder (PTSD), affecting both motivation and attention.

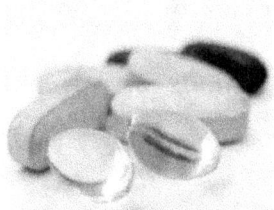

75% of the US population experiences at least some signs of stress in their lives every two weeks.

Stress contributes to heart disease, high blood pressure, strokes, auto-immune disease, and other illnesses.

Stress affects our immune system, leaving us less protected from serious illnesses. Tranquilizers, anti-depressants and ant-anxiety drugs account for ¼ of all prescriptions written in the US.

First you must identify your stressors and eliminate them. Change your attitude or response to the stressor. Don't let it get to you. Re frame your outlook and have an attitude of gratitude. Eat nutritional meals on a regular basis and modify your diet to decrease inflammation. Do gentle exercises like *yoga or tai-chi and pilates*. Incorporate live enzymatic foods to help with inflammation and the proper digestion of foods.

Supplements For Adrenal Health

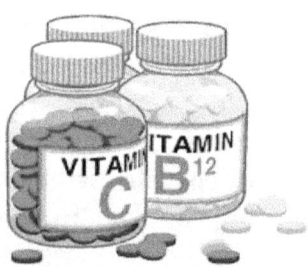

- <u>Vitamin C</u> – the highest concentration of vitamin C in the body resides in the adrenal glands. Vitamin C reduces high cortisol levels, and stimulates the immune system. Is also required by the adrenal glands in the manufacturing of adrenal hormones, along with vitamin B5 (pantothentic acid), vitamin B2 and Magnesium. The quantity of vitamin C also varies from person to person and by stress levels. Stressful events increases the need for more vitamin C and more nutrients. A time release vitamin C would be beneficial in this regard. Also to find out your level of vitamin C your body requires, you can try a very simple test called the **"vitamin C loading test".**

From day one of your vitamin C intake start out with 500mgs with 250mgs of bioflavanoids. Increase your intake of vitamin C by an additional 500mgs and bioflavanoids by 250mgs every hour until your bowl movements become somewhat loose and runny. Once you have achieved this level, then reduce your vitamin C by 500mgs and your bioflavanoids by 250mgs. This usually the amount of vitamin C your body needs at this time. The most common point for this to occur is about 2,500 to 4,000mgs. 2-4 grams for people with adrenal fatigue. Typically, the more chronic your illness of adrenal fatigue is, the more vitamin C you'll need. An interesting read, is a book called *"Why Animals Don't get Heart Attacks, But People Do!" by Dr. Matthias Rath.* Also highly recommended *"Adrenal Fatigue: The 21ˢᵗ Century Stress Syndrome" by James L. Wilson, N.D., D.C., Ph.D.*

- **Pantothenic acid B5** – helps in the production of adrenal hormones and is specific and necessary for adrenal health and function. Vitamin B5 is also considered an anti-stress hormone.

- **Magnesium Glycinate** – is commonly more effective in restoring magnesium levels with in the body than typically other forms of magnesium. It is also involved in over 300 enzymatic functions, reduces ACTH secretion at nigh and helps prevent post exercise hypocortisolism. Excellent also for nervous disorders and stress management.

- **Vitamin B2 (Riboflavin)** – is required in the manufacturing of adrenal hormones and adrenal
health.

- **Adrenal Cortical Extracts***** – Were once the earliest, and still probably the most reliable way of rebuilding the adrenal glands from adrenal fatigue. Made from bovine adrenal glands, they have been used extensively by modern clinics and are considered to be the most important aspect of adrenal treatment.
They provide the essential constituents for adrenal repair that include all the adrenal cell contents, such as RNA/DNA and concentrated nutrients in the form and proportion used by the adrenals to properly function and recover, but contain tiny amounts of the adrenal hormones.

These extracts have been used orally and as injectables since the end of WWI successfully without any side effects. These extracts have also been the corner stone of effective therapy for adrenal fatigue since they were first developed. They can be purchased at health food stores, and online. Good products are –

"Bezwecken Isocort", *"Enzymatic Therapy "ADRENergize", Natural Sources - "Raw Adrenal", Pure Encapulations – ADR- Formula.*

- **Royal Jelly** – A powerhouse of nutrients in a natural form. Loaded with natural vitamins, minerals, enzymes, and hormonal precursors – testosterone, adrenal hormones, and especially high in B5.

Dietary Supplements for Cortisol Control

- **L-Tyrosine** – an amino acid that is the precursor to epinephrine and norepinephrine. Also helps in the manufacture of thyroid hormones. Helps maintain mental performance and concentration during stressful events. Dosages range from 500mgs to 1,000mgs 2x a day.

- **Phosphatidylserine** – has direct cortisol=lowering effects, especially after intense exercise. Dosages are 300mgs 2x a day.

- **Relora*** – A popular herbal formula consisting of magnolia officinalis and Phellodendron amrense, shown to reduce stress and promote relaxation and well-being.

- **Epimedium** – Direct cortisol control, especially following the stress of dieting. Also helps in the manufacturing of testosterone and thyroid hormone modulation.

- **Phytosterols** – Balances cortisol to DHEA ratio, especially following exercise stress.

- **Theanine** – Modulates brain waves for optimal physical and mental performance during stressful times, has a nice calming affect.

- **Omega 3 Fatty acids** – helps to lower cortisol caused by mental stress. Also beneficial for cholesterol levels, memory function and ensures hormonal health.

- **Magnolia Bark*** - helps control cortisol production and the general effects of anxiety. Used also as an anti-stress agent. Also used in the popular anti-stress formula called "Relora."

- **Theanine*** - an amino acid found in green tea that helps to optimize dopamine levels, GABA, and serotonin to deal with stress. The more you take the more your alpha waves increase. It decreases norepinephrine, and lowers blood pressure.

PREGNENOLONE/*DHEA* & THE ADRENAL HORMONES

A natural hormone produced in the body, made from cholesterol, often referred to as the "mother of all hormones". Pregnenolone is also the basic precursor, or starting raw material for the production of all hormones, including <u>DHEA, progesterone, estrogen, testosterone, cortisol and aldosterone</u>, and as such is often referred to as "The Mother Hormone". Pregnenolone shows many of the benefits of cortisol, it reduces allergic reactions, lessens arthritis inflammation and produces a relaxing and mildly euphoric "stress buffer effect" without any of the negative side effects of cortisol. Some patients suffering from Fibromyalgia and CFS have benefited from taking pregnenolone in troche form (allows buccul absorption which enables a lower dose to be prescribed) in doses up to 100mgs daily. Pregnenolone can help balance excess cortisol levels.

Pregnenolone, also called the *"feel good" or "happiness hormone"*. Pregnenolone also affects the balance of serotonin, dopamine, and oxytocin, the bonding, attachment, or "cuddle" hormone. Emotions, fear, anxiety, focus, concentration, memory, trust, endorphins are all directly related to provolone levels.

According to Dr. Ray Peat Ph.D, a renowned nutritional expert, *"pregnenolone very quickly helps fatigued, stressed people regain their ability to handle stress, sometimes with a single dose. It also tends to improve the function of the thyroid and other glands as well. It can have a calming effect on emotions, giving you a mood of resilience and an ability to confront challenges."*

Also people have noticed that pregnenolone has a "face lifting" action, produced by improved circulation to the skin, and by an actual contraction of some muscle like cells in the skin. A similar effect can improve joint mobility in arthritis, tissue elasticity in the lungs, oxygen depletion in emphysema, and even eye conditions, including bulging eyes of Grave's disease. If you are taking adrenal hormones, you may want to take pregnenolone along with it. Pregnenolone comes in pills and creams.

DHEA – (dehydropiandrostene) is an androgen that is produced by both the adrenal glands and the ovaries. DHEA helps to neutralize cortisol's immune-suppressant effect, thereby improving resistance to disease. Cortisol and DHEA are inversely proportional to each other. When one is up, the other goes down. Like norepinephrine and cortisol, DHEA also improves your ability to recover from episodes of stress and trauma, over work, temperature extremes, etc.

And if a women is experiencing a decline in libido due to falling levels of testosterone, often its the declining of DHEA levels that are the root cause of testosterone deficiency, as DHEA is the main ingredient the body uses to manufacture testosterone. If the stress level and frequency of your life becomes too great, then over time your adrenal glands will begin to become exhausted.

 Which means that you will begin to suffer the effects of stress induced fatigue due to insufficient DHEA levels and weak adrenal glands. And interestingly enough the symptoms from weak adrenal glands mirror some of Fibromyalgia and CFS. This will be also characterized by cortisol levels that are too high at night and not high enough levels in the morning hours. Supplementing with DHEA with 10 to 25 mgs once or twice a day will help bring up your DHEA levels back to normal. Some people may need more and some may need less.

An in home saliva test kit will help you to monitor your proper DHEA levels. Typically older people will need more than younger people, as natural levels do decline as we age. Pregnenolone might just be the better choice here to supports adrenal function and health. Pregnenolone is the precursor to both DHEA and cortisol.

Adaptogenic Herb's For Heightened Stress & Physical Well-Being

Adaptogen is a term used in alternative medicine to describe a metabolic regulator which increases the ability of an organism to adapt to environmental factors, and to avoid the potential damage from such factors. Adaptogens are plants (herbs) that are a *__class of therapeutic substances__* that interact with the stress response mediators involved in the *regulation of homeostasis, energy metabolism and the neuro-endocrine immune system*.

Adaptogenic herbs help promote *resistance to stress, fatigue, trauma, and anxiety.* They also are a great addition to help keep cortisol levels under control. Adaptogens also help with restoring the body back to balance by helping to regulate neurotransmitter function and hormonal balance, especially the stress hormones. Their effect is mainly related to the HPTA hypothalamus-pituitary-adrenal-axis. Herbal adaptogens have been employed in traditional Chinese Medicine for thousands of years to maintain the body's vitality, and have also been the most widely studied of all medicinal herbs.

To put it simply, is that adaptogenic herbs help a person *"adapt"* to the stresses of day to day life. They will actually balance various bodily functions, and can be a great asset in assisting those under extreme stress better than any medicine because they target and strengthen the whole body. Used by athletes around the world as a safe and legal performance enhancer, much as the same way we would use food and supplements. For example, it was once strongly suspected that *"Cordyceps"* was used as the *"secret weapon"* by the Chinese Olympic team in recent years to have given them an edge in high level competition in the track & field event, in which they broke world records and won several Gold Medals.

Adaptogens help to reduce the effects of physical, environmental, and psychological stress on the body, and have been shown to boost the heart, liver, adrenal glands, immune system, and mental health of the person taking them.

Herbal Adaptogens

- **Cordyceps** ***– Used by the Chinese in Traditional Oriental Medicine for thousands of years as an important health tonic in debilitating conditions. Is very effective in restoring adrenal gland function and hormonal output. Cordyceps will help increase oxygen uptake therefore increasing energy and stamina. Also helpful with sexual dysfunction problems in men and women. Make sure you purchase the extract form of cordyceps. Dosage: 300 to 400mgs twice a day.

- **Ashwaganda***** – Traditionally described as a great tonic for all weaknesses and rejuvenator, and mild aphrodisiac. Ashwaganda is also a great stress reliever that helps protect you from nervous related symptoms, such as anxiety, depression, and also helps thyroid gland functioning and as a treatment for insomnia where it promotes relaxation. Considered a great adaptogenic herb, ashwaganda can help to lower excessive cortisol levels and raise them if too low. Studies have shown where ashwaganda can help to normalize and balance erratic levels of cortisol. It is especially useful in treating adrenal fatigue and is included in many herbal adrenal support formulas.

- **Rhodiola Rosea***** – excellent anti-depressant, decreases pain, improves mental performance, immune system function, lowers cortisol production, improves adrenal and cardiovascular function, and heals gut inflammation.

- **Jiaogulan***** - Is one of the more powerful herbal adaptogens known. So powerful that locals in China call it "The Herb of Immortality." It's adaptogenic effects benefits the body in two ways. (1) Jiaogulan directly nourishes the internal organs by increasing the blood supply through enhanced cardiac output. (2) Jiaogulan normalizes the nervous systems in the body when they are adversely affected by stress. It's list of benefits are very impressive!

- **Siberian Ginseng **** – helps to energize the body, gives endurance, is an immuno-stimulant, stimulates ACTH production, prevents oxidative stress, normalizes blood pressure and cortisol. It improves the immune system and it suppresses inflammation and DNA damage. One of its components is related to a precursor for DHEA and cortisol. Try one 100mg capsule two times a day. Do not take it at night as it can be a bit stimulating and interfere with sleep.

- **Royal Jelly***** – a nutritional powerhouse with amazing restorative powers. Loaded with natural vitamins, minerals, enzymes, hormone precursors, and especially rich in vitamin B5 an important vitamin for adrenal gland health and stress reduction.

- **Suma Root*** – Named in its native land, South America "Para Toda" (meaning, literally "for everything"). Modern recommendations for suma include an immune system booster, and as a treatment for chronic fatigue, anxiety, and anti-stress agent.

- **Astragalus**** – Normally recommended for the stimulation of the immune system and as for its energy promoting properties. Astragalus may be particularly beneficial for those individuals who feel fatigued due to high levels of emotional and physical stress. A great herbal tonic that has shown many beneficial effects throughout Eastern Traditional medicine.

- **Licorice Root Extract **** – This herb contains plant hormones that mimic the effects of cortisol. Licorice works by partially blocking the conversion of cortisol into cortisone, which can produce higher amounts of circulating cortisol. Start with a small amount and work your way up gradually of licorice root extract 3 x a day. Cortisol will slightly increases the contraction of the medium arteries and heart muscle causing blood pressure to rise. Make sure to also monitor your blood pressure, as licorice may increase your blood pressure in susceptible individuals.

But in any case, people who suffer from hypoadrenia typically have low blood pressure to begin with, so this is not usually a concern. This herb is best known for supporting Adrenal gland function. Known naturally for fortifying cortisone levels, arguably the most important hormone in stress and adrenal fatigue. Licorice root extract has also been used to help decrease symptoms of hypoglycemia, a common side effect of decreased adrenal function. Licorice is available as a tea, capsules, and natural licorice candy, that is always good to keep on hand in case you suddenly feel your adrenal glands giving out and need to temporarily boost yourself.

Note of Caution: Because of it's aldosterone like effects, licorice root may cause sodium retention and thus contribute to high blood pressure in some people.

- <u>Schizandra</u>*** – A traditional classic in traditional Chinese medicine, schizandra has earned it's mark in herbal medicine because of it's life strengthening powers. Because it empowers the mind, and its benefit to the kidneys (adrenal glands), liver, and lungs. It is favored for its ability to counter the effects of stress and fatigue. Scientific studies show it has normalizing effects in cases of insomnia and neurasthenia, and improves mental coordination, concentration, and physical endurance, just to mention some of its health enhancing affects.

<u>References</u> – (Regleson, W., et al. 1994, DHEA –" The Mother Steroid")

(Baschetti, R. 1995, chronic fatigue and licorice (letter)

Murray, M. & Pizzorno, J. Encyclopedia of Natural Medicine: 499. Rocklin, Calif.: Prima Publishing, 1990.

"Radiant Health: The Ancient Wisdom of the Chinese Tonic Herbs. Ron Teeguarden.

"Adaptogens: Herbs for Strength, Stamina, and Stress relief" David Winston and Steven Maimes.

"Adaptogens in Medicinal Herbalism: Elite Herbs and Natural Compounds for Mastering Stress, Aging, and Chronic Disease. Donald R. Yance (August 1, 2013)

American Botanical Council (ABC): A Phytomedical Overview. HerbalGram. 2002; 56:4-52.

- Panossian A, Wikman G. Evidence-based efficacy of adaptogens in fatigue,

and molecular mechanisms related to their stress-protective activity.

Dietary Protocol For Adrenal Health Recovery and Stress Reduction

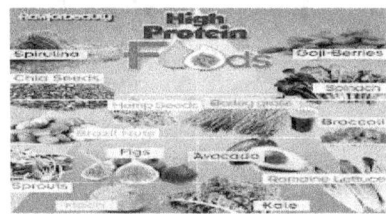

Establishing a healthy dietary protocol can be a very effective measure in restoring adrenal gland health back to normal. Protein meals are one of the keys for maintaining the health of your glandular system, your muscles, and your cells. Foods like fish (mercury free), chicken, beans, and nuts & seeds are a great source of natural protein you should eat on a daily basis. With meats, choose lean cuts of meat from an organic quality like tenderloin or sirloin. Fresh tuna also, salads, nuts and seeds all provide **essential fatty acids, proteins, and vitamins and minerals.**

Learn to snack on almonds, walnuts, sunflower seeds, pumpkin seeds that will nourish you and prevent fatigue when you eat regularly. Drink plenty of water throughout the day to ensure your body is well hydrated. When you feed your body with healthy foods, your adrenal glands will have the nourishment to support your daily lifestyle so they do not have to overwork. You m
You must eliminate processed and refined foods consisting of sugar by products.

A few simple adjustments to your diet may do wonders for you emotional well being. Because a few key foods and supplements will wipe away fatigue, restore balance, and help you to reduce stress without wiping you out (or your wallet).What we eat, has an overwhelming influence on brain chemistry and a direct affect on our response to stress.

By combining the right super foods throughout the day is a great start towards eating right. (1) eat a diet high in complex carbohydrates with a low glycemic index (legumes, and unrefined grains have a balancing effect as they cause fewer blood sugar disturbances. (2) Consume protein three times a day to help with depression and anxiety – proteins will help you to keep your blood sugar levels consistent. (3) Add proteins with high tryptophan amino acids such as pumpkin seeds, sunflower seeds, and parmesan cheese, that aids in the creation of serotonin and endporphins (mood regulating neurotransmitters); and eat foods high in B vitamins, which are necessary for producing SAM-e, a component of serotonin, melatonin and dopamine. B vitamins are often lost in stress, creating a cycle of not having nutrients to make chemicals we need to lift our sprints and strengthen our glands.

To compound this problem, many people often resolve in craving sugary foods as a quick fix junk food to ease their stressors. This type of eating is what got you sick and weak in the first place and often creates a vicious cycle. If you find yourself extremely stressed, eat a diet high in B vitamins and protein that can help you make the switch from resorting to unhealthy junk food. And if you feel your stress is more severe, consider taking a good B complex supplement that is time-released and is of 100mgs in potency or higher.

Super Nutrients For Mood & Stress

Beets - have a number of compounds that have been shown to raise serotonin levels and induce a subsequent calming affect in those who suffer from anxiety, depression and stress. The Betaine found in beets, is also known as *(TMG) trimethylglycine,* which helps raise an important compound called *(SAM-e, S-adenosylmethionine),* that influences **serotonin** metabolism. *SAM-e* can also help relieve the pain and depression from those who suffer from FMS and CFS. There are several scientific studies that can attest to its effectiveness.

Betaine is also a mood enhancer, and in the diet betaine rich foods are pharmacologically active, and can have a positive effect on moods by relaxing the mind. Beets or Beet root, because it contains Betaine (TMG) and increases the production of SAM-e, is therefore considered a "Mood-Food". Beets have a unique chemical make-up with high levels of important micronutrients. Betaine is also a dietary anti-oxidant with a particularly high bio-availability, with a very little being excreted under normal conditions. It also has other anti-oxidant nutrients including vitamin C and beta-carotene which help fight free radical build-up.

Black beans are another super food that is high in fiber, complex carbohydrates and protein. This is an all in one combination that prevents blood sugar levels from rising too fast, supplies protein that helps to stop the cravings for sugar and junk foods, and contributes to stabilizing stress. One cup alone of black beans will supply you with 15 grams of protein. Black beans are also filled with nutrients that directly contribute to brain health, giving you the ability to cope with stress.

Dark Chocolate is the number one food craved by American women that causes the brain to release *endorphins*, brain chemicals that make us feel good and help to control pain. Chocolate contains chemical compounds called *"flavonoids"*, also found in wine, that have anti-oxidant properties and reduce serum cholesterol. The best chemical producing chocolate is dark chocolate, also high in fat, so eating as little as one ounce is enough to be beneficial. The human body produces at least 20 different endorphins. Which produce four key effects on the body/mind; (1) enhance the immune system, (2) relieve pain, (3) reduce stress, and (4) post pone the aging process. Science has also found that beta-endorphins can activate human NK (Natural Killer) cells and boost the immune system.

Gruyere Cheese (groo-YEHR) is similar to Swiss cheese, is high in the amino acid tryptophan that produces serotonin, an important neurotransmitter in the brain that keeps us focused and calm. It is also rich in calcium, just half a cup provides

(667mgs) and magnesium (24mgs) known to help prevent anxiety. A perfect protein source that contains B vitamins and zinc which is often found low in people who are in depressed states.

Mustard Greens, this nutritional power house, may not be liked by many people as their first choice of food, but they are extremely nutritious, offering you a high amount of B vitamins needed to promote a steady supply of healthy neurotransmitter production for controlling stress levels, mustard greens are also high in minerals managanese, copper, magnesium, calcium, potassium, and phosphorus which are all necessary for relaxed muscles, anti-depressant, and memory enhancement. In addition to all the nutrients listed, mustard greens are extremely high in vitamin A, the anti-oxidant lutein and Zeaxanthin and vitamin C.

Nutritional Yeast is a great way in getting all of your necessary B vitamins needed to keep stress under control and provides the nutrients to make SAM-e, necessary for serotonin, melatonin and dopamine production. In addition, nutritional yeast is also high in protein, niacin B3, and B6 which lessens irritability and keeps the mind focused. It can be bought at any health food store, but ask for the best tasting nutritional yeast they carry, like (Red Star). But don't confuse nutritional yeast with Brewer's yeast. Two table spoons a day, which can be added to any beverage, add stir and drink!

Nutritional yeast can also be sprinkled on pop corn, over spaghetti, pizza, or any other dishes as a great healthy snack, or it can also be used as a seasoning for salads, gravies, soups, casseroles, burgers, and spreads.

Quinoa (Keen-wah), a grain that supplies a complete protein, providing all nine essential amino acids, and is a great source of complex carbohydrates. This combination helps to keep the blood sugar levels balanced throughout the day. This super food is a favorite among many who value its nutritional content. Quinoa is high in minerals such as magnesium, copper, calcium, and iron. Quinoa is an excellent source of magnesium, a mineral that helps relax blood vessels, preventing the constriction and rebound dilation characteristic of migraines. Quinoa is also a good source of Riboflavin B2, which is also shown to reduce the frequency of migraine attacks.

Pumpkin Seeds are one of the richest source of minerals. They are also high in tryptophan for serotonin production and contain good monunsaturated fats for brain health creating the perfect snack food for brain health. Pumpkin seeds are a well balanced source of the minerals magnesium, manganese, phosphorus, iron, copper, and a high content of zinc.

Tuna fish, a nutrient dense food, high in protein, B vitamins, B3, B1, and B6 – necessary nutrients to make SAM-e, a needed component for serotonin and melatonin production. Plus tuna is also rich in the minerals magnesium and Omega-3 fatty acids that contribute to optimal brain function.

Eating fish, like tuna, as little as one to three times a month has been found to protect against *"ischemic stroke"*, a stroke caused by the lack of blood flow to the brain. One interesting study found in the "Journal of European Clinical Nutrition" - in the 2004 issue, there was a significant relationship between consuming fish rich in Omega 3 fats, lowered hostility scores in 3,581 young urban adults. Those with the highest intake of Omega 3 fatty acids had only a 10% likelihood of having the highest scores. Hostility, has been shown in human studies to predict the development of heart disease.

<u>Winter Squash</u>, is one of the only many vegetables that can lay claim to a high content of B vitamins, and omega 3 fatty acids that are quickly lost when under severe stress. Winter squash is also rich in anti-oxidants vitamins A, C, and E.

<u>Water</u>, a very under estimated liquid that many people take for granted not realizing the important significant value to human life. Studies have linked many health related issue's due to the deficiency of water. What is not realized by many people, dehydration can cause decreased energy levels, mental dysfunction (depression), fatigue, joint and muscle pain, constipation, and once that backs up, waste will build up and cause a host of other ailments. A lack of water can be the unknown culprit in many disorders, and is the number one cause of daytime disease. 80% of the brain tissue consists of water.

Just a 2% drop in water can trigger fuzzy, short-term memory, trouble with basic math and difficulty focusing. The basic requirement consumption of water is, drinking at least half of your body weight in ounces, i.e., 150 pounds divided in half = 75lbs; next convert that into ounces=75 ounce/day. A medium size bottle of water is approximately 25 ounces. Try and drink three of those each day. And remember, its perfectly safe to drink to drink more!

Realize that if the body is dehydrated, several types of anxiety disorders and nervousness can be induced, the most common one is Generalized Anxiety disorder (GAD). Beverages with caffeine also increase anxiety. Trying to replace soda, coffee, and tea with water will be a great start in reducing anxiety and improving your stress levels,

Ways to Relieve Stress

In your general learning to help yourself relieve stress influences ability to deal with pain and other symptoms of your condition. The more relaxed you become, the better the results in pain management and discomfort of fibroblast. Here are a few ways you can relieve stress and help yourself relax.

<u>Exercise</u> – Regular exercise can be a great way in relieving your stress level. Exercise helps your body create more endorphins, your feel good body chemicals, exercise also helps the body to produce more of growth hormone in which most FMS and CFS are deficient in, Make it a habit of exercising several times a week and you'll begin to

notice your stress levels start to diminish. You can start out slowly in the beginning by doing some walking and eventually increase this to aerobics and then to a more progressive style of resistance training. You will find that exercise can elevate your moods, relax your muscles,, and even give you a feeling of being in more control over your symptoms.

<u>Take a warm bath with Epsom salt.</u>
Epsom salt is magnesium based and can help you relax tense muscles that may have been in a knot for quite some time. And also helps to remove toxins and impurities from your body.

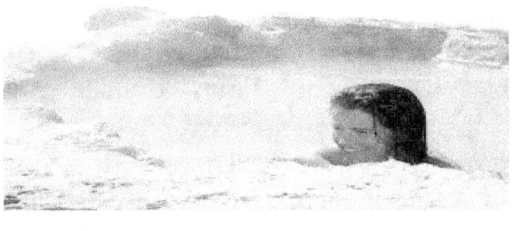

<u>Know your limitations</u> – try and not to over commit yourself to work, family, or friend. Finding balance in your life is a key to overcoming fibromylgia, and is one of the best ways to do
 that is to make sure you take enough time for yourself.

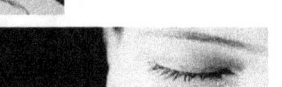

<u>Get a good night sleep</u> – Fibromyalgia and sleep disorders can go hand in hand. Solving this problem can be a key towards recovery from CFS and FMS. Learning some of the sleep resolutions discussed in the section of solving fibroblast sleep disorder.

Uncovering The <u>Role Players</u> in FM & CFS: Supporting Hormonal Balance

Because fibromyalgia is a syndrome with varied symptomatology it is very difficult to pinpoint a specific cause of location within the body. It affects the glandular system of the body such as the hypothalamus-Pituitary-Axis, pituitary, thyroid, and adrenal glands. With each gland contributing to it's own set of symptoms.

• **Fibromyalgia and CFS are both associated with <u>highly sensitive nerve cells</u> in the spinal <u>cord and brain</u>. The exaggerated sensitivity levels may result from chemical changes in the brain from the neurotransmitters or/and the spinal cord that controls pain. As a result of these changes, the person feels pain more quickly and diffuse muscle pain is present.**

• **Fibromyalgia is linked to brain chemical (Neurotransmitters) imbalances that leads to lower tolerance to pain and restless sleep with daytime fatigue, <u>especially serotonin</u>. From here, there is only one step to a decreased physical activity, muscles become more sensitive, more painful and more easily irritable.**

• **Fibromyalgia and CFS is caused by hormonal imbalances between cortisol and growth hormone. The release of these hormones is controlled by the pituitary gland and the hypothalamus. Hormonal imbalances lead to fatigue, mood changes, memory problems, low pain tolerance and other symptoms.**

With chronic stress being the underlying factor in here, several studies have demonstrated how chronic stress undermines normal hormonal function. Poor sleep, chronic stress, nutritional deficiencies, prescription drugs, and other stressors take their toll when accumulated over a number of years. Research shows that a large majority of Fibro sufferers are deficient in **serotonin, dopamine, and norepinephrine**. These three neurotransmitters are essential for optimal mood and mental functioning.

Serotonin also helps regulate moods, sleep, digestion, bowl movements, pain, and mental clarity. Additionally, individuals with Fibro have low levels of the amino acid tryptophane, as well as 5-hydroxytryptophan (5-HTP), which are needed for the production of serotonin. There are some nutritional supplements that can help restore optimal neurotransmitter balance, especially serotonin and norepinephrine levels, which is critical for Fibro sufferers. While the exact cause of Fibro is still not known to science today, we do know that individuals with FM and CFS have a hormonal imbalance related to the hypothalamus, pituitary, thyroid and adrenal glands which can create a host of detrimental health conditions.

The main function of the hypothalamus is to maintain the body's status quo (homeostasis). Because of its wide range of influence, the hypothalamus could be considered the body's master gland (computer). The hypothalamus receives continuous input about the state of health of the body and must then be able to initiate changes if anything goes wrong.

The hypothalamus regulates blood pressure, digestion, (bloating, gas, indigestion, and reflux), sleep/wake cycle, sex drive, body temperature, balance, and coordination, heart rate, and sweating; all of which can be problematic in Fibromyalgia sufferers. If these hormone levels fluctuate, it has effects on the whole body. It has been fairly obvious by now that stress is thee main contributing factor to these underlying hormonal imbalances affecting the function of the hypothalamus-pituitary-adrenal gland-axis (HPTA). That is why Fibromyalgia has been referred to as a "stress-related disorder" because stress both precedes its onset and aggravates its symptoms causing stress-induced changes in the hippocampal area of the brain.

This causes a cascade of disturbances and malfunctions with unbalanced neurotransmitters and hormonal levels. Thus causing controversies of belief among doctors in treating and/or diagnosing Fibromalgia/CFS. Some site that a **thyroid** deficiency as being the main cause of FM and CFS, other doctors may claim that a deficiency in the hormone **"Relaxin"** a hormone found in pregnant women, in which relaxin receptors can be found in all connective tissues disrupting connective tissue function.

And other supporting theories believed by other doctors that may contribute to the cause and/or start of FM/CFS are: *Leaky Gut Syndrome, Insulin imbalance, Progesterone deficiency, Serotonin deficiency/imbalance, Estrogen dominance, Cortisol insufficiency, Low Adrenal/Thyroid function, Enzyme Insufficiency, etc* Now you can see why this particular problem has gone undiagnosed without the exact contributing cause for all these years.

The Hypothalamus-Pituitary-Adrenal-Axis (HTPA) Dysfunction
"How It Affects FMS & CFS"

The main function of the hypothalamus is "homeostasis", or maintaining the body's status quo. The hypothalamus receives and transmits messages from the nervous system and hormonally through the circulatory system. Considered also as the body's "master computer system" it has a broad sphere of influence on the whole functioning of the human body. It receives continuous input about the state of the body on a daily level, 24/7 basis and must be able to initiate compensatory changes if anything drifts out of line.

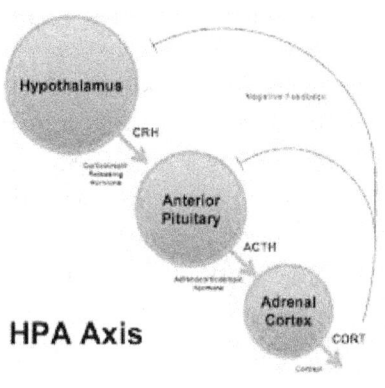

One of the most destructive ways that can great affect the workings of the hypothalamus gland and its communicating co-parts (pituitary-adrenal and thyroid glands) is chronic emotional and physical stress. Surveys have revealed by the Fibromyalgia Network, that over 62% of Fibromylagic and CFS listed chronic emotional and physical stress as being the initiating factor in acquiring FMS. This in my belief and experience, leads me to believe that chronic stress serves as the underlying catalyst in the onset of hypothalamic-pituitary-adrenal axis (HPTA) dysfunction.

Regulatory Function of The Hypothalamus
In Relation To FMS/CFS

- Blood pressure – (found low in FMS and CFS)
- Body temperature – (Often low in FMS)
- Sweating – (experienced in those with FMS)
- Circadian rhythm – (sleep-wake cycle, constant problem with FMS)
- Sex drive – (sexual dysfunction is a common problem in FMS and CFS)
- Digestion - (stomach distress also common in FMS patients)
- Balance and coordination - (problem with FMS patients)
- Heart rate – (heart arrhythmias and mitral valve prolapse (MVP) common finding in FMS)
- Adrenal Hormones – (constantly low in FMS and CFS patients)
- Thyroid hormones – (hypothyroidism and metabolism problem also common in those FMS and CFS) and recent studies have shown that the majority of FMS and CFS patients suffer from low thyroid and adrenal problems.

Symptoms Created From HPTA Dysfunction
Vicious Cycle

- Chronic stress disrupts the HPTA homeostasis
- Chronic pain disrupts the circadian rhythm
- Dysfunction in the circadian rhythm results in poor sleep-wake poor sleep

reduces growth hormone production, leading to poor memory, fatigue, suppressed immune function, and more pain.

- Increased pain resulting from lack of sleep and GH production further leads to disrupting sleep and depletion of stress coping chemicals including serotonin.
- A reduction in serotonin now causes an increase in the neurotransmitter, substance P, which also enhances pain receptors, creating even more pain.
- Poor sleep and ongoing stress from lack of sleep and rest leads to more fatigue, mood disorders, IBS, and may cause thyroid dysfunction.
- Chronic stress now contributes to adrenal fatigue, decreased DHEA levels, a lowered resistance to stress, and a decreased stress coping ability then leads to a compromised immune system function.
- Lowered blood volume circulation from adrenal dysfunction and a resultant low blood pressure state, leads to further fatigue.

And thus the cycle continues on until gland function no longer exists!

This is a vicious cycle that leads to destruction, so please take care of your body and it will take care of you! <u>Remember, the body always strives to heal itself, this is the way it was designed.</u> But it can not do that if we don't try and help the healing affects to take place, and how we do that is by starting to clean things up that have gone astray, <u>by changing our lifestyle, managing stress, eating healthy foods, adding nutritional support (supplements), detoxifying and cleansing, and by using the muscles you were born with to exercise!</u>

The Thyroid: Adrenal Connection In Fibromyalgia

About 80% of those who suffer from adrenal fatigue also have a number of symptoms of low thyroid as well. They both work together in the body regulating vital everyday functions that take place. Usually when one gland is affected, the other one normally follows. Left unresolved, a chain reaction of other symptoms soon follows. The thyroid is another gland that is easily sensitive to the affects of stress. Both of these glands are ultimately regulated by the hypothalamus-pituitary-adrenal axis and easily burdened by stressful situations. Taking a hypothalamus extract may help to normalize your thyroid and adrenal functioning when they both need a little fine tuning.

The key to determining underlying bodily burdens is to look at your health history time line and note things that have occurred within the past few months of the onset of adrenal fatigue. Once the body burden is discovered, find a way to limit or remove it.

Thyroid system

The Thyroid Gland / Fibromyalgia Relationship

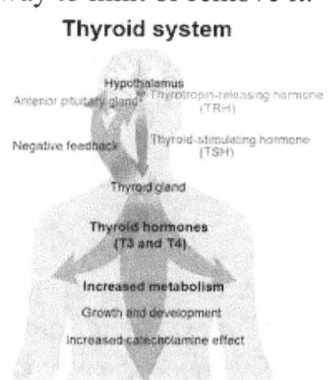

I find that over 50% of Fibromyalgia and CFS patients are suffering with low thyroid function, with nearly more than half of them have undiagnosed thyroid issue's.
Both conditions share similar symptoms, including fatigue, exhaustion, depression, brain fog, and varying degrees of muscle and joint pain.

In addition these thyroid issues could also be amplifying your CFS or Fibromyalgia symptoms, making them worse than they would be if your thyroid was functioning properly. And if it's not functioning properly, then treating your thyroid could improve your Fibromylagia.

However, if left unresolved, hypothyroidism will create an auto-immune reaction that can lead to an inflammation and destruction of the thyroid gland caused by anti-bodies against the thyroid tissue. Resulting in an auto-immune condition called "Hashimoto's Thyroiditis".

This happens when anti-bodies direct white blood cells to invade and destroy the thyroid gland. Eventually the thyroid gland can be destroyed in which now the person becomes hypothyroid. Hashimoto's may also be associated with auto-immune disorders especially against other endocrine glands (diabetes, low adrenal function, low parathyroid function, B12 deficiency). Anti-bodies attack and will disable various organs including the intestines, the adrenals, and the pancreas. There is also a high incidence of "Gluten" allergies with Hashimoto's. Gluten may produce a flare up of thyroid anti-bodies when allergies co-exist.

Auto-immune reactions are the primary cause of thyroid disorders. When there are symptoms of either hypothyroidism or hyperthyroidism, screen for thyroid anti-bodies (TPO and TBG). TSH (thyroid stimulating hormone) is not the best test to measure thyroid function. T4 does not adequately convert into T3. Reference ranges do not reflect if the thyroid hormone level is too high or low for you. The pituitary gland may also be sluggish and not increase sufficient TSH even though the peripheral tissues need more thyroid hormone. It is therefore better to use clinical symptoms and a physical exam to diagnose thyroid insufficiency. Testing confirms the diagnoses and may help indicate the source of the symptoms. Thyroid hormones may be sub-optimal, even though TSH numbers are in the normal range of.5 to 5. It is more important to evaluate the T3 and the free T4 levels and bring them into optimal range.

To diagnose thyroid auto-immunity (Hashimoto's), measure the thyroid peroxidase (TPO) anti-bodies. TPO is positive in 85 to 100% of cases in Hashimoto's disorder. Iodine has also been claimed to be a major co-factor and stimulator for the enzyme TPO. It may also increase levels of TPO anti bodies resulting in auto-immune flare-ups. Thus it is very important to be careful when using iodine with Hashimoto's thyroiditis.

Hyperthyroidism is a condition where the thyroid gland is overactive, and produces an excess of thyroid hormone. The gland becomes overactive primarily due to auto-immune Grave's disease, or in some cases due to thyroid nodules that produce excess thyroid hormone, or viral illness. Hyperthyroidism (overactive thyroid) disease will also commonly increase muscle tension and cause agitation and sleep disruption – a perfect recipe for Fibromyalgia. The gender of people who have experienced hyperthyroidism and Fibromyalgia are mostly women 100% of the time as opposed to men 0.00%. But it is hypothyroidism that is more commonly associated with Fibromyalgia and CFS with many of the same symptoms.

The primary 3 symptoms that they share with fibro and CFS are severe fatigue, brain fog, and muscle and joint pain, which usually isn't quite as severe as with Fibromyalgia. With Fibromyalgia, blood tests are usually negative, with a thyroid condition this is sometimes true as well, and many times you can't rely on positive thyroid blood tests even when the thyroid blood tests are accurate, they don't tell you anything about the underlying cause of the condition.

AS a result other tests are usually necessary to help the doctor find the actual cause of the disorder. And usually when the thyroid gland is affected you will find the adrenal glands to be compromised as well. When this happens you can also be sure that there will be a hormone imbalance which can contribute to a condition called estrogen dominance which involves an imbalance in estrogen and progesterone. This can involve an excess in estrogen and usually a deficiency in progesterone.

This can cause a lot of problems, and can contribute to many of the symptoms associated with Fibromyalgia and thyroid condition. And just is the case with weak adrenal glands, any existing hormone imbalance will need to be corrected in order to restore the health of someone with Fibromyalgia or a thyroid condition. In addition to the estrogen and progesterone, imbalances in other hormones can also be causing or contributing to their condition. For this reason it might be necessary to obtain a hormone panel to determine if there is an imbalance, and if so, to find out which hormones are involved.

This of course will help the doctor put together a necessary protocol to help correct this imbalance. Sometimes this involves giving natural progesterone to the patient without resorting to prescription hormones. Most people who follow through with a natural health protocol to restore their health, find it is well worth the effort. I find that many people with Fibromyalgia are willing to follow such a health protocol because most people with this condition experience severe pain and debilitating fatigue, and on the average the symptoms are worse than people with thyroid conditions.
Also, for both Fibromyalgia and thyroid conditions it is wise to consult with a competent doctor endocrine doctor or a naturopathic one that have experience with Fibromyalgia. Many people attempt to try and self-treat these conditions, but are so complex that it is extremely difficult to achieve maximum results on your own. Treating these conditions requires a strict natural treatment protocol which definitely involves modifying certain lifestyle factors, dietary changes, specific nutritional supplements and herbs. And if there are any specific underlying hormonal imbalances, which is always frequently the case, this will also need to be detected and addressed. Truth be told this is a very complex process that is challenging enough in order to restore your health.

For most people that have Fibromyalgia with a thyroid and adrenal condition, your goal will be to find the underlying condition through the necessary testing of a complete thyroid panel test (not a simple TSH test) – Adrenal stress index test, hormonal panel test, hair analysis test for nutritional deficiencies, etc., then address these causes as necessary. When I have consulted with people who had Fibro who were taking over a dozen medications, I've discovered that in all the cases the medications did a poor job of managing their pain and their symptoms. But for those who followed a natural treatment protocol found the answer in getting their life back together again in achieving a complete recovery from their horrible condition.

Symptoms <u>Low Thyroid</u> Can Mimic Fibromyalgia

- **Fatigue**
- **Brain Fog**
- **Muscle and joint pain**
- **Insomnia**
- **Depression**
- **Muscle weakness**
- **Pain stiffness, or swelling in your joints**
- **Difficulty concentrating**
- **Constipation**
- **Puffy face**
- **Hoarse voice**
- **Unexplained weight gain**
- **Heavier than normal menstrual periods**
- **Pale, dry skin**
- **Cold extremities**
- **Hair loss**
- **Digestive problems**
- **Trouble swallowing pills**

<u>**In summary**</u>, it is definitely possible to restore the health of someone with Fibromyalgia, as well as many people who have had <u>thyroid and auto-immune thyroid conditions</u>. But one must first detect the cause of these conditions, and then take the necessary measures to restore the person's health back to normal. <u>Doing this will take time and commitment on the person's behalf, but if it means there's a possibility of restoring their health back to normal then most people will find this "sacrifice" well worth it</u>!

<u>**Note:**</u> When treating a thyroid condition, there are two options; synthetic medication and natural Glandulars. Most doctors will prescribe medications such as ***Synthroid*** or ***Levothyroxine*** to treat your hypothyroidism. These medications only contain T4 thyroid hormone. I believe glandulars are a much better option. Using a natural glandular, such as ***Armour Thyroid***, gives you both T3 and T4 thyroid hormones. They are made from pig thyroid, which is similar to human thyroid. However, if you go with a natural glandular, choose Armour Thyroid. Because they think that the natural glandulars are standardized, meaning that you may not get a consistent amount of thyroid hormone in a natural pill.

In addition, natural glandulars have been proven to work better on depression than many anti-depressants! Synthetic thyroid medicines can not make this claim. Natural glandulars also contain both T3 and T4 hormones which your thyroid produces naturally; the synthetics most doctors prescribe do not contain both. Plus natural products are utilized by the body better than do synthetics.

If you would like to read more about diagnosing thyroid disorder, and auto-immune disease, and how an undiagnosed thyroid disorder could be affecting you, I highly recommended that you read - ***"Why Do I Still Have Thyroid Symptoms?" by Datis Kharrazian.***

Optimizing Thyroid Function

You can't make thyroid hormone without <u>iodine.</u> Most Americans are terribly deficient in iodine, as they don't get enough from their diets. Iodized salt provides only about 400mcgs per teaspoon. You can get iodine by eating seafood and iodine supplements. Taking 12.5 to 25mgs daily will help you to metabolize excess estrogen, reduce breast tenderness caused by estrogen dominance, and clear halogen (chlorine, bromine, fluoride) toxicity.

Causes of Hypothyroidism

The epidemic of thyroid under activity is largely caused by <u>chronic stress,</u> poor lifestyle, nutritional deficiencies (iodine), and environmental toxicity. <u>Iodine deficiency is the primary cause worldwide,</u> *other possible causes for primary hypothyroidism are excessive iodine and drugs, congenital, and diseases that infiltrate the thyroid.* Thyroid function also decreases with age, and the failure of the thyroid to bounce back after an acute stress may cause thyroid deficiency after the stressor.

Thyroid gland failure may also be caused by a *<u>diet lacking B6, B2, niacin, magnesium, selenium, zinc, and copper, which are co-factors in thyroid hormone production</u>*. A lack of tyrosine is also common in vegetarians, vegans, and bodybuilders. Other possible causes may be the pituitary may not be producing enough TSH to stimulate the thyroid. <u>This is secondary hypothyroidism.</u> *Chronic stress may also fatigue the pituitary gland* which may include *lifestyle, pregnancy, medications, and unneeded thyroid replacement therapy.* Failure of the hypothalamic control may not be stimulating the pituitary enough which is frequently associated with cortisol and stress hormones that adversely affect the functioning of the hypothalamus.

Hypothalamic glandulars may be helpful in this regard with stress management to reduce the frequency of damage caused by stress. The conversion of T4 to T3 that the cells can use, is something to be a ware of concerning thyroid supplementation, especially with medications that are often prescribed. Your TSH (thyroid stimulating hormone), T4, and T3 blood tests may be within normal limits, but a hypothyroid condition may still exist unknowingly to you. Look for low body temperature and hypothyroid symptoms with normal blood tests. ***Below you will find a helpful list which states what interferes with T4 to T3 conversions:***

<u>Substances That Can Interfere With The Absorption of Thyroid Hormone Medication</u>

- **Inadequate protein intake**
- **Low progesterone levels**
- **Deficiencies in selenium, chromium, zinc, iodine iron, copper, vitamin A, B2, B6, B12, and vitamin E.**
- **Beta blockers**
- **Heavy metal toxicity**
- **Smoking**
- **Too much iodine**
- **Theophylline**
- **GH deficiency**
- **Soy**
- **Too much or too little cortisol**
- **Stress-related**
- **SSRI's**
- **Lithium**
- **Opiates**
- **Alcohol**
- **Obesity**
- **Trauma**
- **Inflammation**
- **Fasting, dieting**
- **Glucocorticoids**
- **High glucose and insulin**
- **Calcium supplements**
- **Anti-acid's**
- **Iron supplements**
- **Food in general, do not take your thyroid med's with any food in general. Dairy products also.**

Interference with the conversion of receptor uptake failure results in thyroid resistance. Just like insulin resistance, where cells shut off their receptor doors to insulin, in receptor-resistant hypothyroidism the cells shut their doors to T3. Vitamin D levels that are too low may be also associated with this problem, and either high or too low cortisol may also decrease thyroid receptor responsiveness.

Adrenal insufficiency may also contribute. Thyroid hormones won't work efficiently without cortisol. Elevated and lowered cortisol levels (as in adrenal exhaustion) affects thyroid production, conversion, and receptor uptake, Correcting adrenal dysfunction first will help to resolve any thyroid related issue's.

Thyroid Tests You Can do At Home

The Thyroid Neck Check – **This test is advocated by the American Association of Clinical Endocrinologists. To perform the test you will need a glass of water and a hand held mirror. Hold the mirror out in front of you so you can clearly see the area of your neck just below your Adam's apple and above your collar bone.**

Tip your head back, while continuing to look at this area, take a sip of water and continue on swallowing.

Look at your neck while swallowing. Check for any lumps or bulges while you swallow. Don't focus on your Adam's apple; your thyroid gland is located further down your neck, closer to your collar bone. Take a few sips of water and repeat this process.

If you see or feel any lumps or bulges in this area, see your doctor. A thyroid nodule is likely to move when you swallow, where as a lump elsewhere on your neck will not.

The Broda O. Barnes Basal Temperature Test –

This test was first discovered by a famous thyroidologist Dr. Broda Barnes, that found out out that the basal (resting) body temperature is a good indicator of thyroid function. An under active thyroid can produce a drop in body temperature, where as an overactive thyroid can increase body temperature. Measuring your body temperature is a great tool you can use to diagnose a problem with your thyroid gland. It should also be used in conjunction with medical tests, specifically a complete thyroid panel.

Instructions for Performing the Thyroid Temperature Test
Use a mercury thermometer. Clean the thermometer with cool soapy water. Gripping the end opposite of the bulb, shake down the thermometer until it reaches 96 degrees fahrenheit or lower. Place the thermometer beside your bed within easy reach, so you can pick it up while still lying down the next morning.

The next morning, as soon as you wake up, place the thermometer in your armpit. Make sure that there is no clothing in between your armpit and the thermometer. Hold and place the thermometer there for ten minutes and continue lying still for that time.. Write down your temperature. You must do this for 4 consecutive days.

Important Tips: *Women should do this test on the second day of their menstrual cycle for a more accurate reading*. It is important to take this test first thing in the morning hours upon waking up without moving from your bed, eaten anything or having anything to drink. This way you will be recording your lowest body temperature of the day.

Treatment For Thyroid Dysfunctions

Treatment for thyroid disorders depend on what type thyroid disease you have, and in some cases, the severity of the condition. The normal treatment for auto-immune thyroid conditions are:

- **Gluten free diet** for at least 60 days if positive for gliadin anti-bodies-substances.

- **Remove processed foods from diet.**

- Include pure <u>sea salt</u> which is the kind the body naturally excepts and utilizes. Discard and stop using <u>regular table salt that has been bleached and heavily refined.</u>

- Correct hormonal imbalances, especially DHEA\ insufficiency and adrenal dysfunctional. Use enough thyroid hormones to keep TSH around 1.0

- Restore proper intestinal function and GI flora.

- Avoid iodine supplementation with high TPO.

- Rectify any iodine deficiency (with caution).

- Supplement with Magnesium.

<u>TREAT THE ADRENAL GLANDS FIRST!</u>

<u>Important:</u> The thyroid gland will not function properly without <u>treating the</u> <u>adrenal</u> <u>glands first and the hypothalamus and pituitary</u> <u>gland.</u>

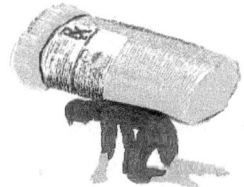

Conventional Medical Thyroid: T3 Treatment Choices

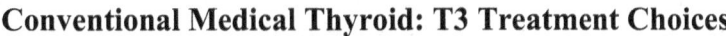

T3 has a short half life about 7 hours, vs T4 (Levothyroxine or Synthyroid) of 7 days. Use a 12 hour extended release type, twice a day to keep T3 levels steady. Also available in multiples of 7.5 mcg.

- Cytomel – is a T3 hormone and is available in 5, 25, and 50mcgs.

- <u>Armour Thyroid* - has 20% T3: Armour equivalent 9 mcg T3 and 38mcg T4. (Best one to use)</u> is made from natural sources, works very effectively.

- Bio-Thyroid – is available with various combinations of T4:T3. Bio-Throid is a sustained release capsule (12 to 24 hours based on the size of the capsule).

- **Levothyroxine (T4)** – composed of thyroxine sodium and come in a dose of 50, 100 or 200mcgs. Considered the primary medical treatment and is identical to the hormone thyroxine that your own thyroid makes.

Natural Thyroid Treatment

Once you have determined that there's enough evidence to support a low functioning thyroid gland, you can begin to try the recommended supplementation. Below is a list of over the counter products (OTC) that will help stimulate your thyroid. Most of the recommended supplements can be found on line at www.notmedicine.com or www.amazon.com, which have all been used with an excellent success rate.

- **Iodine** – This nutrient is critical for the production of thyroid hormones. The best sources of supplemental iodine come from iodine rich seaweeds such as Bladderwrack, kelp, or dulse.

- **Natural Sea Salt** – this type of salt contains naturally occurring trace minerals such as iodine, magnesium, potassium, and iron. The minerals contained in this type of salt is similar to the salt our body needs, and hasn't been refined as regular table salt(sodium chloride) which should not be used. Our bodies will absorb natural sea salt much more easily, and the minetals they contain will help support your thyroid gland. Look for "real salt from www.realsalt.com or from www.seasalt.com. This is the most healthiest type of salt to consume.

- **Tyrosine** – is the basic building block of all thyroid hormones, a deficiency in tyrosine will most certainly make it difficult for a person's thyroid to make adequate amounts of T4 and T3 hormone. However, because of its availability in the diet, a shortage will most likely stem from an inability to properly breakdown amino acids because of stomach related problems or a problem from absorption.

Malabsorption is a common problem with FMS and CFS patients. One good combo formula to try is from - *(Enzymatic Therapy's Thyroid & Tyrosine and Thorne Research's Thyrocsin)* can be found at www.vitaminshoppe.com.
Tyrosine is also a precursor to the neurotransmitter dopamine, norepinephrine, and epinephrine(adrenaline). And is also needed for healthy adrenal support and pituitary gland function. Dosage 500 to 1,000mgs two times a day upon rising in the am hrs and no later than 5 pm. Taking any later in the evening hours may keep you awake.

- **Glandular extracts** – derived from the glands of animal tissue, cows and pigs, contains everything required for a healthy thyroid gland function. Glandular extracts are a very effective method for restoring a low functioning thyroid.

Thyro-Complex – has a multi-glandular formula with supporting nutrients. This product has been used successfully for many thyroid patients to come off their prescription thyroid medications.

- **Thyroid-120** – this supplement is one of MBI Nutraceuticals products that has also been a very effective glandular support supplement for hypothyroidism. This glandular product is similar to the prescription version of Armour desiccated extract, except that it contains a bovine thyroid in stead of porcine.

- **T-100** – is a very powerful thyroid booster that is used when the thyroid gland needs a great deal of stimulation when normal supplements do not respond. Should be used carefully as it can make your thyroid over shoot into hyperthyroidism. T-100 is a multi-glandular supplement with added supporting nutrients including tyrosine, iodine herbs – Irish moss, dulse, bladderwrack, and homeopathic ingredients as well.

- **Selenium** – This is the best mineral that you can take if you suffer from low thyroid. Selenium can help to ease thyroid disorders that are related to auto-immune disorders. It also helps with the removal of mercury removal from the body. Selenium is also a required mineral for the production of thyroid hormones and a deficiency can cause thyroid disorders. Selenium is also an important anti-oxidant that helps the body fight off disease and inflammation. Look for selenium citrate or selenium picolinate. Dosage: 200mcg every morning with meals, and can also be taken in the evening for an additional dose if you feel a lack of energy.

Note: In all my years of practice, I have found out that it doesn't necessarily matter which kind of thyroid hormone product you start out with so much, as which kind you end up with after trying several different types to see which one works best for you. Sometimes it takes a combination of two or three of the above medicines that may prove to be the magic combination for a particular person to get a response.

Chapter 8

Fibromyalgia
Serotonin, and Neurotransmitters

There is one thing for certain, and that is when you have fibromyalgia and CFS your brain neurotransmitters are certainly out of whack. The human brain is made up of billions of neurons that communicate with each other to control everything that goes on your body. Communication between these neurons are called neurotransmitters, which create and control signals. Each bodily function and emotional response is linked to the operation of specific neurotransmitters. Every time you feel happy, sad, depressed, in pain, hungry, anxious, or cry tears of joy, neurotransmitters are the ones responsible.

However, when they are not in balance and levels of particular neurotransmitters are too high or too low, things can get in out of order and create psychological and physical disorders. In 1989, I.J. Russell found low serum levels of serotonin in a group of FMS patients. Studies have found that too much stress can lead to permanently low levels of serotonin. FMS and Chronic Fatigue syndrome have been associated with irregular levels of several neurotransmitters, including:

- **Serotonin** – (Found mainly in central nervous system & in the intestinal tract) - Affects the sleep cycle, body temperature, hunger, appetite, sex drive, regulates mood and behavior, pain processing, and addicted personalities.

- **Dopamine** – (Neurotransmitter and neurohormone) Controls motor function and drive, movement disorders, motivation, mental focus, pleasure, addiction, elation and euphoria.

- **Norepinephrine** – (Functions as a stress hormone and neurotransmitter) Affects the Fight or flight response, alertness, memory, response action, heart rate, and blood pressure.

- **GABA** – (Chief inhibitory neurotransmitter/Central Nervous system) Braking system of the Brain, calms the mind, sleep, relaxation, and anxiety.

- **Acetylcholine** – (Located in both the central nervous system & peripheral nervous system) – Acts as a neuromodulator in the CNS & PNS, plays a role in memory recall, cognitive function, attention and arousal.

Neurotransmitters play a vital part in relation to some of the more chronic symptoms that FMS and CFS patients often experience. Research has also focused on how to regulate these brain chemicals in order to alleviate the symptoms of FMS/CFS. Although the exact definite cause has not yet been determined from FMS, many scientists relate the disorder to the low levels of serotonin. It is estimated through research and study that women normally have one third less serotonin than men do. Interesting enough it also no wonder that the majority of patients with FMS and CFS are women, hmmm......interesting connection?

And ongoing body of evidence and of emotional stress further depletes the serotonin levels and reserves from the body, leading to many similar symptoms that FMS and CFS often experience.
This also helps to explain the intense food cravings – particularly for refined carbohydrates, that when eaten mimic the sense of well being created by serotonin.

Low Serotonin Deficiency Questionnaire

Throughout your life, have you ever had periods of significant depression, anxiety, panic, obsessive-compulsive disorder, an eating disorder, or social anxiety for you considered or had professional counseling?

Have you ever taken anti-depressant medication?

Did the anti-depressant significantly help your symptoms?

Have you ever been diagnosed with any of the following: fibromyalgia, chronic fatigue syndrome, irritable bowl syndrome, migraine headaches?

Were any of your blood relatives treated for any of the disorders listed so far?

Do you feel a sense of depression when the days start getting shorter or the sky is overcast for weeks at a time?

Are you especially sensitive or uncomfortable when exposed to perfumes or chemical smells?

If you're given a prescription medicine, do you frequently have to stop taking it because of side effects?

Have you discovered that the smallest dose of medicine(one half or even one quarter of a tablet) is often adequate for you?

Do you crave carbohydrates, sugar, or chocolate, especially during the days before your period?

Serotonin Deficiency Signs/Symptoms

- Depression, Nervousness, Anxiousness.
- Fears, Phobias
- Obsessive compulsive tendency.
- Sleep problems
- Low self-esteem/confidence.
- Anger/rage/explosive behavior/assaultive.
- Crave sugar/carbohydrates/alcohol/marijuana/ used substances to improve mood & relaxation.
- Feel worse in and dislike dark weather.
- Self destructive/masochistic or suicidal thoughts/plans.
- Worrier
- Chronic pain/migraines/headaches/fibromyalgia/chronic fatigue.
- Family history of depression/anxiety/OCD/eating disorder.

Serotonin levels may be low due to a combination of factors and reasons such as *genetics, chronic stress, poor diet, inadequate sleep, nutritional deficiencies, and metabolic disorders.* Serotonin can also be raised effectively using nutrient based therapies or medications. Serotonin is also synthesized from the amino acid Tryptophan.

Factors which reduce serotonin levels:

- Stress
- PCB's, pesticides, and plastic chemicals exposure
- Under-methylation
- Inadequate sun exposure
- Tryptophan deficiency -(direct precursor)

- **Iron, calcium, mahnesium, zinc, B3, B6, folate & vitamin C deficiency**
- **Inadequate sleep**
- **Glutathione deficiency**
- **Chronic infections**
- **Food allergies**
- **Genetic serotonin receptors abnormalties**
- **Chronic opiod use, alcohol, amphetamine & marijuana use**
- **Human growth hormone deficiency**
- **Progesterone deficiency Impaired blood flow to the brain**
- **Insulin resistance or deficiency**

Pain and Low Serotonin with Fibromyalgia

Since serotonin is an inhibitory neurotransmitter that calms the nervous system to relieve tension and anxiety, its deficiency is thought to be the reason for the lowering of the pain threshold that occurs in fibroblast patients.

The use of (SSR's) serotonin re-uptake inhibitors by physicians have also been a productive treatment program. Serotonin does much more than regulating mood and behavior, It's multi-faceted health consequences on deficiency is based on its complex functions as a neurotransmitter, adequate brain levels of serotonin are therefore critical for promoting feelings of well being, satiety, and relaxation.

It is also possible that women's lack of serotonin is responsible for fibromyalgia's muscle pain and brain fog symptoms. Along with extreme sensitivity to orders like perfume or chemicals, and extreme sensitivity to the side effects of medications. Serotonin's activity, for mood and pain control, is at its maximum during the awake state and at minimum during sleep. Which could be the reason why FMS and CFS patients sleep so little. In any case, the body has other uses for serotonin other than for sleep when you have FMS and CFS, which is pain regulation. If you are in constant pain, it stands for reason for the body to stay in a higher serotonin state, meaning awake, than in the lower producing state of asleep, as it needs the chemical to regulate pain.

Know that, when in a chronic state of pain, and pain is considered a survival mechanism, which means, pain control, is going to take precedence over the body's need for sleep. The body knows it can do with less sleep, however, it perceives pain as a major threat to the body's well being, so it is most likely going to give handling the pain, a priority. When in a chronic state of pain, what occurs is the body, rather rapidly depletes its store of serotonin, so now the mechanism of pain control fails. But, the body is persistent, in that it will keep trying to maintain the awake state, in order to try to increase serotonin availability. This creates a vicious cycle that is almost inevitable, since serotonin is also needed to regulate sleep.

So, between the body's depleted levels and the brains persistence, we do not sleep, which perpetuates the pain-fatigue cycle, we are all familiar with. Raising serotonin levels not only has a powerful muscle relaxing effect, it can also powerfully stimulate our natural painkillers, the endorphins. That's part of why the serotonin specific nutrients I'm about to reveal can be so useful and effective with painful conditions like migraines and arthritic pain, particularly in combination with a good mood diet, the basic supplements, and the elimination of allergy foods.

Chapter 9

ESTROGEN DOMINANCE AND FMS/CFS

Studies have shown that as many 80% of women suffer from from Fibromyalgia and CFS. And with factors in mind, is there a connection to female hormones and Fibromyalgia? According to Dr. John Lee, in his book *"What Your Doctor May Not tell You About Premenopause"* Estrogen dominance is defined as a condition where a women can have deficient, normal, or 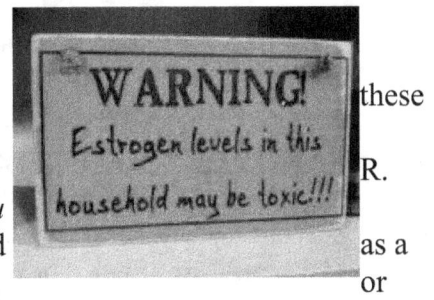 these R. excess estrogen but has little or no progesterone to balance its effects in the body. This also occurs when women experience a drop in estrogen levels during menopause, regardless of progesterone balance. Estrogen dominance is becoming one of the more common causes of hormonal imbalances today among women.

The problem with estrogen in most women is that estrogen is stored in body fat, so most women who suffer from obesity can also experience the symptoms of estrogen dominance even when the body stops making estrogen. However, low estrogen levels can also cause some Fibromyalgia symptoms, and doctors often will prescribe natural progesterone when a women is placed on Hormone Replacement Therapy (HRT).

Progesterone is the hormone that helps to modulate the negative effects of estrogen, and keep in mind that even a low amount of estrogen will dominate if it is not properly balanced by adequate levels of progesterone. If you find that you wind up continuously battling cyclic depression, anger, or deep-seated resentment, you be suffering from PMS, a condition that is directly related to estrogen overload (estrogen dominance). Look for the following lists of both physical and emotional signs of estrogen dominance to see if you fit this profile:

Physical Signs of Estrogen Dominance

- **Brain Fog**   Fibromyalgia   Slowed Metabolism
- Adrenal exhaustion   Fat gain around the midsection
- Cold hands and feet   Uterine cramping
- **Decreased sex drive**   Water retention
- Breast enlargement   Infertility
- **Carbohydrate cravings**   **Irritability**
- Certain types of acne   Auto-Immune disorders
- Magnesium deficiency   Hair loss
- **Headaches**   **Emotional Symptoms of Estrogen Dominance**
- Heavy menstrual flow
- Hypoglycemia   Depression and anxiety

- Weight gain around the hips and thighs   Inability to focus and concentrate
- **Insomnia**   **Loss of libido**
- **Fatigue**   **Mood swings**
- **Thyroid dysfunction**   **Quick to anger**
- **Allergy symptoms**

Direct & Indirect Causes of Estrogen Dominance

1. **Commercially fed cattle and poultry** – these are fed estrogen like hormones and growth hormones.

2. <u>**Xenoestrogen**</u> **exposure such as petrochemical products found in every day beauty and personal care products, car exhaust, pesticides, herbicides, solvents, adhesives, dry cleaning chemicals, and synthetic estrogen from HRT and birth control pills.**

3. **Chronic stress due to adrenal gland exhaustion. (see adrenal support supplements)**

4. **Obesity – Fat converts to estrogen.**

5. **High coffee consumption – caffeine is linked to higher estrogen levels.**

6. **Diet of trans fatty acids (pastries, cookies, and processed foods).**

7. <u>**Canned foods and bottled water**</u>**. (known to contain a chemical called Bisphenol A (BPA) classified as xenoestrogens. Which can increase your abdominal fat.**

8. **Lack of anti-oxidants.**

9. **Cigarette smoking.**

10. **Zinc deficiency.**

11. **Progesterone deficiency.**

12. **Insulin resistance (from excessive use of starches & sugar).**

13. **Sleep deprivation.**

14. **Fluoridated water and tooth paste.**

15. **Magnesium deficiency.**

16. **Using drugs that impair liver function.**

17. **Lack of sulfur-containing amino acids (SAMe, Methionine, NAC, Cysteine)**

Remedy For Counteracting Xenoestrogens

Take <u>NAC</u> (*N-acetylcysteine*), it can help to break down pesticides in your body. Recommended dosage- 500mg twice a day.

<u>Chlorophyll supplements</u> (*chlorella/spirolina*) can also help with detoxifying your body of xenoestrogens. Eating a diet consisting of green and cruciferious vegetables (kale, spinach, broccoli, cauliflower, brussel sprouts, bok choy, cabbage, chard, turnip greens) or you can supplement with drinkable greens sold as powdered mixed green drinks (Perfect Food byGarden of Life, Pro Greens byAllergy Research, and Greens + by Greens Plus). They all contain specific phytonutrients (indole-3-carbinol) that helps to fight against estrogenic chemical compounds.

Chamomile tea.

Garlic and Onions.

<u>Curcumin</u> – use as a supplement or as a spice (tumeric) in your cooking. Curcumin can block xenoestrogens from entering your cells that might allow xenobiotics.

<u>Note:</u> The symptoms of estrogen dominance can mimic other diseases such as **hypothyroidism**, **diabetes**, and even **multiple sclerosis**. So check with your health-care practitioner to rule out these serious conditions.

As you can see from list above, the presence of estrogen overload can cause a number of distressing symptoms that can include both emotional and physical problems. Estrogen is a central nervous system stimulant while progesterone has the opposite effects. Maintaining the right balance between these two hormones is a complex and delicate process. And the recommended solution is to supply an adequate amount of progesterone to balance the body's excess estrogen levels.

Other recommended treatments should be included is <u>dietary adjustments, detoxification, maintaining an ideal weight, and exercise</u>. These positive and much needed adjustments along with **natural progesterone** can do much to counter act the effects of excess estrogen dominance.

A person with estrogen issues (high levels) may also be suffering from Fibromyalgia as well and can be more symptomatic making these two conditions much more difficult for the doctors to diagnose. And doctors will usually treat estrogen dominance with synthetic progestin which only brings on more of the side effects which can be at least as miserable as Fibromyalgia and include joint pain, muscle pain, weight gain, bloating, fatigue, depression, irritability, and so on.

When estrogen levels soar, they create a shortage of the amino acid *Tryptophan and*

Vitamin B6. The result is often drastic changes in mood and physical well being, as too much estrogen can block the action of *Vitamin B6* and force it to be eliminated from the body. This can also speed up the production of Tryptophan, which, ironically, makes it less likely to convert Tryptophan to serotonin. Synthetic estrogen replacement therapy to relieve symptoms of menopausal symptoms may also develop a vitamin B6 deficiency that contributes to a depressed mental state. Dramatic fluctuations in mood and extreme irritability are common side effects of excess estrogen stimulated disorders.

The Tryptophan link to serotonin is also influenced by estrogen. In order to have enough serotonin, you need to consume adequate amounts of tryptophan - *protein-based foods like chocolate, oats, dried dates, milk, yogurt, cottage cheese, red meat, turkey, poultry(white meat), eggs, fish, spirulina, bananas, peanuts, pumpkin seeds, and sunflower seeds.* Studies have also shown us that women are more sensitive to serotonin fluctuations than men are. This also explains why during their menstrual cycle when estrogen levels fluctuate the carvings for carbohydrates increase.

Estrogen Metabolism & Progesterone Balance

Supplementing with estrogen metabolizers can help promote proper estrogen balance throughout a person's life cycle, and may be particularly helpful during the pre- and peri-menopausal years. Estrogen metabolizers can be very helpful for various estrogen dominant related conditions including lessening Fibromyalgia and the related mental and physical symptoms associated with it. A proper diet adjustment free of hormones (organic based) with helpful natural hormonal plant based supplements should be in order in balancing estrogen dominance.

- Supplement of choice **DIM (Diindolylmethane)** – a naturally occurring phytonutrient found in cruciferous vegetables such as – broccoli, cauliflower, cabbage, and brussel sprouts. DIM helps increase the specific aerobic metabolism for estrogen, multpling the chance for estrogen to be broken down into its beneficial form or "good" estrogen metabolites. While simultaneously reducing the levels of 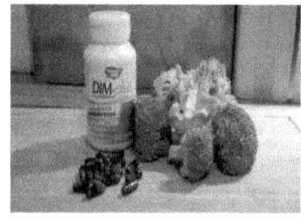 undesirable or "bad" estrogen metabolites which may actually cause cancer.

- **Natural progesterone Cream (Progesta-Care)** – A bio-identical progesterone product from Life-Flo provides natural progesterone supplementation that will natural supplement low progesterone levels, helping to balance the ratio between estrogen and progesterone.

- **Chaste Berry (Vitex Agnus Castus)** Used as a supreme hormonal tonic for women, and backed by extensive clinical studies, as well as over two thousand years of use in folk medicine, have proved the effectiveness of this remedy. Vitex is not a hormone, but works with your body to regulate hormones. According to Nancy Dunne, ND, vitex raises progesterone levels and helps your body reach a hormonal balance that is right for you. Vitex acts on the pituitary gland and hypothalamus by increasing luteinizing hormone production, and very gently inhibits the release of follicule stimulating hormones. Vitex will help to balance the ratio of estrogen to progesterone with the ratio shifting in favor of progesterone, and your hormones normalize. For estrogen dominance, this progesterone shift makes Vitex a God send.

Vitex is also a slow acting herb, and is considered a long term solution, rather than a quick fix to mask symptoms. But regardless, it works very effectively and has been used in Europe for all of the hormonal needs of women, and has resolved over 90% of female gynecological problems. Make sure the Vitex that you buy is standardized for 0.5% of agnusides and take 175 to 225 mg daily. Vitex also comes in liquid extract form and in capsules, and has a very good safety track record.

- **Balanced diet** consisting of organic products, should include more vegetables, especially the cruciferous kind listed above, **high fiber food**s to leach out excess estrogen body, plenty of fish and seafood, poultry, fruits, nuts and seeds. And avoid all processed and refined foods, junk foods, and sugar by products.

- **Any popular <u>Anti-oxidant supplements.</u>**

- **A good <u>Multi-Vitamin/Mineral</u> supplement.**

No matter what your age or individual levels of hormones, there are ways to give your body the natural support it needs to build better hormonal health. For most women, a combination approach works beautifully. And there is no need to suffer the consequential affect of raging hormones, especially when it combines and worsens with health conditions such as Fibromyalgia and CFS.

The four simple elements that you need to start with are

(1) Limit your exposure to xenoestrogens, and choose organic foods when possible, wash your produce, avoid plastics for storing food, and limit body care and cleaning products to those with all natural ingredients.

(2) Try and eat a natural, plant based diet, eating lots of veggies to provide fiber to leach out excess estrogen residue, and avoid foods that offer no nutritional value, like junk foods, processed foods, sugar by products and definitely stay away from bad fatty foods that can contribute to estrogen build up.

(3) Restore balance with supplements that will help balance your hormones such as vitex, and progest cream, and a multi-mineral supplement, anti-oxidants also are helpful to counter potential problems. (4) Apply an exercise program to help speed up health and manage stress levels, exercising is a very effective way to help release toxins and create more endorphins, your feel good chemicals. And most importantly, manage your stress levels by taking a good herbal adaptogen like Rhodiola Rosea, because stress has a big impact on hormonal cycles, as excessive stress is known to cause a shift in estrogen levels.

The Hormone Connection: Estrogen & Serotonin

In women, the levels of serotonin are also very much related to their levels of estrogen. During the few days to a week before menstruation, estrogen slowly drops and continues to drop until your first day of flow, when the next cycle begins and estrogen begins to rise again (usually toward the end of menstruation). As estrogen drops, so flows serotonin, and you enter PMS land, where you are irritable, moody, and cry. Some women will notice that the week after their period ends, when estrogen and serotonin are on the rise, is the only time of the month their Fibromyalgia actually seems to improve.

The Tryptophan link to serotonin is also influenced by estrogen. In order to have enough serotonin, you need to consume adequate amounts of Tryptophan (an amino acid). To maintain optimal levels of Tryptophan in the body, it must be supplied with certain amounts of vitamin B6. Estrogen can block the action of vitamin B6. Estrogen can block the action of vitamin B6 and force it to be eliminated from the body. It can also speed up the production of Tryptophan, which, ironically, makes it less likely to convert to into serotonin.

This connection between low serotonin and Fibromyalgia is also very known by many physicians that will prescribe serotonin boosting anti-depressants right after the start. Optimization of serotonin and dopamine levels seem to be the right choice in relief from pain and sleep disturbances. People with Fibromyalgia and CFS typically have 3 or more other neurotransmitter problems that are active simultaneously. That when treated with the correct neurotransmitters, patients often reported 100% relief of Fibromyalgia. This is Fibromyalgia treatment at its best with virtually no drugs or drug side effects.

Important Physical Clues of Serotonin Deficiency

Serotonin deficiency can be linked to several health related issues that often goes undetected and unrecognized. It's deficiency is a common denominator in the etiology of a number of health disorder such as irritability bowl syndrome, asthma, sleep disturbances, migraines, fatigue, carbohydrate cravings, and obesity. Under normal conditions, neurons in the brain release serotonin to carry messages to other to other neurons: for example, to alter some aspect of mood, appetite, confidence, or sleep. Serotonin is then returned to the parent neuron to be reused for signaling.

 In people with low serotonin levels, however, the available serotonin is recaptured too quickly, leaving it insufficient time to adequately activate neuron and allow the signal to sufficiently continue along the neural network. This can result in a number of disorders.

Serotonins Impact on Sleeping Disorder

One of the **"key"** findings in patients with Fibromyalgia is an altered sleep pattern, presumably as a result of the *low serotonin levels.* The main problem that was discovered, is that the deeper levels of sleep (Stages 3 & 4 are not achieved for long periods of time. As a result, people with FMS wake up feeling tired, worn out and in pain. The severity of of the pain of FMS correlates with the rating of sleep quality. But when Fibromyalgia patients get a good nights sleep, they have less pain.

Conversely, when they sleep poorly, they're symptoms are more severe. The analogy of this sleep cycle is similar to a battery charger, if the body is not being re-charged properly, the muscles of the body result in pain. With a good positive full charge (a restful sleep), there is no pain and it can function normally. Supplements that have been shown to be effective in this regard for a proper restful sleeping patterns include – *Tryptophan, 5-HTP, SAM-e, St. John's Wort, Calcium and Magnesium* can all improve the quality of sleep and long needed relief for those who have suffered with FMS/CFS.

Normal sleeping habits will vary from person to person. With the average time being around 8 hours, some people need a much longer time, while others may only require several hours or so. It is also important to remember that as you get older you require less sleep. Fibromyalgia
is one of the conditions that are known as "low serotonin syndrome". Regulation of serotonin metabolism takes place during the deep or therapeutic sleep patterns which are discussed in another section. With the disturbances of Fibromyalgia, the metabolic regulation is disrupted. This causes further immune system dysfunction due to the role serotonin play in the activation of killer cells.

Recent scientific tests have found that people with Fibromyalgia suffer from decreased cerebral blood flow and have higher levels of substance P in their system. Substance P is a chemical involved in pain transmission in the nervous system. It is also thought to play a role in pain, inflammation and mood disorders.

 Substance P which works together with serotonin, and is responsible for transmitting painful impulses to the brain and spinal cord. It produces a nerve generated impulse that dilates blood vessels, and in addition, can cause fluid and proteins to migrate from cells to outside the cells. Low serotonin levels can cause elevated substance P levels. These elevated substance P levels are 3 times higher in people with Fibromyalgia, which could explain the enhancement of pain perception which is experienced in those with FMS and CFS. Because of this, people with fibroblast have a lower pain threshold and that they had more trouble with anxiety and depression.

While much research is still being conducted, it would appear clearly that there is some evidence that "low serotonin syndrome" and symptoms of Fibromyalgia are strongly related. And the fact that females have a lower capacity to produce serotonin than men may help explain the fact that over 90% of Fibromyalgics are female. When events occur that produce the "low serotonin syndrome", this lessened capability to produce serotonin could be a crucial component in the greater female susceptibility to the onset of symptoms.

Scientists have recently concluded that serotonin levels determine sleeping and waking cycles. This fact alone explains to some degree why sleeping habits and mood are so tightly interwoven. If you don't make or utilize enough serotonin, you may sleep for shorter intervals or not at all.

Serotonin inducing drugs like the SSRI's (Prozac) actually inhibit Rem sleep due to their unnatural action on serotonin levels. One of the common side effects of Prozac is the inability to sleep well. This points out that when we artificially manipulate serotonin through chemical agents, we can change sleeping patterns. Tryptophan, being the natural precursor to serotonin, is often recommended for disturbed sleeping patterns (as well as depression). 5-HTP (5-Hydroxytryptophan) is a chemical the body makes from tryptophan (an essential amino acid you get from foods). Tryptophan is converted into 5-HTP, then to serotonin, which basically means it is one step away from conversion into serotonin.

Tryptophan and 5-HTP are both dietary supplements that can be purchased in health stores. They both can increase the levels of serotonin quite effectively. Tryptophan can be found in certain foods such as *milk, bananas, turkey, chicken, pumpkin, sunflower seeds, turnips, and collard greens, and seaweed.* 5-HTP on the other hand is not found in any foods, but is derived from the seeds of Griffonia Simplicifolia. <u>Vitamins B6 and vitamin C are both required in the metabolism of serotonin.</u>

Natural Ways to Boost Serotonin Levels

Here are some ways that your body can make serotonin that may free you from needing to rely on long-term use of prescription drugs. Here are some helpful hints:

- **Get enough vitamin B6** – can be acquired from food or supplementation, B6 options are- spinach, turnip greens, garlic, cauliflower, mustard greens, celery, fish (especially tuna, halibut, salmon, cod and snapper), chicken, turkey, and lean beef.
- **Eat -Amaranth, buckwheat, millet and quinoa seeds,** are all healthy carbohydrates and small amounts of the right carbohydrates are critical to boosting serotonin.
- **Focus on eating high quality protein foods** – that specifically have a higher percentage of tryptophan (like turkey, sunflower seeds, and pumpkin seeds) will provide much needed tryptophan, the precursor of serotonin. (research shows that eating protein with carbohydrates actually works against your ability to make serotonin).

- **Get plenty of exercise** – researchers have found that exercise boosts serotonin and your endorphin levels.
- **Get some sun exposure** – early morning sun exposure can boost your body's production of melatonin in the evening. Serotonin converts into melatonin for a great night sleep.
- **Reduce stress** – prolonged physical or emotional stress produces adrenaline and cortisol, which can interfere with serotonin.
- **Eliminate Sugar** – If you have low serotonin, you may have intense cravings for sugar. This is your body's way of trying to increase serotonin because eating

sugar produces insulin, which helps Tryptophan go into your brain. However too much sugar can eventually cause addiction to sugar, insulin resistance, hypoglycemia and type 2 diabetes.

Focus on Emotional healing – reducing stress and focusing on spending more time relaxing is a first step in boosting your serotonin levels. Meditation exercises like yoga are a great way of boosting your brains level of neurotransmitters and hormones. It is also found to be a great stress reliever.

Serotonin Boosting Supplements

- **5-HTP** - **5-hydroxytryptophan** is naturally produced in the body from tryptophan, an essential amino acid. 5-HTP can increase the level of serotonin the brain produces and reverse serotonin deficiency. Although there has been no established safe dose regimen yet, anything from 50 to 300mgs has been used in clinical trials shown to be effective. Dosages may vary among individuals taking 5-HTP, finding your optimal dose is recommended. Start off with a low dose of 50mgs and judge as you go along increasing the amount slowly.

Along with helping people manage depression, sleep and eating disorders, 5-HTP also

appears to offer relief from various symptoms associated with CFS and FMS. According to fibromyalgia researchers *H. Moldofsky and J.J. Warsh,* theorize that primary FMS may arise from a deficiency of circulating tryptophan. In a study published in pain; *(1978;5:65 71;Moldofsky and Warsh*) reported that the higher the concentration of unbound tryptophan in the plasma of FMS patients, the more profound the symptoms.

Many fibromyalgia people may be interested to know that clinical studies published in peer reviewed medical journals report that 5 HTP can be effective in relieving musculoskeletal and other symptoms in those diagnosed with FMS and CFS. Also the (The Journal of International Medical Research;1992; 20:182 – 1189) concluded that "good" or fair" clinical improvement occurred in 50% of Fibromyalgia patients.

5-HTP effectively improved the symptoms of FMS/CFS by helping to mediate slow-wave sleep as well as influence how pain is perceived by the body/mind *(1978; 5:65 71 Modoldofsky and Warsh)*

Tryptophan – In peer reviewed scientific studies Tryptophan had been repeatedly proven to – *reduce or eliminate depression, relieve insomnia, reduce the tendency to over eat, reduce pain (FMS/CFS) reduce the compulsion to commit suicide, and reduce the tendency towards angry or violent outbursts*.

Tryptophan may be a better choice for Fibromyalgia patients than 5-HTP, as 5-HTP lacks the many of Tryptophan's beneficial actions on pain control and muscular relaxation which are very important in reducing many of the complaints fibroblast patients have.

As a patient deals with the myraid of concerns that FMS/CFS produces, tryptophan can clear and calm the mind/body and also allow for a more restful period of sleep at night. Tryptophan helps to control muscle stiffness and spasms, the twitches that tend to wake up a person at night are greatly reduced. When used in lower doses during the day, tryptophan can smooth out the rough spots, lower tempers, frustrations, calm stress levels, and provide for a better sense of well being.

Fibromylagia patients not finding relief from medication or support from family and friends tend to over eat comfort foods which are high in carbohydrates and therefore fattening. By combining the over consumption of carbohydrates with the sedentary nature of Fibromyalgia, one will have the recipe for creating obesity.

By raising serotonin levels through Tryptophan use, you can increase the sense of comfort and well being and decrease the appetite. Pure pharmaceutical Tryptophan (the purest form) has no side-effects and is essential to proper brain function and to life! Dosage is usually one 500mg capsule for each 50lbs of body weight when taken before bed time, taken always on an empty stomach or at least one hour away from food. You can also freely experiment in taking less than that amount and work your way up to the full dose if needed.

During the day you may try one to two capsules in-between meals to maintain a higher production of serotonin during your waking hours. Try adding vitamin B6 and vitamin C to help with the metabolism and conversion of serotonin. Tryptophan will provide all of the benefits a higher level of serotonin brings, however when combined to a comprehensive program or protocol to over come FMS/CFS, such as outlined in this book, your road towards wellness and healing will add a fuller more pain free life.

(References -*Liberman, J., et al; Mood, performance & pain sensitivity: changes induced by food constituents. J. Psychiat. Res., 17(2): 135-145, 11982-83), (Braverman, E., R, Pfeiffer, C., C. :Suicide and biochemistry. Biol. Psych., 20: 123124, 1985.)*

Natural Food sources - The highest dietary food source of **Tryptophan** are protein foods that include – chicken, turkey, tuna, soybeans, beef, lamb, halibut, salmon, shrimp, snapper, dairy products, nuts, seeds, and bananas.

Natural Homemade Serotonin Boost (Recipe) - This is a simple recipe that you can make at home with ingredients that are normally found in the kitchen of the average American home: Get one whole banana, one cup of warm to hot milk, 2 tablespoons of pure un-refined honey, a pinch of nutmeg, and blend all together in a blender, let it cool down so it is warm but not too hot and then drink and enjoy!

This drink/recipe will provide you with a nice calmness (serotonin induced) to help relive stress or anxiety, or take it before bed for a nice deep relaxing sleep!

SAM-e – **(S-Adenosylmethionine - pronounced "sammy")** Not a prescription drug or an herb, SAM-e is a natural substance produced by the body from (ATP) and the amino acid Methionine. Fibromyalgia patients get the best of all worlds with relief from depression and muscle soreness and stiffness without no side-effects or possible adverse interactions with other medications. SAM-e has been used in Europe for over 20 years and is just beginning to make the headlines in publications like "Newsweek

Magazine: Los Angeles Times" and in books, and in major television networks.

SAM-e is one of the "key" components in any treatment protocol for FMS and CFS. It's benefits towards healing are amazing, it's effectiveness in treating depression is just as effective as anti-depressant drugs without any side-effects. SAM-e works under the process called "methylation". Methylation is a natural function that happens ever second throughout the body and is responsible for the regulation of brain function, preserving bone health, and protecting against heart disease. SAM-e also helps the body produce and break down brain chemicals such as serotonin, melatonin, dopamine and adrenaline as well as vitamin B12. It is involved in almost everything the body does on a daily level, regulating the various hormones and brain neurotransmitters.

In 1987 a double blind crossover study involving 17 patients at the Institute of Medical Pathology I, Rheumatic Disease Unit, University of Pisa, Italy, doctors first reported that SAM-e could help reduce the symptoms of FMS. One group of patients were given 200mgs of SAM-e per day while another group were given placebos. Two weeks later, the results were dramatic! Patients noticed significant improvement in mood, outlook and the relief of trigger points, pain , decreased tenderness, and stiffness of the muscles. *(American Journal of Medicine, Nov.20, 1987, Vol. 83, supp.5A.)*

SAME-e is must have supplement in your arsenal for the therapy of FMS and CFS, and should be included most definitely. Low levels of SAM-e have been connected with FMS and can be a very effective treatment for the variety of symptoms FMS/CFS often experience. **(Note)** when purchasing SAM-e, make sure your product is a full-strength SAM-e, and tablets must be enteric coated, meaning the tablets pass through the acidic environment of the stomach intact, and can be absorbed most efficiently by the body.

The amounts used in various studies may vary widely, but for the many patients who have taken SAM-e for Fibromyalgia relief reported that SAM-e has helped them more than anything else. <u>Dosages for them that used SAM-e were 200mgs to 800mgs a day, and in some cases even more.</u> Because of the no side-effects dosages can be increased when necessary, and consider that this is something that normally you couldn't do with prescription drugs (increasing the dosage without side effects).

(Important) – FMS and CFS are difficult syndromes which now medical science is beginning to grasp on it being better understood. We are lucky to have something (SAM-e) as natural and effective from nature to be made available for those of us that suffer from crippling and annoying diseases.

St.John's Wort - This herb has received much attention for its natural anti-depressant effects. It has been used extensively in Europe to treat depression and has recently become very popular in the United States for improving anxiety, fear, sleep & appetite, apathy, depression, and nerve pain in those with Fibromyalgia and Chronic fatigue. St. John's Wort is one of the best non-narcotic herbs for dealing with nerve pain, and is thus very useful as a Fibromyalgia herb. Laboratory results show that it contains different <u>compounds that have effects on GABA receptors, serotonin, dopamine, and monoamine oxidase.</u> The extract of St. John's Wort has been reported to improve sleep, in part because it increases brain output of serotonin and melatonin when taken at night time. It has also shown to have immune system modulating effects, stimulating the immune response when it is low, and suppressing it when it in some conditions when it is overactive.

St. John's Wort also works on the brains serotonin levels by preventing its breakdown, which results in a steady rise of serotonin levels. Taking B vitamins along with St. John's Wort will help increase its metabolism within the body. Used to treat a variety of illnesses, it is becoming one of the most widely purchased herbal products in the United States. The extract is often helpful in treating FMS and CFS because of its ability to relieve depression and improve sleep quality. When purchasing the product make sure its standardized for its (0.3 % hypericin content). <u>Dosages are 900mgs to 1,350mgs per day divided into two doses. St. John's Wort can also be used in combination with 5-HTP and Magnesium.</u>

(Important) St. John's Wort should not be taken with any medications, especially prescription anti-deppressants and women who are pregnant.

<u>Passion Flower (Tea)</u>– Since its introduction into European herbal medicine systems, passion flower has been used as a sedative, anti-spasmodic, and a nerve tonic. In many countries in Europe, the US and Canada, the use of passion flower leaves have been used to tranquilize and settle edgy nerves that has been documented for over 200 years. It's other use's have been in the relief of insomnia, dysentery, menstrual difficulties, neuralgia, epilepsy and muscle spasms and pain. Passion flower also contains naturally occurring serotonin as well as a chemical called maltol which has been documented to have sedative effects inducing natural calming properties. It has also been the subject of much scientific research of it's sedative, anti-spasmodic and analgesic effects, after almost 100 years.

Passion flower **tea** can help induce a calm state, demonstrate anti-inflammatory action, pain relieving attributes in a variety of conditions. Because of its natural containing serotonin qualities, passion flower tea can be of great help in helping those who suffer from the symptoms of FMS and CFS.

<u>It's main actions in order</u> are – *anti-depressant, analgesic (pain reliever), anti-spasmodic, sedative, and central nervous system* depressant. <u>Properties/Actions Documented by research</u>: **pain reliever, anti-inflammatory, anti-anxiety, anti-spasmodic, cough suppressant, central nervous system depressant, diuretic, hypotensive (lowers blood pressure), and sedative.**

<u>Note:</u> Anti-depressant drugs do not produce serotonin, <u>they merely recycle it</u>. Nature depends on replenishing these brain chemicals not recycling them. That's why the side effects of anti-depressant drugs are so severe and can include – suicide, mania, violent behavior, and aggression. Prozac manufacturers know that more than 10% of people who took the drug **"Prozac"** with episodes of mania. With only one exception all of the school shootings from 1993, when they started prescribing anti-depressants for children, until now involved **"Ritalin"**, an anti-depressants or both! Yet there is so much money involved with selling the number one drug in the world that you've likely never heard of those facts until today.

Chapter 10

Melatonin The Stress Relief & Sleep Aid For FMS/CFS

With sleep being one of the major problems of FMS and CFS, you have to look at one of nature's natural sleep producing hormones, *Melatonin*. Produced in the pineal gland of the brain that regulates the sleep wake cycle of the body, and other important body functions. Melatonin is a sleep hormone that is secreted by the pineal gland in a circadian rhythm. It basically tells your body that it's night and it's time to go to bed. It is also naturally produced in the brain from the *amino acid Tryptophan*, and can be found in dietary sources such as *tart cherry juice, tomatoes, grape skins, and seeds from fennel, celery, poppy and sunflower.* Melatonin has become a popular therapy, used to promote sleep or flight-jet lag, it can treat your circadian rhythm where you sleep the right amount of time but your body clock is at the wrong time.

Shift workers with abnormal work hours, and people making frequent overseas trips all deal with the timing of their need to sleep. Melatonin works with your biological clock by telling your brain when it is time to sleep. Sometimes called the *"vampire hormone"* because it is produced primarily by darkness and inhibited by light. The levels of your melatonin increase in the middle of the night and gradually fall as the night turns into day. So the less exposure to night time (darkness) and the more exposure to day time (light), can really push your biological clock in the wrong direction. By re-setting your circadian rhythm (biological clock) you can help yourself in making the corrective action in eliminating an important part of healing towards Fibromylagia. Correct sleeping habits in those who have FMS and CFS is the first step in recovery of FMS and CFS.

Although it is best known as a sleeping aid, melatonin may also help relieve, and benefit other known health conditions such as:

- **Fibromyalgia and CFS -**
- **IBS relief -**
- **Chronic Migraines -**
- **Stress Relief -**
- **Anti-Aging -**
- **Cardiovascular disease -**
- **Immune system -**
- **Sex enhancing -**
- **Anti-Cancer -**
- **Anti-oxidant -**

According to Dr. Walter Pierpaoli, PH.D., and Dr. Williamson, M.D., in their groundbreaking book - "The Melatonin Miracle", who did the original research on melatonin discovered that melatonin is more than just a sleeping hormone. Current research is now revealing that melatonin may be affective in treating Fibromyalgia pain. As most patients with Fibromyalgia and CFS have sleep problems and fatigue, melatonin may also help these problems through the serotonin path way by resetting the body's sleep wake cycle and through it's involvement in the manufacturing of growth hormone production while sleeping undisturbed.

One small study suggested that Fibromyalgia patients may have lower levels of melatonin during dark hours and theorized that these reduced levels of melatonin may in fact contribute to the sleep disturbances commonly experienced by Fibromylagia patients (Wikber et al., 1998). A 2000 study by Criteria et al. Investigated the effects of melatonin on pain, sleep, disturbances, fatigue, depression, anxiety, and overall ability to function in 21 patients with Fibromyalgia.

It was further concluded that the patients tender points and sleep quality both improved. A recent article posted in the journal "Current Pain and Headache" Reports discusses the use of melatonin as a treatment for FMS. Two small open studies testing the use of melatonin as a treatment for FMS reported significant improvement. One study used 3mgs of melatonin and the other used 6mgs. Following the second study, researchers concluded that 10mgs of melatonin taken nightly brought more relief.

Most of the health issues, conditions and diseases of today are caused by the rising levels of stress. And if you are already suffering from some kind of disease or health condition such as diabetes, hypertension, heart disease, IBS, Thyroid, FMS and CFS, elevated stress is likely to magnify your health condition even more. According to the American Academy of family physicians, more than two thirds of all doctor visits are due to stress related ailments.

Numerous studies have also documented the link between severe stress and the various health disorders that are triggered by a particularly traumatic or stressful event. The stress of life which no doubt has taken its toll on likely victims that suffer and cope with illness, it is no wonder that our life expectancy has dropped. And no matter how far we advance in technology, stress will always be a fact of life!

Fortunately, melatonin can help protect us against the ravages of stress by blunting the negative effects of stress hormones, and by doing so can prevent a myriad of common diseases. Melatonin has been shown to prevent the negative effects of corticosteroids by normalizing the high levels of corticosteroids in our body. It is the prolonged exposure to these stress hormones that can injure every organ system in our body, from our hearts to our brain that causes the many illnesses that you may not even have thought of as being related to stress or exacerbated by stress.

Melatonin is effective in reducing the stress response in individuals associated with excessive cortisol, by helping protect the body against stress induced damage. Melatonin produces this effect by enhancing your body's production of endorphins, which are neuro-chemicals that relieve pain and reduce anxiety. Melatonin also functions as a potent anti-oxidant by reducing oxidative stress in protecting the nucleus of your cells that contains genetic materials, against the damage done by free radicals.

A restful sound night's sleep is one of the basic foundations for good health and stronger immunity. Sleep has two purposes, and that is to allow our bodies to rest and to refuel itself. Melatonin supplements can help normalize your disturbed sleeping habits which are absolutely critical to having a restorative and rejuvenating sleep. The failure to get sufficient sleep can adversely affect virtually every system of the body including the immune system, the brain system, impair the proper functioning of our glandular system, create unapparent anxieties, create depression, impair our judgment, and impair our ability to manage stress. Melatonin can help ease the burden of stress by regulating one of life's important functions, sound sleep!

Possible Causes of Low Melatonin in FMS & CFS

There are several factors that can contribute to low levels of melatonin which can impair its production, which are:

- **Excess exposure to light during evening hours**
- **Stress – chronic levels of stress deplete levels of melatonin, too much induced cortisol, (Fibromylagia/Chronic Fatigue) – one of the possible causes, by excess cortisol levels generated by stress.**
- **Anxiety (brought on by stress related effects)**
- **Improper intake of proteins from diet (lack of Tryptophan, precursor to melatonin)**
- **Cancer, decreased blood flow, Alzheimer's disease, other dementia's**
- **Excess intake of vitamin B12, over 3,000mcgs**
- **General Aging – levels of melatonin decline rapidly with aging, and are minimal by age 70**
- **Excess intake of caffeine (depletes levels of melatonin), alcohol (impairs the production of melatonin), nicotine(depletes levels also), beta-blocker medications, anti-depressants, sleeping pills, tranquilizers.**
- **Lack of sleep impairs the production of melatonin**

Because FMS and CFS people have various sleep disturbances and lower levels of melatonin, this can cause the disruption of their circadian rhythm which frequently occurs with FMS patients. When sufficient levels of melatonin are present it has been known to synchronize circadian rhythms and thus improve sleep.

Symptoms Of Low Melatonin

Low levels of melatonin is evident by having sleep related problems and poor dream recall. Low levels are also found in those with seasonal affective disorder, schizophrenia, and even those poor souls of suicide who commit suicide at night are also known to have low levels of melatonin as well. These conditions should be of no surprise because low levels of Tryptophan are associated with a higher incidence of suicide, and Tryptophan is a precursor to melatonin.

Indicators that may help you distinguish low levels of melatonin are – *eating during sleep hours (high cortisol levels), a constant of fatigue, forgetting your dreams upon awaking, a history of disturbed sleeping patterns, cluster headaches, depression and anxiety, pms, and low levels of hormones, low progesterone or estrogen dominance.*

And like most hormones in the body, melatonin appears to be most beneficial to those individuals who are not producing adequate levels themselves.

Melatonin levels can also be tested through blood tests, urine and saliva test. And at times, just like everything else in life, there exists a logical solution to common health related problems, as the body can not function as it was meant to without adequate levels of vital controlling substances that stimulate their target cells properly. Melatonin is just one piece of the puzzle that can influence many of the body's processes, from hormones to neurotransmitters.

Dosage: The correct dosage of melatonin, according to research conducted at MIT, for it to be effective is 0.3 to 1.0mgs in a sub lingual tablet for proper absorption, 30 minutes before bed time. A slow time release formula works best. Many of the commercial forms of melatonin are 3 to 10 times the amount your body would need. As higher dosages would less affective and recommended. It is a hormone and can have negative side effects if abused. In fact in Europe, high doses of melatonin have been used as a contraceptive.

Chapter 11

Sexual Dysfunction in Fibromyalgia & CFS

I am sure that many of those who suffer from FM and CFS that have had sex on their mind, know that is the last thing on their mind to be had. This inability to have normal sexual relations 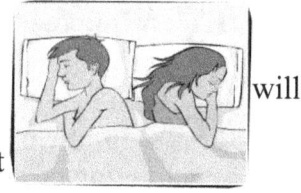will have a negative impact on anyone. A study that was done in 2008 determined that up to 78% of women with FMS stated that their <u>desire</u> limited their sexual life in one way or another, and 97% of Fibro' patients experienced sexual dysfunction overall. Their sexual problems pertain to – *desire, arousal, lubrication, inability to have an orgasm, and pain during intercourse.*

Furthermore, the researchers concluded that coexisting depression was significantly associated with sexual dysfunction *(Orellana et al.. 2008)*. Given the impact these implications have on a woman's life and their relationship and marriage it is surprising, and somewhat sad, that the first actual report did not appear in the scientific literature until 2004, and the first clinical study was not published until 2005. <u>Below are some of the ways FM can affect your sex life as well as some **"tips"** on how to deal with the changes.</u>

- Joint and/or muscle pain can make sex painful or uncomfortable.
- Relentless fatigue can make sex not possible
- Depression and chronic pain can reduce sex drive or cause erectile dysfunction (ED)
- Medications often prescribed for FM can reduce libido and cause vaginal dryness.
- Medications used to treat FM can cause erectile dysfunction(ED) in men.
- Skin rashes can make sex painful or uncomfortable.

- FM and medications can cause a multi-tude of physical changes such as rashes, scars, weight gain, or loss, hair loss, et. These changes can make a person feel ugly, uncomfortable, not themselves, insecure, unwanted, etc. It can also make some partners attraction change.
- FM and medications used to treat can cause hormonal imbalances that effect libido, and orgasms.
- Partners can also feel insecure, rejected, and frustrated by the reduced amount of sex which can strain the relationship or marriage.
- Partners can feel confused and insecure on, when it is and isn't ok to initiate sex.
- Brain chemistry abnormalities of neurotransmitter imbalance of FMS can affect sexual desire.
- Partners can feel insecure, rejected, and frustrated by the reduced amount of sex.

TIPS: To Improve Sexual Dysfunction

- **Keep an accurate and consistent symptom record**s is a fundamental part of an effective management treatment plan. As <u>symptoms</u> tend to vary greatly from patient to patient as a result of a negative reactions to new medical treatments (medications).
- **Apply the recommended FM healing protocol** to reset and restore hormonal balance.
- **Your change in diet and supplement support** will also help heal your FM symptoms.
- **Use the recommended supplements for pain and inflammation.**
- **Try a warm bath with Epsom Salt** to loosen up and soothe tight & tender sore muscles before having sexual intercourse.
- **Use a natural lubricant for dryness.**
- **Monitor your hormonal levels** and if needed talk to your health-care physician about supplementation, or try the recommended remedies for <u>restoring hormone balance</u>.
- Try cuddling and other ways of being intimate with your partner to substitute when intercourse is not possible.
- **Try a gentle massage with Aromatherapy oils (lavender),** to relax your mind and muscles and ease tension.
- Remind yourself that this is condition is only temporary and is not forever to allow healing to take place.
- Always keep the lines of communication open in building a secure relationship so that when there are temporary problems or dry spells, you have a solid relationship to get you through it.
- Partners should reassure their Fibromyalgia counter part that they are still attractive no matter what.

There have not been many published studies given the magnitude of this problem (sexual dysfunction) and which the results have been conflicting with those who suffer from FMS and CFS with sexual intercourse. Every person that may suffer with this dilemma is a little bit different, because in some patients there may be more pain than fatigue and depressed, while others may be more fatigued and in pain, and not anxious at all to contemplate sexual intercourse. Most people who reported widespread pain had the most difficulties with sexual issues. *(Tikiz et al., 2005)*

One pain disorder that did garner enough interest to warrant its own study was that of a condition called *"vulvodynia", meaning from the latin words "pain in the vulva" or the soft tissue surrounding the opening of the vagina, including the labia, clitoris, and the vaginal opening.* Most women reported discomfort ranging from a stinging pain, to burning, stabbing, or itching, and at times can be so severe that sexual intercourse is not possible. This specific discomfort may be a type of pain syndrome called *"neuropathic pain", which translates to "pain wthin the nerves".* And if its due to pain nerves that have become more sensitized, it is then termed *"peripheral neuropathy".*

This also occurs in the central nervous system where normal sensations are instead interpreted as being painful, and known as *"central neuropathic pain".* The most common medications used to treat this condition are actually drugs originally intended to treat epilepsy, referred to as *anti-convulsants.* Two other conditions that also seem to be more prevalent in patients with FMS are *"pelvic pain and coccydynia".* In a study of 499 females, 66% of females and 68% of male patients with FMS, all reported pain in the pelvic area. Coccydynia is a pain in your tail bone, and the same study also revealed coccyx pain in 38% and 10.5% of females and males, respectively.

Pelvic pain itself may also increase the pain you feel from other parts of the body by acting as an "amplifier" to your nervous system. Pelvic pain in those with FMS, is strongly associated with a condition called *"primary dysmenorrhea"*, or the pain that women normally feel around the time of menstruation.

Most women who suffer from these symptoms of sexual dysfunction are often reluctant to bring up these issues with their health-care practitioners because they feel it is embarrassed or ashamed. Pain is nothing to be ashamed of simply because it occurs in a different part of the body. Fatigue is always an issue with FMS, and often is related to sexual dysfunction. And interestingly, patients with CFS seem to report less sexual dysfunction than patients with FMS, at least according to the patients in the study.*(Clinical rheumatol. 2009 Apr;28(4):365-9. Doi: 10.1007/s 10067-009-1093. Epub 2009 Jan 23.)*

Fibromyalgia and Sexual Dysfunction in Men

Fibromyalgia occurs disproportionately among women and men, at a rate of 9 to 1 in favor of women. And the reasons for this discrepancy are still uncertainly clear. Some health experts suggest that these differences are likely the result of an interaction between numerous biological, psychological, and sociocultural factors *(Yunus 2001).*

However, men also who suffer from the debilitating affects of FMS share the same consequences in sexual dysfunction as women do. Men with FMS that suffer from erectile dysfunction may often feel as if their masculinity has been taken away, and may even feel broken and even suicidal. In men an increased definite correlation between FMS and erectile dysfunction has been documented, and has also been on the rise.

Fibromyalgia can be a direct, as well as an indirect, result of this disorder. The pain caused by Fibromyalgia, particularly in the testicles and penis area, is the most direct and immediate cause of erectile dysfunction. Many sufferer's of FMS both male and female also report reduced sexual drive. This leads to performance anxiety, depression, and ultimately impotence in male patients. Add to that the excessive physical and mental fatigue caused by sleep deprivation and muscle and joint pains are also instrumental in reducing the libido and rendering the patient unable to perform sexually.

Conventional treatment for men with Ed may result in the use of PDE-5 inhibitors such as **Viagra or Cialis,** and possible anti-depressant medication such as **Prozac, Zoloft, Paxil,** etc. Which normally complicates the issue even worse by creating additional problems. Harvard Medical School's Dr. Joseph Glenmullen recently reported on the many dreadful side effects associated with conventional anti-depressant medications. That include neurological disorders, sexual dysfunction (in up to 60% of its user's), debilitating withdrawal symptoms (including hallucinations, dizziness, nausea, and anxiety).

Other recommended medicines often prescribed that can make matters much worse in those suffering from sexual dysfunction of FMS are *anti-convulsant medications like "Neurontin, Gabitril, and Lyrica".* And the listed side effects of these medications sound like some of the symptoms associated with FMS and CFS, include - *"fatigue, brain fog, muscle aches, poor mental clarity, mood disorders, weakness, sexual dysfunction, prolonged drowsiness, fluid retention, weight gain, thought disorder, double vision, etc., etc,.* Shall I go on? Cause there are a lot more side effects! And for a complete list of the current medication normally prescribed for FMS, see the section "Conventional Treatments For FMS and CFS".

In general cases of FMS in men (ED) and in women with sexual dysfunction, it is easy to see and understand how when sleep is affected by FMS you will experience a loss of growth hormone (GH) and low levels of serotonin/melatonin, which helps to initiate a correct sound sleeping pattern, vitally important in the production of growth hormone and muscle pain and tenderness. An effective treatment would be to balance serotonin levels through diet and supplementation (5-HTP precursor to serotonin), and employ a suitable physical resistance type exercise program, which also helps to boost your natural pain chemical (endorphins) and growth hormone, and testosterone levels, and follow the recommended natural treatment protocol for healing FMS and CFS. (Also see sections on reversing and treating FMS and CFS)

Conventional Treatment of Sexual Dysfunction in FM

Overall, women with FMS say they have less sexual arousal, more pain with sex, fewer orgasms, and less sexual activity. Sometimes, with these issues, it may also be due to side effects of medications given which can reduce the ability of a women to achieve sexual orgasms. Unfortunately this also occurs with medications such as, anti-depressants that have side effects of decreased libido, causing a neurotransmitter imbalance, in *serotonin, dopamine, and norepinephrine,* which can all play a huge part in affecting sexual function in women. **(Note: *See section on serotonin and FMS/CFS)***

However, truth be told, considering all the related issues and symptoms with FMS, sex may be the least thing on your mind. With Fibromyalgia, based on my experience with past FMS and CFS clients, it is perfectly clear that in order to restore sexual function, hormonal and neurotransmitter balance must be in place, by achieving this with a specific dietary protocol, body-detoxification, and also by reducing or eliminating the amount of so many different medications given with all of their conflicting side effects. Sexual function can be restored once again.

Issue's To Correct With Sexual Dysfunction of FMS

Decreased sexual desire (hormonal imbalance(testosterone) & neurotransmitter imbalance (serotonin & dopamine)

Decreased arousal (circulatory impairment & neurotransmitter/hormonal imbalances) same as above.

Lessening of orgasmic experience (insufficient hormones - testosterone-oxytocin & amino acid-histidine)

Increase in genital pain (due to vulvodynia -(pain, irritation or rawness of female genital area) could be due to insufficient secretion or lubrication of female hormone levels, especially estrogens, and acetylcholine which is needed in the female arousal response *(References – Kalichman L. Association between FM and sexual dysfunction in women. Clin. Rheumatoid. 2009 Jan. 23.).*

Insufficient Sleeping Patterns (due to low serotonin levels and growth hormone (GH) and insufficient nutrient uptake, possible malabsorption of nutrients – vitamins, minerals, and amino acids).

Sexual dysfunction becomes much worse for women who have FM and/or CFS especially if menopausal. With so many factors involving Fibromyalgia and CFS, which can include and impair sexual function, can all be broken down to understand the complexity of sexual function, when malfunctions occur, and they are:

Possible Causes of Sexual Dysfunction in FM & CFS

- **Hormonal imbalance** of estrogen, progesterone, testosterone, and growth hormone. All need to be in balance for sexual activity. Can cause decreased arousal response and low sex drive.

- **Neurotransmitter imbalance** which includes dopamine, acetylcholine, norepinephrine resulting from poor nutrition and stress. Can cause depression, anxieties, and lack of desire and no interest in sexual activity.

- **Glandular insufficiency** (weak adrenal & thyroid hormones) excess cortisol or insufficient amounts of cortisol, affecting thyroid output of T4 and T3 thyroid hormones. (same as above)

- **Malabsorption** (due to a digestive enzyme deficiency) causing foods not to be absorbed for nutritional uptake. Lack of vitamins, minerals, and amino acids, needed for hormonal production and neurotransmitter functioning and balance.

- **Possible undetected yeast over growth** (candida infection) possibly due to poor dietary habits of consuming large quantities of carbohydrates (sugar), and saturated fats. Yeast infection can affect all of the above.

- **Heavy Metal Toxicity** - Can also cause cause hormonal and neurotransmitter imbalances affecting sexual function.

Several studies have also linked sexual dysfunction in patients with Fibromyalgia. All reports agree that sexual dysfunction seems frequently impaired in this condition. The dysfunction is also usually severe and may affect all domains of sexuality. Given the complexity of factors involved in human sexual function and intricacy of the physiopathology of FM, many factors and mechanisms have been implicated as well. As mentioned above.*(Sexual Dysfunction in patients with FM; Current Rheumatology Reports, Dec. 2009, Vol. 11, Issue 6, pp 437-442)*

Chapter 12

THE YEAST CONNECTION AND FMS/CFS

There are two controversial diagnosis associated with Fibromyalgia are food sensitivities and candida over growth syndrome. With fibromylagia and chronic fatigue patients this often results from a chronic craving for carbohydrates and sweets that can contribute to yeast over growth which results in a condition called Candida Albicans. There are also many patients of FM and FCS that usually test positive for candida lead to fibroblast and hypothyroid symptoms.

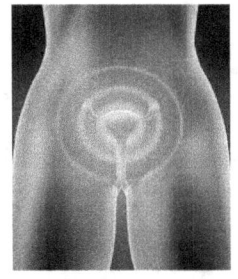

And it is often found that Fibromyalgia and hypothyroid symptoms also improve after a candida infection is treated.

Candida Albicans can cause a host of various symptoms and a yeast over growth can interfere with the absorption of nutrients in the gut, which is where we absorb most of the beneficial components of the food we eat. This may also explain the phenomena such as the inability of some people with FM and CFS to get the benefit of Tryptophan in foods they eat from a malabsorption problem. It may just as well have a great deal to do with their hormonal imbalances in general.

It is also interesting that once the diet has been changed to a low carb' diet and including more protein and vegetables, by depriving the yeasts of the starches and sugars it needs to grow and reproduce, Fibromyalgia patients then often start to feel better. I also don't want to leave you with the impression that FMS is caused by a yeast over growth, but do think and have noticed that people who have FMS and CFS and excess yeast build up do feel much more worse than those who do have FMS and don't have a yeast over growth.

Research does show that there is a common link that associates a yeast problem in many people that have FM and CFS. There are many studies that explain the common connection of malabsorpton and nutrient deficiencies like Tryptophan which is the precursor to serotonin that affects sleeping patterns, and many other nutrient deficiencies because of malabsorption of not getting the proper nutritional balance to offset disease and allow the healing process to occur. And how FMS and CFS people never seem to get better when on medication from doctors, but instead are on a crash course to no where!

Candidiasis is Widespread

Some doctors may also scoff of this idea, so don't be surprised if you mention it to your doctor and are told to forget about the idea. But yet, just show them the research, cause there are many studies out there linking the two associated conditions. Candida or systemic yeast over growth has always been an epidemic in America.

Approximately 80% of Americans (mostly females) have the over growth, and Practitioners in the natural health field are giving Candida the blame for virtually every health problem under the sun. From skin rashes to cancer, while candida over growth is a legitimate health issue. What many people fail to realize is that systemic yeast over growth has been with us since there were yeasts and people on earth.

The escalation of systemic yeast over growth occurred and spread with the use of *anti-biotics* since World War II; the utilization of high doses of cortisone; the vast increases of consuming refined carbohydrates, particularly refined sugar (an estimated 120 pounds per capita each year) and the wide spread use of the birth-control pill. It is also estimated that roughly half of the world's population will suffer from a candida-related condition in their lifetime.

There are over 30 million people who suffer from over growth of candida albicans, and that's only the number in North America. More and more anti-biotics are being prescribed for children than ever before. From 1977 to 1986, anti-biotic prescriptions for children under the age of ten increased an alarming 51%, while the number of children in this age group grew by only 9%, and anti-biotic prescriptions for children under the age of 3 showed the most dramatic increase *(Dr. Michael Schmidt, in Childhood Ear Infections- North Atlantic Books, Berkely, CA.)*

Yeast pioneers first alerted the world to this now common condition, in a series of articles in the **Journal of Orthomolecular Psychiatry from 1978 through 1984** and also in his enlightened book, **"The Missing Diagnosis" (Birmingham, Alabama, 1983)** Dr. Truss revealed the relationship of Candida albicans to a myriad of chronic illnesses that defied diagnosis.

Additionally, pioneering work by Sidney M Baker, M.D., of New Haven Connecticut, and the clinical discoveries by Dr. William G. Cook, M.D., in his famous best seller *"The Yeast Connection"*, both that have helped make the world aware of the many symptoms of this mysterious destroyer of good health attributed to Candida albicans. Systemic yeast over growth is a serious illness that can make your life very miserable, and even in some cases cause death.

But now that you have been made well aware of Candida albicans, you may be wondering whether or not this is your problem? This questionnaire taken out from Dr. Crook's Candida Questionnaire and score sheet from his run away best seller *"The*

Yeast Connection" can help you determine if you might have a yeast over growth problem.

Candida Health Questionnaire and Score Sheet
Section A: History

1. Have you taken tetracyclines (Sumycin), Panmycin, Vibramycin, Minocin, etc., or any other anti-biotics for acne for 1 month or longer? Point/score 35
2. Have you, at any time in your life, taken other broad spectrum anti-biotics for respiratory, urinary or other infections (for 2 months or longer) or in shorter courses 4 or more times in a year? Point/score 35
3. Have you taken a broad spectrum anti-biotic drug – even in a single course? Point/score 6
4. Have you, at any time in your life been bothered by persistent prostatis, vaginitis, or other problems affecting your reproductive organs? Point/score 25
5. Have you been pregnant 2 or more times? Point/score 5 or 1 time? Point/score 3
6. Have you taken birth control pills for 2 years? Point/score 15 or for 6 months to 2 years? Point/score 8
7. Have you taken prednisone, decadron or other cortisone drugs for more than 2 weeks? Point/score 15 or for 2 weeks or less point/score 6
8. Does exposure to perfumes, insecticides, fabric shop odors and other chemicals provoke moderate to severe symptoms? Point score 20
9. Are symptoms worse on damp, muggy days or in moldy places? Point/score 20
10. Have you had athlete's foot, ring worm, "jock itch" or other chronic fungous infections of the skin or nails? Have such infections been severe or persistent? Point/score 20 or mild or moderate? Point/score 10
11. Do you crave sugar? Point score 10
12. Do you crave bread? Point score 10
13. Do you crave alcoholic beverages? Point score 120
14. Does tobacco smoke really bother you? Point score 10

Total score for section A _____

Section B: Major Symptoms

For each of your symptoms, enter the appropriate figure in the point score column:

- If a symptom is occasional or mild score 3 points
- If a symptom is frequent and/or moderately severe score 6 points
- If a symptom is severe and/or disabling score 9 points
- Add the total score and then record it at the end of this section.

1. Fatigue or lethargy____
2. Feeling of being drained____
3. Poor memory____

4. Feeling spacy or unreal____
5. Inability to make decisions____
6. Numbness, burning or tingling____
7. Insomnia____
8. Muscle aches____
9. Muscle weakness____
10. Pain and/or swelling in joints____
11. Abdominal pain____
12. Constipation____
13. Diarrhea____
14. Bloating, belching or intestinal gas____
15. Trouble vaginal burning, itching or discharge____
16. Prostatitis____
17. Impotence____
18. Loss of sex drive or feeling____
19. Endometriosis or infertility____
20. Cramps and/or other menstrual irregularities____
21. Premenstrual tension____
22. Attacks of anxiety or crying____
23. Cold hands and feet and/or chilliness____
24. Shaking or irritable when hungry____

Total score – Section B_____

Section C: Other Symptoms

For each of your symptoms, enter the appropriate figure in the point score column:
If your symptom is occasional or mild score 1 points
If your symptom is frequent and/or moderately severe score 2 points
If a symptom is severe and/or disabling score 3 points
Add the total score in the box at the end of this section.

1. Drowsiness____
2. Irritability or jitteriness____
3. Incoordination____
4. Inability to concentrate____
5. Frequent mood swings____
6. Headaches____
7. Dizziness/ loss of balance____
8. Pressure above ears, and feeling of head swelling____
9. Tendency to bruise easily____
10. Chronic rashes or itching____
11. Numbness, tingling____
12. Indigestion or heartburn____
13. Food sensitivities or intolerance____
14. Mucus in stools____

15. Rectal itching____
16. Dry mouth or throat____
17. Rash or blisters in mouth____
18. Bad breath____
19. Foot, hair or body odor not relieved by washing Nasal congestion or post nasal drip____
20. Nasal congestion or post nasal drip____
21. Nasal itching___
22. Sore throat____
23. Laryngitis loss of voice____
24. Cough or recurrent bronchitis____
25. Pain or tightness in chest____
26. Wheezing or shortness of breath____
27. Urinary frequency or urgency____
28. Burning on urination____
29. Spots in front of eyes or erratic vision_____
30. Burning or tearing of eyes____
31. recurrent infections or fluid in ears____
32. Ear pain or deafness____

Total score Section C_____
Total score Section A _____
Total score Section B_____
Grand total score_____

Note: the grand total score will help you and your physician decide if your health problems are yeast connected. Scores will run higher as 7 items in the questionnaire pertain to women, while only 2 apply to men. Yeast-connected problems are almost certainly present in women with scores over 180, and 140 in men. Yeast connected problems are probably present in women with scores over 120, and 90 in men. Yeast connected problems are prossibly present in women with scores over 60 and scores over 40 in men. And with scores of less than 60 in women and 40 in men, yeasts are less apt to cause health problems.

If your questionnaire score shows that you might have candida, there are several corrective measures that you can take. Preferably under the guidance of a health care practitioner that understands candida albicans would be advised or you could follow the recommended procedure on how to eliminate candida through diet and supplementation. You could also take a saliva or stool test to be sure. To test for candida albicans the best out there right now are - A Serum or Saliva D-arabintol levels – D-arabintol is a toxic by product of systemic candida and the levels can be quantitatively measured to determine the extent of the infection, or a Candida Elisa blood test that detects antibodies, and a comprehensive digestive stool analysis can also help to determine for candida albicans.

These tests can be quite expensive and even if you have medical coverage, insurance companies might be reluctant to pay up. If that's the case with you, diagnose it yourself and just use your common sense and think back over your medical history. Take note of how many candida symptoms you have and what their severity is.

Candida Yeast Infection Self Exam Test

This test can help you to determine if candida yeast overgrowth is likely. If you find yourself eating these kinds of foods several times a week, much less everyday or several times a day, then it definitely indicates trouble. That "sweet" tooth could indicate a deeper underlying health problem like candida albicans yeast infection overgrowth. With the exception of fruit, most of these are not even considered real foods. They are packaged, processed, refined and lifeless. They are loaded with sugar. And if you are craving sugar (and if you eat these types of foods) then the chances are high that you are feeding the yeast beastie. These lifeless foods include:

- **Colas, juices, candies, alcohol, fast food snacks, ice cream, french fries, puddings, desserts, cakes, pies, breads, donuts, etc.,**

Self-Test – Your Body Fluids: (A Saliva – Spit Test) - This test is best done upon waking first thing in the morning before you put anything in your mouth, so before you rinse out your mouth, get a glass of water (*a clear glass*), and now start to build up an amount of saliva (*spit*) your mouth saliva, do not cough up anything and spit in the glass of water. Observe what happens. The saliva will float which is OK and normal, If withing 15 minutes you see thin projections extending downward into the water, it is a positive sign for candida.

The projections may look like hair, or small strings, like a jelly fish or spider legs, moving down into the water from the saliva floating on the top. Other positive indications might be very "cloudy" saliva that will sink to the bottom of the glass within a few minutes or particles that slowly sink or suspend below the saliva glob. What you are seeing are colonies of yeast which band together to form the strings.

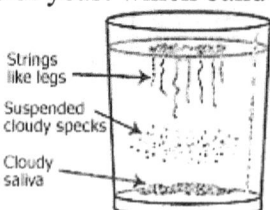

Candid Saliva characteristics of yeast overgrowth: *(1) Strings of saliva traveling down to the bottom of the glass. (2) Cloudy saliva that sinks to the bottom of the glass. (3) Cloudy specks of saliva suspended in the water.*

If you can not find a local physician to work with you on testing for candida albicans, you can also order an online Candida Immune Complexes test at Evenstar.com. Or look through your local phone book directory and seek out a health care practitioner that specializes in yeast over growths and infections.

Conquering Candid, The Dietary Do's and Don'ts

If your diagnosis is confirmed, you can start a three month, anti yeast food and supplement plan, which usually stops yeast related symptoms very quickly, even in the first week. This also calls for a radical change in lifestyle that should be followed diligently. Candida is a serious infection which can spread throughout the body and cause serious harm and complications, especially if you other health related issues. The first course of action would be to -

- **Stop eating sugar products** – white, brown, corn syrup, honey, maple syrup, or molasses – and sugared products, as well as milk, cheese, fruit, bakery goods made with white flower. Milk and yeast containing foods do not always cause or encourage overgrowth of candida, but they often cause food sensitivities and allergies, which can produce symptoms similar to those of candida. They should be omitted from the diet for at least 3 weeks and then add them singly and monitored to see if they produce any marked physiological reactions before reinstating them back to your diet.
- **Eat plenty of vegetables,** whole grains, meat(chicken and lamb), fish, nuts(except peanuts), seeds, cold pressed oils, and sugarless fruitless yogurts to reinforce your defending beneficial intestinal bacteria.(many milk-intolerants can tolerate yogurt). Include papayas they contain natural enzymes.
- **Add food supplements to your daily diet.** Two tablespoons of liquid lactobacillus acidophilus before each meal. This is one type of friendly bacteria (lactobacillus acidopholis) that helps to keep candida in check. Also add **Kyolic Garlic** two times a day with meals. Two 500mg of (GLA) gamma-linoenic acid tablets 3 times a day, a good multivitamin and mineral supplement, a good vitamin B complex pill (50mg) of the major B vitamins to compensate for the reduced declining levels of friendly bacteria. Add 4 grams of vitamin C powder (Emergen-C) start out out with 2grams of the vitamin C powder and slowly build up to the 4 grams daily. And last consume 2 cups of **Pau D' Arco te**a a day, commonly called **Taheebo tea.**

Caprylic Acid – One of the most potent non-drug or natural yeast fighting agents derived from coconut oil. It is commonly sold as a dietary supplement in health food stores.

- **Abstain from all forms of alcohol.** Refrain from smoking and abuse of drugs. Purchase Capristan or Caprilic acid for 1 tablet 3 x a day..
- **Add an exercise program to boost your immune system.**
- **Eliminate all processed foods** during your therapy anti-candida diet which includes all boxed, and canned goods. Absolutely *no cheeses* and *peanuts (often contaminated with aspergillus mold)* should in your diet. Also avoid brewer's yeast -packaged foods that include yeast. Cheese is a fermented food and a mold, is to be avoided also. Yeast by products, breads, cakes, cookies, pizza, sandwiches.

The emergence of yeast as a major cause of food cravings has been a hidden indicative factor in the 20th century. Eventually this has caused it to multiply quite rapidly and affect the whole body which can cause a multitude of health problems. Yeasts can multiply very rapidly in your body and can go by undetected creating symptoms that mimic other diseases. As you have read thus far that the use of *anti-biotic, drugs and medications (birth control pills, spermicidal creams and foams, cortisone-predispose, and similar steroids; nutritional deficiencies, poor digestion, poor diets, excessive carbohydrates and sugar intake, anti-biotic residues in commercial meats, a weakened immune system, use of recreational drugs -alcohol, marijuana, tobacco, can all stress your internal organs the liver, adrenal glands and the immune system spreading and* multiplying rendering your body helplessly to it's deadly affects.

It is the poor digestion and malabsorption that set the stage for yeast over growth. And if you don't have enough digestive juices (hydrochloric acid) in your stomach, and friendly intestinal bacteria to keep it in check, yeast is then more likely to to over grow and multiply. Preventing its over growth when these three following conditions are met, will normally render the yeast harmless and cease it's harmful effects on the body. The three conditions to employ are:

1. **Provide a staple of friendly bacteria in your intestines. (B complex vitamins 100mgs, include Probiotic supplements like - lactobacillus acidipholus, bulgaris bifidus)**

2. **Boost your immune system by keeping strong and intact. (Colostrum supplements-Excellent for Immune system build up and for killing yeast over growth)**

3. **Keep a diet that is balanced with adequate proteins (** *preferably organic poultry, chicken, turkey, lean red meats, fish, beans),* **vegetables** *(especially the cruciferious kind-broccoli, cauliflower, cabbage),* **and essential fattty acids** *(omega 3's, olive oil, primrose oil, flax seed oil, and fish oils),* **and your not over eating simple carbohydrates** *(particularly sugar, and refined carbohydrates, and grains.*

Pro-Biotics and Candida Albicans

Pro-biotics are one of the most important 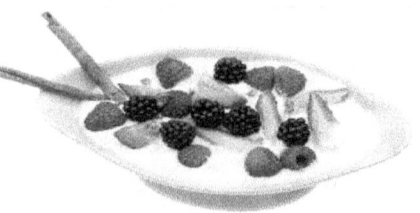 parts of a candid albicans cure. They are the good bacteria that live in your intestines and digest your food for you. They produce many beneficial chemicals and help process the waste for elimination. With them you are strong and healthy and full of energy. Without them you would die!

Basically your intestines are like your second brain, they determine how you feel, if they (intestines) are unhappy, you are unhappy. Just try to smile and enjoy yourself when you have heartburn, gas, diarrhea or constipation. There are an estimated of 400 types of bacteria that live in your gut, composed of three pounds (nearly 100 trillion) of bacteria inside your digestive system. And there also ten times more bacteria in your gut than there are cells in your body. So, you can see the importance of how friendly bacteria has such a big influence on our health. When the intestines are unhappy, they are not functioning up to their full capacity. Which means that a lot of the nutrients are not being digested fully and not all of the toxins are being cleared from the body.

Many of the candida albicans kill off the friendly bacteria, and it is the poor food choices that feed the bad bacteria and harm the good bacteria. You already know how and why yeast over growth can occur and multiplies rapidly, how also anti-biotics and other medicines can kill or limit the growth of the good or friendly bacteria. It is all of these things adding together that can lead to a candida over growth.

Probiotics work to restore the normal flora in your intestines by competing with other organisms for nutrients. They also produce other beneficial chemicals which help to increase your body's immunity or make the environment less favorable for the bad bacteria to live.

Pro-biotics help to produce B vitamins such as **niacin B3**, **folic acid, B6, biotin, vitamin k, butryic acid (may help to prevent cancer), lactic acid, acetic acid, short chain fatty acids** (lowers intestinal pH making it too acidic for candida to survive), hydrogen peroxide(makes the gut inhospitable to the candida), and bacteriocins (anti-microble compounds that kill yeasts, viruses and bad bacteria.

And in addition to helping you treat candida albicans, probiotics can also help treat many other health conditions that may or may not be related to a candida over growth. Other conditions that probiotics can treat or help cure are:

- **Allergies, auto-immune disease, weak immune system.**
- **Digestive problems – acid reflux, bloating, constipation, diarrhea, heart burn, gas, nausea, traverler's diarrhea.**
- **Eczema in children, food allergies, infections, parasites, and Uro-genital problems.**
- **May also improve skin health and treat herpes infections.**

Instructions For Taking Pro-biotics

- **Best taken 30 minutes before eating**
- **choose a brand that contains live mixtures (a broad spectrum multi-probiotics is best)**
- **Choose a brand that has an expiration date on the label.**
- **Avoid extreme heat or freezing as it will kill the bacteria.**
- **Certain brands must be kept refrigerated to keep the bacteria viable.**
- **Prebiotics are food for the probiotic – they ensure the bacteria thrive.**

You can also get probiotics by eating fermented foods. Many of these fermented foods contain massive quantities of probiotics, so try to have some with your foods with your meals to help keep the healthy bacteria in your gut. Whether you are taking probiotics to cure a candida over growth or simply for overall health, the important thing to remember is that you take them. They are virtually important to the health of your immune system which can kill off the yeast over growth. Do yourself a favor and include them in your daily diet. _**Remember, all disease manifests in the stomach, and when your stomach doesn't feel good , then you don't feel good !**_

A good brand and product is Swanson's Signature line called "Ultimate Probiotic Formula".

Golden Rules To Apply For Candida Albicans Control

Systemic yeast over growth has been plaguing the American public for generations now and it is important that we realize how and why this disease can grow and impair the health of so many people. And by applying certain rules to better protect yourself and your loved ones, you can then be better prepared to prevent yeast over growth from happening to you. Rules to follow are:

1. **Wear cotton**, white under garments like night gowns and pajamas. Avoid plastic and synthetic clothing which causes perspiration to be trapped and cause bacteria. Change under clothing and stockings daily. Wash all white clothing in a bleach solution. For women it is better to wear skirts instead of slacks, to allow for better air circulation to the genital area. And if slacks are worn they should definitely not be tight.

2. **Personal Hygiene** is important when urinating and defecating. Frequent bathing is also important. Women who use tampons should change them every few hours, as tampons can cause increased fungal activity. Feminine pads should be preferred. Learn to disinfect your toothbrush with diluted H_2O_2. Use a new tooth brush every two weeks or so. When wearing shoes sprinkle some medicated powder in shoes to feet from bacteria build up. Rub some on your feet and in between toes.

3. **Follow your candida recommended diet.** Learn to eliminate harmful foods (sugar, and sugar by products) that can impair your immune system. Add more fiber to your diet, probiotics and protein based foods. A proper anti-candida diet can help speed up the elimination of yeasts.

4. **Take the appropriate supplements that are recommended for candida.**

5. **Get the 7 essentials**: fresh air, natural foods(organic if possible), exercise, water(distilled) for drinking, daily showers, swim in the ocean if possible, get moderates amount of sunshine, get sufficient amounts of sleep and rest, prayer and meditation, and apply positive thinking in stress management.

6. **Avoid drugs and anti-biotics** that can destroy the beneficial intestinal flora and weaken your immune system that can cause yeast over growth.

7. **Build up the strength of your adrenal glands** to help you conquer food allergies that can weaken your adrenal glands. Take specific herbal adaptogens for adrenal health (Rhodiola Rosea and Schizandria).

8. **Learn to disinfect your food preparation items** like your cutting board (lemon

rub), knives, spoons, and forks, soak them in distilled water with fresh lemon juice or wash them thoroughly in hot water.

9.   **Bring disposable plastic eating utensils** with you when eating in restaurants, also carry with you straws for drinking.

10. **Have a hair analysis** done by a health care practitioner that specializes in hair tissue mineral analysis, to look for vital mineral deficiencies and toxic heavy metals.

11. **Exercise** at least 20 minutes or more for several days of the week. Exercise is a great way to restore health and vitality and stimulate your blood circulation.

12. **Avoid regular store bought meats that are not organic.** Which are normally laced with hormones and anti-biotics. Research has also shown that almost half of all anti-biotics used in the US are fed to farm animals, which has led to the growth of drug resistent bacteria that are hazardous to humans (New England Journal of Medicine.)

13. **Using pro-biotics** has benefited most individuals in eliminating yeast over growths. A very important requirement for Candida albicans.

<u>Important</u>: before employing and following the recommended course of treating for candida albicans, it will be a good idea to utilize a sufficient body cleanse to rid your body of toxins and start off fresh with the recommended candida plan or protocol.

Candida Yeast Infection Protocol

<u>Nutritional Support</u>: Foods that have proven to help with yeast (candidiasis) & fungal infections are: *Yogurt with Probiotic Cultures, Garlic and Flax Seeds.*

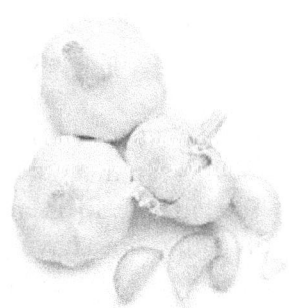

<u>Avoid</u> – *refined white flour and refined white sugars and large amounts of honey, maple syrup, and fruit juices. Avoid milk and other dairy products. Avoid alcoholic beverages, cheeses, dried fruits, and peanuts.*

<u>Nutrients</u> that have been proven to help with Yeast (candidiasis) & fungal infections are: *Probiotics, Plant Source Digestive enzymes, Cat's claw, Olive Leaf extract, Garlic, Tea tree oil, Grape Seed extract, Caprylic Acid(very effective against candida) and Larch Arabinogalactan.*

<u>Exercises</u> have also been proven to be helpful in candida infections by stimulating the immune system and prevent you from further yeast infections.

Chapter 13

Curing FM & CFS: In Search of The Cure!

Amazingly enough, as of late 1982, Fibromyalgia was not even recognized or entered in the doctor's standard clinical reference bible, the Merck Manual. The closest 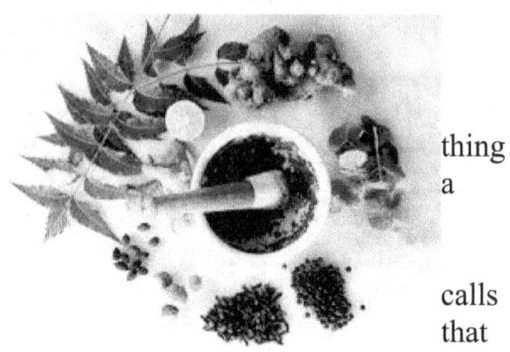 thing you'll find is *"Myalgia"* which is described as a muscular pain. For which the recommended procedure implied aspirin and anti-inflammatory's. Today, conventional treatment calls for a wide variety of prescription medications that include:

- Anti-depressants *(Cymbalta)*
- Anti-anxiety scripts *(Xanax)*
- SSRI's (serotonin re-uptake inhibitors-*Prozac)*
- Pain med's **(Opiates-Vicodin,)**
- Nerve pain *(Lyrica)*
- Anti-inflammatory pills *(Prednisone)*
- Muscle relaxants/spasms (**Flexeril**)
- Sleeping pills *(Seroquel)*
- Hypothyroid medicine *(Synthyroid & Cytomel)*

The list of these medications goes on and on, and some of these medicines include very powerful drugs that often bring on serious side effects that require additional prescriptions for just the side effects, which create a vicious cycle. It's no wonder that conventional medicine has never found a cure for an illness that has been around since the early 1980's. How can one find a cure for an illness that is treated with synthetic drugs that the body normally rejects and only creates harm within the body. What modern science fails to realize, and is taught in holistic health schools, the body will always try to heal itself on a natural level, Homeostasis.

Also what ever happened to - "Let Thy Food Be Thy Medicine?" a sol-gen that is put on banners in most medical schools, taught by the father of natural medicine, "Hippocrates". Please, do not miss interpret my beliefs, conventional medicine (Allopathy) does have it's place in healing, some drugs and medicines do save lives and are necessary in healing. But when it pertains to certain diseases that do not respond to drugs, and only gets worse because of it, it is time to employ a different method of healing, and that is natural healing.

And to this day, doctors acknowledge they have no idea "What causes" Fibromyalgia, don't know how to cure it, but yet prescriptions are dispensed with an authoritarian attitude, stating *"This will help you feel better"*. Now, does that make sense to you? Why would you take drugs if doctors don't know what fibromyalgia is, what caused it, or how to cure (heal) it? Yet people do just that for every physical ailment. The interesting part is, in other parts of the world, there are incidences of diseases that practically don't exist in "undeveloped" parts of the world. But now, Western scientists have recently acknowledged what Traditional Chinese Medicine (TCM) really is. The sad part, is traditional Chinese medicine has known for centuries that Fibromyalgia and all bodily functions can be reversed with natural means.

Countries that acknowledge the natural way of healing by applying food, herbs, and a mind-body connection (meditation & yoga), that our (the US) modern lifestyle that is causing these diseases and that Western Medicine's theory and doctrines fail to recognize that diseases are not separate from the person. *In fact every disease can be more accurately called an expression of the patient's lifestyle, beliefs, and energies.* Our body was designed to heal itself, given that it has the proper care-nutrition, herbal supplements, spiritual and emotional well-being. For example, cancer is not a tumor, it is a systemic disorder that can only truly be healed by helping to support the body, not by attacking it with chemical bombs (radiation, chemo) or knives. The manifestation of a tumor is a physical expression of the systemic disorder, and simply removing the tumor does nothing to cure the disease.

Why is it that other countries around the world, except the US, employ the healing of diseases through the means of both Naturopathy and Allopathy medicine? When for thousands of years many ill fated disease have been cured by components of traditional medicine, herbal and nutritional therapy, restorative physical exercise, meditation, acupuncture, and remedial massage. Our concept in this country only see's the monetary value of disease manifestations, developing powerful drugs that cure nothing but create symptoms and side effects only to prescribe more prescriptions. And to this day, even the common cold has no cure, diabetes no cure, cancers no cure, but yet you can find medication for any possible disease that you can think of from A to Z. And to say the least, there has not been one single cure for many of the listed diseases. ***The reason in my belief, is that here is no money in the cure, but the money is in the medicine!***

We develop medicines to treat symptoms only and to just keep you alive long enough to keep on buying the medicine that you need to stay alive. We have lost the basic concept of healing, but in stead have resorted to making profits from disease and illnesses. Could it be that modern medicine is a **"Two Trillion Dollar"** a year business in America, and that large pharmaceutical drug companies are making more money than the drug cartels ever thought of, sickness is big business.

As a nation we lead the world in diseases that do not exist in other countries and if they do they are treated by the simple means of diet and physical exercise. The body is designed to heal itself provided it has the proper support to do its job. Holistic healing is now being recognized regardless of what any one chooses to believe or think.

By using a combination of a healthy mind (psyche), body, spirit (spiritual) lifestyle you can prevent or heal any and all body malfunctions. Your diet is one of the major influences on healing and reversing Fibromylagia. Every vitamin, mineral, trace mineral, amino acid, enzyme,
and nutrient within our body required for us to thrive, and be healthy and disease free, can be found on earth

So it makes sense, when the father of natural medicine "Hippocrate's 400BC" stated –

<u>Let Thy Food Be Thy Medicine,</u> he was referring to "we are what we eat." The medicine is found in foods, plants, herb's, and the earth where it comes from and where we go back to. An example of this, is nature's wild animals like the mongoose who can with stand the bite of one of the world's deadliest snakes, the 'Cobra', one bite of the cobra's venom can kill 20 men, but the mongoose is not affected. Why? Because they eat a plant (herb) that counter acts the poison of the cobra's bite (an anti-venom) that neutralizes the cobra's highly toxic venom, called "plantain", in which it will sort out to eat if bitten by the deadly snake.

This example just proves how we can look into nature and discover it amazing life giving substances that we as people are a part of. And the cure's for almost every disease and ailment can be found in nature. Other countries like India, China, Japan, and Europe throughout the ages have all resorted to natural healing as far back as 6,000 years ago, and even to this day they still use herb's, food, meditation, and exercise as the basic frame work for healing disease. Many years ago, in the US, you would of found herbal elixirs in most of the drugstores in America. As Herbal medicine, and Homeopathy were the primary forms of healing here in the US.

In 1985, the World Health Organization estimated about 80% of the world's population relied on herbs for their primary health care needs. And of the drugs in today's modern pharmaceutical armamentarium, approximately 65% were originally derived from plant-based chemicals. Still to this day, 25% of prescription drugs and over the counter (OTC) drugs continue to be derived from plant materials. However, over the last 100 years, Americans have lost touch with their herbal medicines, and sadly the United States is unique in being one of the only nations to have almost completely lost its herbal tradition. In the midst of the herbal renaissance, it is estimated that 70% of all medical doctors in France and Germany regularly still prescribe herbal preparations.

It is also beyond me why we have lost this natural way of healing where other countries still practice to this day. Herbal medicines have the potential of providing the American people with a lower cost and safer alternative to many of the excessively expensive, and often dangerous pharmaceuticals commonly used today. The adverse effects caused by pharmaceuticals are responsible for approximately one third of all hospital admissions. And once in the hospital, 35% of the patients can expect an adverse drug effect.

The development of pharmaceutical drugs some 100 years ago changed our focus from natural healing to the new "wonder drugs". That is when medical practice turned away from herbal botanicals and embraced these chemical-based medicines.

 Losing the sight of an important concept of nature, that man-made chemicals of synthetic matter do little to support over all health. Medicines made from plants on the other hand, tend to nourish the body without taxing it, supporting the body system rather than suppressing it.

There is a passage in the bible, in Genesis 1:29:30 that says it all pertaining to natural medicine and it reads -*"**And God said, behold, I have given you every herb bearing seed, which is upon the face of the earth, and every tree, in which is the fruit of a*** *tree yielding seed; to you it shall be for meat."*

"And to every beast of the earth, and to every fowl of the air, and to everything that creepeth upon the earth, wherein there is life, I have given every green herb for meat; and it was so."

This simple and acknowledged truth about all diseases and healing, is that it is important to know and understand that nature has provided everything we need to sustain health and well-being, that for every sickness, there's a cure, and for every cause, there's an explanation.

When millions of people start experiencing the same health problem, something is seriously wrong. Something is unbalanced, causing your body to become diseased by poor nutrition and a poor lifestyle. <u>Fibromyalgia is just that, a product of the modern lifestyle that caused your body to become a toxic wasteland due to an over-acidification of the body from an inverted way of living, thinking, and eating</u>. Therefore there can only be one way of healing, and that is to alkalize the body and break the cycle of imbalance, in allowing you to regain what you have lost, your energy and vitality.

The first order of healing is to neutralize the toxic levels of acid within your body and give it a rest from its acidic state. When you cleanse the body from the overflow of acids, it starts to heal and rebuild itself, it starts to heal and recover slowly but surely. It's important to attend to what you put in your inside your body when dealing with diseases. The solution is to get your body back to it's natural state by cleansing yourself from the inside, physically and mentally. You also have to remember, your body can restore every wound, diseased organ or damaged cell that comes your way, but it can not do that if you keep polluting it with toxic food, toxic thinking and a toxic lifestyle.

Chapter 14

The Importance of Acid & Alkaline Balance

"The pH balance of the blood stream is one of the most important biochemical balances in all of the human body chemistry."
(Dr. Robert O. Young)

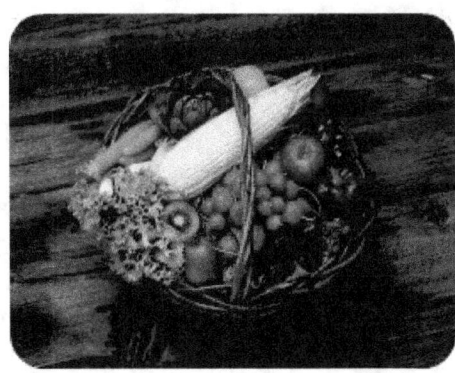

It is known that all diseases known to man, run in an acidic state. Over acidity, which can become a dangerous condition that weakens all body systems, is very common today. It gives rise to an internal environment conducive to disease, as opposed to a pH-balanced environment which allows normal body function necessary for the body to resist disease. A healthy body maintains an adequate alkaline reserves to meet emergency demands. When excess acids must be neutralized, our alkaline reserves are depleted leaving the body in a weakened condition.

The concept of acid alkaline imbalance as the cause of disease is not new. In 1933 a New York doctor named William Howard Hay published a ground breaking book, "A New Health Era" in which he maintains that all disease is a caused by auto toxification (or "self-poisoning") due to acid accumulation in the body.

Understanding pH & Disease Manifestation

PH (potential of hydrogen) is a measure of the acidity or alkalinity of a solution. It is a measure on a scale of 0 to 14 with the lower the pH the more the acid the solution, the higher the pH the more alkaline (or base) the solution. When a solution is neither acidic nor alkaline it has a pH of 7 which is neutral.

Water is the most abundant compound in the human body, compromising 70% of the body. The body has an acid-alkaline (or acid-base) ratio called the pH which is a balance between positively charged ions (alkaline-forming). The body continually strives to balance the pH. When the balance is compromised many problems can occur. This refers to the pH of the body's fluids and tissues, not the pH of the stomach.

Acidic conditions in the body often result in health problems such as *cancer, chronic fatigue, fibromyalgia, arthritis, osteoporosis, viruses, ALS and MLS, weight gain, skin conditions, and many more other diseases.* An acidic condition (acidosis) decreases the bodies ability to properly absorb minerals and other nutrients, decreases the energy production in cells, decreases its ability to repair damaged cells, decreases its ability to detoxify heavy metals, allows tumor cells to grow and thrive, and creates fatigue and disease. According to experts, over acidity is also one of the major seven causes of inflammation, especially in arthritic conditions.

Causes of Acidosis

The body can be come acid due to a number of reasons, generally from a combination of the following, - eating a diet mainly of acid forming foods that create a high acid pH in your body, Emotional stress also creates an acid environment within the body, smoking cigarettes is another factor, lack of oxygenated blood due to shallow breathing from a lack of exercise, environmental pollution, water additives (chlorine and fluoride) build up levels in the blood, cosmetic and personal care products also helps to contribute to an acidic state as well, *such as tooth paste, amalgam fillings, deodorants, baking soda, and also many food products.* Due to being in an acid state, people do not get enough minerals in their diet due to the loss of mineral content of the soil where plants are grown.

One of the main reasons people become overly acidic is due to the standard American diet, which is far too high in acid-producing animal products like meat, eggs, and dairy, and far too low in alkaline producing foods like fresh vegetables. Additionally we also eat acid producing foods like white flour products and sugar, and drink acid producing beverages like coffee and soft drinks. We use way too many drugs which are also acid forming, and we use artificial chemical sweeteners like NutraSweet, Equal, or Aspartame, which are all extremely acid forming. One of the healthiest things we can do is to correct an overly acid body by cleaning up our diet and lifestyle.

When the body becomes acidic, it will do all what it can to balance itself. In order to do this, it will use the alkaline minerals in the blood or stored in tissues, the acids will build up in the cells, creating acidosis and setting the stage for a variety of maladies. The result is, toxic over load with in the body's tissue's with the end result being a manifestation of disease. Most people who suffer from from disease have an unbalanced pH and are overly acidic. This condition forces the body to borrow minerals – *including calcium, sodium, potassium, and magnesium from vital organs and bones to buffer (neutralize) the acid and safely remove it from the body*.

Because of this strain, the body can suffer severe and prolong damage due to high acidity, a condition that may go undetected for years. Some of the health conditions that are a result of an overly acidic body are:

- **Cardiovascular disease due to the constriction of blood vessels and the reduction of blood oxygen.**
- **Weight gain, obesity, and diabetes**
- **Bladder and kidney conditions, and kidney stones**
- **Immune deficiency problems, allergies**
- **Acceleration of free radical damage that can contribute to cancer conditions**
- **Premature aging**
- **Osteoporosis, weak brittle bones, bone spurs, and bone fractures**
- **Joint pain, aching muscles and lactic acid build up**
- **Low energy and chronic fatigue**
- **Candida (yeast infection)**
- **Excitability of nervous system, sciatica**
- **Tendency to depressive illnesses, anxiety, panic disorders**
- **Weakening of the skin, hair, nails, tooth decay, and bones**

If Cells Die, We Die

Having a pH level slightly more alkaline is crucial towards good health and bodily function. The ph levels of your internal fluids (especially blood) directly affects every cell in your body. If your pH levels become too acidic, the body takes extreme measures to stabilize it. Most often the blood will pull alkaline minerals (sodium, calcium, & magnesium) from tissues to neutralize strong acids. However, if your pH deviates too far from the acidic side of the scale, oxygen levels decrease, and cellular metabolism will stop.

Now, that was not an attempt to scare you into an alkaline diet (although the benefits are great). All bodily functions have acidic affects on the blood and tissues. Your body is equipped to self regulate your pH levels, however our diets and our environment make maintaining a healthy pH balance a more difficult task. These external factors can lead to over acidity, which can wreak havoc on tissues and cellular function, including heart beat and brain function. Scientists even believe that an extremely acidic body is the root-cause of all disease manifestations. Disease always will manifest in the stomach, we are what we eat period!

According to Dr. Robert O. Young, author of "The pH Miracle", he states - "Physiological diseases are almost always the result of too much acid stressing the body's pH balance, to the point where it provokes the body into producing symptoms we call disease." Virtually all chronic diseases known to science -*Aids, Cancer, Diabetes, MLS, AlS, FMS, CFS, Lupus, Lyme disease, Psoriasis, Arthritis, IBS, etc., etc.,* will all most certainly be in an acidic state, and this is how disease escalates into it's full blown state.

Being overly acidic, usually there are warning signs that indicate the body is becoming to acidic. These symptoms" are generally the body's attempt to stabilize pH, but not all symptoms will be noticeable at times. But here are a few common indicators that indicate stages of acidity within the body:

- **Loss of energy**
- **Sensitivity and irritation -(IBS)**
- **Mucus and congestion**
- **Inflammation**
- **Hardening of soft tissue - (Lupus, Lyme, Fibromyalgia)**
- **Ulceration**
- **Degeneration – (Cancer, Heart Disease, Stroke, Aids)**

(Source: The pH Miracle – Dr. Robert O. Young)

Balance pH Levels For Excellent Health

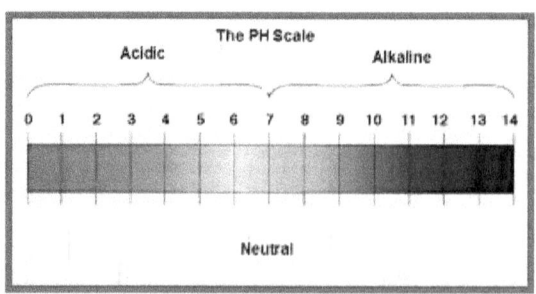

Keeping your body in the proper pH balance is one of the keys in maintaining superior health and warding off disease. By doing doing so, you will be allowing your body to assimilate minerals and nutrients properly only when its pH is balanced. If you are not getting the results you expect from your nutritional or herbal program, look for an acid alkaline imbalance. Even the right herbal program may not work if your body's pH is out of balance. Testing your pH levels can easily be determined in the privacy of your own home with pH test-strips that you can buy at your local pharmacy. Testing your morning urine pH would be the ideal time and moment for an accurate reading. Anything before 7.0 is considered acidic, and anything above 7.45 is slightly alkaline.

Saliva & Urine-pH Testing

Your saliva is also a very good indicator of blood pH readings and should be tested along with the morning urine reading. But when testing your saliva, the best time would be early morning upon awakening from sleep right before you brush your teeth or gargling with mouthwash, as this will give a false reading. Make sure your mouth is just rinsed out with water before you check your saliva

Healthy saliva levels should be in the range of 6.4 to 7.4 on the pH scale. Any readings within this scale indicates you have a good pH balance and plenty of mineral reserves. Readings of 6.25 to 6.75 means that the body is slightly more acidic than it should be.

Shifting your diet towards alkaline forming foods should bring your pH back to normal. Readings lower than 6.25 means your body is severely acidic and very low in mineral reserves. And your body is struggling with an acid environment that is toxic and your placing your internal organs under severe stress. This can cause a metabolic decline within your glandular system creating all sorts of metabolic havoc.

Urine and saliva readings should neutral between 6.8 to 7.2, and your blood pH should always be within a range of 7.35 and 7.45, slightly alkaline is always better than being in an acidic state. According to Dr. Robert O. Young "The pH Miracle", maintaining a saliva and urine pH of 7.2 or above will be an ideal level, in keeping your body from sickness and disease. You will never get sick!

Diet To Balance Proper pH Levels

To correct any extreme imbalance, you will need to shift your diet towards alkaline forming foods and shift away from acid forming foods. You don't want to totally eliminate these foods because your body needs the proteins and fats, but do limit them (especially processed foods). Eating lots more fruits and vegetables and drinking lots of pure water is incredibly important when trying to achieve body pH balance. Also, always remember to test your saliva before meals or at least 30 minutes to an hour after eating. Otherwise your pH levels will give a different reading because of the reaction with foods.

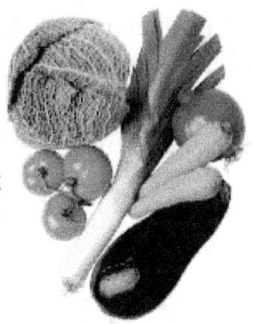

The rise of disease's, cancer, obesity, malnutrition is sky-rocketing. It is the failure of mankind in not recognizing that most diseases can be cured and prevented through proper nutrition. So, it is therefore vitally important to maintain a proper ratio between acid and alkaline foods in the diet. To maintain health and prevent disease, the diet should consistent of 80% alkaline forming foods and 20% acid forming foods.

Common Symptoms of Alkaline Urine (pH 7-8)
- **Possible urinary tract infections**
- **Vegetarian diet**

- **Alkalosis**
- **Vomiting**
- **Alkalizing drugs**
- **Pyloric stenosis/obstruction**

Common Symptoms of an Acid Urine (pH 5 - 6)
- **Gout**
- **Fever**
- **Candida parasites**
- **Excess alcohol**
- **Excess hcl supplements or too high protein/dairy or meat**
- **Predisposition to uric acid calculi (kidney stones)**
- **Phenacetin intake**

This helps maintain a healthy balance and strong resistance against disease. Most importantly, to assist in the curing of any disease, the higher the ratio of alkaline elements in the diet, the faster your recovery will be from disease. Alkaline's neutralizes acids, so therefore it is imperative that your diet includes plenty of alkaline foods to offset the effects of acid forming foods. Consider adding *green leafy vegetables*, *spirulina* and *hemp protein powders* as a natural and alkaline meal replacement. Below is a list of some of the most common alkaline and acid foods that you should be aware of:

Alkalized Foods To Help Control High Acid Levels

Almonds, apples, apricots, avocados, bananas, beans, beet greens, beets, blackberries, broccoli, brussel sprouts, cabbage, carrots, celery, cauliflower, chard leaves, cherries, cucumbers, dried dates, figs, grapefruit, grapes, green beans, green peas, lemons, lettuce, lima beans, limes, millet, molasses, mushrooms, onions, oranges, parsnips, peaches, pears, pineapples, potatoes, yams, radishes, raisins, raspberries, sauerkraut, soy beans, spinach, straw berries, tangerines, tomatoes, water cress, watermelon.

Common Acid Forming Foods

Bacon, barley grains, beef, blueberries, bran wheat, bran oats, white bread, whole wheat bread, butter, carob, cheese, chicken, cod, corn, eggs, white flour, whole wheat flour, haddock, honey, lamb, lobster, milk, macaroni, oatmeal, oysters, peanut butter, peanuts, pork, prunes, brown rice, white rice, salmon, sardines, sausage, scallops, shrimp, spaghetti, squash, sunflower seeds, turkey, veal.

Your blood ph may vary from day to day, because of certain foods that may be eaten, and fluctuations may vary according to your readings. But hopefully you get the general idea of how important your blood pH can be in sickness and in health. To get a better understanding of body pH levels, I recommend you read the books *"The pH Miracle" by Robert O. Young,* and the book *"Alkalize or Die" by Dr. Theodore A. Baroody*, two excellent books that will open your eye's on how important pH levels are to maintaining a healthy lifestyle.

What To Do For Cancer, Candida Albicans, CFS/FMS, & Other Diseases

When the body's pH level reaches an alkaline state of 7.4, cancer cells become dormant. When the body's pH level reaches 8.5, cancer cells die! Cancer can be cured simply by maintaining your pH level at 8.5 or higher! An alkaline pH means an increase in oxygenated blood. And many diseases such as cancer, viruses and candida albicans cannot exist in a highly oxygenated, alkaline environment. If your body is seriously compromised by disease, you would do well to research the works of professionals who specialize in this specific area. And in the meantime you can begin by changing your diet and learning how to safely release the accumulation of toxic substances in your body. Often these toxins inhibit the body's ability to properly absorb nutrients, especially minerals needed to balance pH levels.

Important Points To Remember on Your pH Level Tests: Testing the pH level of your saliva or urine is only going to give you a general trend. Unfortunately, there is no way to determine the Exact pH level of the blood without undergoing a live blood analysis. However, they can still give you a good indication – so test, and then take the average and then follow this trend over time noticing the difference any changes in your diet can make.

Important:
To check your urine and saliva readings, I recommend you look into a home test kit that is available on line from (www.findingmyphbalance.com) that comes with a complete booklet of explanation and a 15 foot roll of test strips to help you take the confusion out of pH testing. Home pH testing is a great and valuable tool in helping you determine a healthy and proper diet, especially if your in the habit of overly consuming high acid foods.

Chapter 15

HEAVY METAL TOXICITY AND FMS/CFS

Toxic metals play a key role in diseased conditions such as FMS and CFS. They undermine the immune system and can cause a multitude of other physical, mental, emotional and behavioral symptoms which have been recognized for many years. However, we do need some metals in our body in a biological form for the many different body functions and these metals are known as minerals.

But too large a quantity, of the wrong form and certain metals can have a detrimental effect. Today, we are exposed to toxic metals every day in our modern world, for example: aluminum from foil packages, deodorants, mercury in vaccinations and amalgam fillings, copper from water piping intake, fluoride in tooth paste, lead in petrol and nickel in hydrogenated fats. And some to occupational exposure to toxic metals

(Chronic fatigue syndrome, Fibromyalgia, Lupus, Rheumatoid Arthritis,

Scleroderma, MCS: the mercury connection. B. Windham, (ED.) 2009).
Today, toxic metals are also being recognized as being the major cause of many illnesses and are the hidden reason behind chronic and frequent infections (especially Candida Albicans over growth and parasitic infections) and chronic fatigue syndrome, Fibromyalgia, and auto-immune diseases. High metal toxicity also plays a large part in many of the psychological conditions such as depression and anxiety because metals, and in particular mercury, are highly attracted to, and have a very deleterious and persistent effect on the central nervous system. Toxic metals primarily cause damage by blocking receptor sites on cells and by poisoning enzymes and thus generally reduce the biochemical function of the individual and the ability to detoxify. Toxic metals can and do effect any bodily system, but are particularly damaging to the:

- **Endocrine system** – poisons the process of the thyroid, adrenal glands, pancreas and controlling glands in the brain.
- **Nervous system** – (affecting the nerves that govern 'automatic functions') that supply the organs and track up to the brain and central nervous system disrupting function of the organs supplied in the process.
- **Lymphatic system** – impairs the proper circulation of the lymph causing it to become sluggish and toxic.
- **Immune system** – Impairs the delicate and complex immune response giving rise to secondary viral, candida, bacterial or parasitic infections that are responsible for many of the sufferer's symptoms.

The point here is to just show you how toxins can accumulate within the body and explain to you how and why other factors can cause disease in the body. There is only so much that the body can take of toxic stress and of how our bodies can deal with this toxic over load before it breaks down. Because now, people are no longer getting sick from one or toxins, but rather a myriad of toxins that doctors often are unable to isolate a single cause of illness and believe that it is all in the patient's head.

Regaining Your Health From Toxic Over Load

In order to truly start down the road of regaining your health, it is important to be brutally honest with yourself and detoxify your body, mind and spirit. The foundation to a truly effective healing approach is to promote detoxification. This can also be done in a variety of ways, including improving your diet, appropriate exercise, and appropriate use of detoxifying nutritional supplements and herbs. It is also a key to address mental and emotional stressors through an appropriate avenue such as counseling, meditation, journaling, tai chi, yoga, and qi gong.

Detoxification & Cleansing

Typical diets today, in the Us, consistent of so many foods that contribute to an unhealthy state. Example, the the world in Diabetes, Cancer, Heart disease, Auto- disease and its enough to make you wonder why and this be so for a country that's considered to be a great wrongful US leads immune how can super

TOXIC HAZARD

power would make you believe that we have our things in order, especially with health. But that subject is for maybe another book!

But seriously speaking, detoxification all begins with diet, and a cleanse to jump start yourself into a sort of whole body spring cleaning, just like the earth renews itself after a long winter. A cleanse is basically a juice fast, although not actually a fast, which technically involves nothing more than water and requires close medical supervision. Think of this cleanse as a liquid fest, rather than a fast. Typically this cleanse will take three to 7 days and it will give you the results you want. Sometimes the length of the cleanse will vary from person to person, depending upon the persons current situation and how one tolerates the cleanse.

The cleanse helps to eliminate acid wastes and negative micro forms throughout your body, detoxifying your blood, tissues, and digestive system along with toxic metal build up. This will also get rid of pollutants that were built up in your body, especially your colon, from eating all those poorly combined processed foods, fried foods, starches, sugars, and over cooked foods. It is recommended to do a 2 to a 3 day cleanse (liquid) and up to 10 days if seriously ill (though you should seek supervision for an extended cleanse). Up to 7 days is good for everyone who can manage it.

While on this cleanse you should drink at least four liters of purified water, with pH drops (CIO2), a day (with lemon or lime juice if you like). Include if you like, as part of or in addition to those 4 liters, 6 to 8 ounce glasses of fresh green vegetable juice, to help clear the toxins out of your system and make your body more alkaline. Some examples to try juicing are - *cucumber, kale, broccoli, celery, lettuce, collards, okra, wheat grass, barley grass, watercress, parsley, cabbage, spinach, alfalfa sprouts or just about any other green vegetables.* You can also search online for many of the available recipes that include juice fasts and whole body cleanse to give you more of a broader spectrum of some fun and enjoying combinations.

It will also be easier in the beginning for some people to basically start out with something simple for the first few days like carrots and beets just to get used to drinking fresh vegetable juices, then eventually wean off the carrot and beets and gradually start up the amounts of greens. If you do decide to use the carrot and beets, use half of the beets at first a day to begin with, as it can add considerably to the bowl cleansing effect of the juice. Also make sure that you always dilute the juice with water, whether or not you are on a cleanse. Use ten times the amount of water (purified) as juice and add four drops of CIO2 per cup. This will increase the alkalinity of your juice from 6.2 to 9.5.

For those who can not make fresh juice, you can use the concentrated green powder mixed into water instead, use one quarter teaspoon per 8 ounces of water plus 4 drops of CIO2. You can also add or take one to two green capsule of powder with your fluids if you need the added convenience. Your meals should consistent of soups, mostly broth's of chicken or beef, or vegetable soup. Teas are also great to employ during your cleanse for the few days, and good ones to use are – Red clover, Chaparral, Pau D'Arco, and Essiac – a special blend (excellent choice) and Raspberry leaf. You can also add 3 tablespoons of essential oils (cold pressed flax seed oil), virgin olive oil, borage oil, primrose oil, or a blend like Udo's Oil that you can take by the spoonful.

It is also normal to feel hunger pangs during the cleanse, which is normally the result of those little pesky micro forms screaming to be fed, so resist any urge to break your cleanse and continue on cause the results will be well worth it. Those initial hunger pangs are the worst, and if the urge approaches you, just snack on some carrots or celery sticks to fill the void. Once you are over the hump of hunger pangs you will begin to notice a new renowned sense of energy. If hunger seems to be a problem, a supplement use of the mineral chromium, may help or try drinking in more water with a teaspoon of green powder per cup to help take the edge off. And besides the water will also help to wash away the impurities in your system. Supplements can also help you to maximize the effect of a good body cleanse that will quickly bring the body back into balance.

During the cleanse the two most crucial things are the pH drops (CIO2 or hydrogen peroxide) and the concentrated green powder. Add your CIO2 drops, 4 total per cup of water into all your pure water. Mix one-quarter teaspoon of the concentrated green powder into 8 ounces of pure water 3 times a day, or take one capsule 3 times a day with a meal" or drink. While on the cleanse diet, add a complete multi-mineral supplement, as minerals are particularly important because all other nutrients, including vitamins, proteins, enzymes, amino acids, and carbohydrates, require minerals for normal biochemical functioning.

It is also recommended during this fast to add a [*chlorophyll* supplement along with *noni fruit concentrate* for its anti-fungal and anti-parsitic properties and enzyme activation. Note that all of these general recommendations can have a laxative effect, green juice alone can do it too. But that is the way your body physically gets rid of the waste. If say by chance your body does not a laxative effect due to the cleanse, you might want to add a mild natural laxative formula to your program. Look for one including butternut root bark, cascara sagrada bark, rhubarb root, ginger root, licorice root, irish moss, and cayenne. Aloe vera is another cleansing aid that can help break up pockets of protein, especially in the small intestines. Add one teaspoon of cold pressed, whole-leaf juice to your green juice, or take it with a meal.

NOTE: It is also a good idea while on any cleansing formula to keep a journal and record your results and reactions.

"Key" Points in Detoxification

A great deal more can be achieved in detoxification is to restore the intestinal flora and reestablish intestinal peristalsis. The important various methods of cleansing include fasting (short or long term), juicing, detoxification diets(including high fiber, enzyme rich diets, exercise, and hydrotherapy. Colonic irrigation should also be used only in exceptional cases, and then under the supervision of a well trained physician.

These techniques can help rid your body of many toxins, heavy metals, pollutants, parasites, and chemicals that your body has accumulated throughout the years. Supplements should also be used regularly to rebuild your defense barriers, such as mucosa and skin. Anti oxidants should be included as well, including vitamins A, E, C, selenium, Zinc, and the enzyme (SOD); minerals; and other certain enzyme mixtures to provide support for circulation to (and function of) mucosa; to promote waste detoxification and disposal; and to help heal chronic infections; and accelerate the inflammatory process, thus expediting return to healthy tissue. The primary goal of detoxification is to:

- **Break up wastes and toxins in the body**
- **Eliminate wastes and toxins**
- **Improve excretion**
- **Invigorate the body's detoxification mechanism**
- **Provide relief when the immune system is depressed.**

To Watch Out For Basic Principles

<u>Motivations & Reasons to Fast</u> – **Detoxification, healing, break addictions, weight loss, glandular health.**

<u>Conditions Fasting Has Helped</u> – **Allergies, asthma, hay fever, hives, migraines, obesity, insomnia, high and low blood pressure, acne, rheumatism, ulcers, liver problems, kidney problems, gall stones, constipation, diarrhea, and diseases.**

<u>Criteria for Choosing the Length of the Fast</u> – **Fasting experience, physical strength & condition, nature of illness, previous diet and level of toxicity, age and mental attitude, schedule of work and activities, environment and weather**

<u>Detoxification Techniques</u> – **Massage, bath of Epsom salt and skin brushing, steam baths, colonics and enemas, psyllium seed or flax seed bulk laxative drinks, exercise.**

<u>Organs of Elimination</u> – **Lungs, liver, kidneys, skin, eyes, colon, tongue.**

Symptoms of a Healing Effect

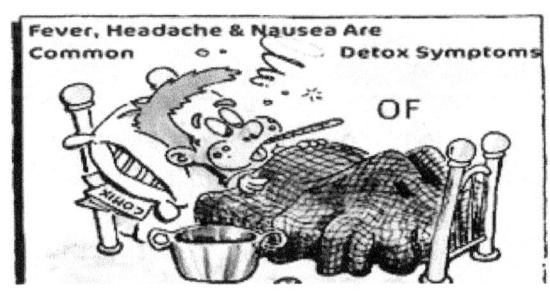

During a cleanse, toxins are dumped from where they've been stored in the tissues into the blood so they can be eliminated. That means you may feel before you feel better.

This is what is called the healing effect or healing crisis, which may affect some people and then again may not, different people tend to experience varying degrees of unpleasantness, or not at all. Some of these symptoms include:

Rash, eczema, acne, nausea, weakness, dizziness, hot flashes, fatigue, bronchitis, asthma, headaches, faintness, fever, diarrhea, muscle aches, bad breath, stuffed nose, running nose, irregular heartbeat, irregular menstruation, light headedness, flu like feelings.

If and when this happens, use lots of water with pH drops and fresh lemon or lime juice will help flush out the toxins and their negative effects out quickly. So, if you are having symptoms, just increase your daily water intake. A healing affect is actually a good sign and nothing to really worry about.

Making The Transition Back To A Full Diet

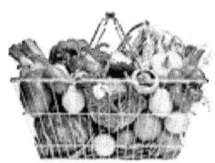

Now that you are cleansed and removed the stock pile of debris and toxins from your body, you have now cleared the way for optimal health. The next step is to provide your body with what it needs to stay healthy. If you give your body the vital materials it needs to construct and form new healthy cells, your body will then heal itself and restore balance and harmony to your new well being of life.

The proper diet is now going to be essential going back to solid foods and keeping clear of certain foods. Keep your diet on low carbohydrates and focus on dark green and yellow vegetables, seeds, nuts, grains and essential fatty acids and include also healthy oils, low sugar fruits (tomatoes, avocados, lemon, and limes), soybeans, tofu, lentils, and raw seeds and nuts. At least 40% of your diet should be raw. The higher the level of enzymes in your food the faster you will repair and rebuild your body, and cooking destroys your foods vital natural enzymes and life force. You may also still want to keep your green juice mix every now and then. You should focus on your diet being 80% alkaline also.

The combination of a cleansing when necessary and a good diet is designed to keep your body in balance over the long term. It will restore ph balance, stop over growth of negative micro forms, and heal the damage resulting from the toxins they emit. Please note, to truly achieve optimal health, you also need to break the pattern of negativity that feeds sickness in disease. The acid diet you are leaving behind is just one step in creating good health.

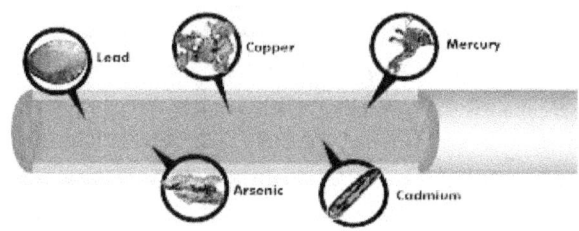

Today, with the environment being overly polluted with toxic chemicals from our ever growing society, ranging from the foods we eat on a daily basis to the chemical air we breathe from industrial factories that pollute the air, and may enter the body via industrial food processing, water we drink, contaminated air, absorption through the skin in agriculture, manufacturing, pharmaceutical, cosmetics, industrial, or in residential settings. So, in general we basically become in contact with heavy toxic metals from breathing polluted air, skin absorption from contact with cosmetics and personal hygiene items, foods we eat from grocery markets (boxed and can foods), house hold chemicals we buy, and those who live in old homes that have lead and copper piping.

And the question one may ask in this is "how toxic are we?" metal toxicity is quickly becoming a serious matter and a growing concern as more and more chemicals and toxins are used in products that increase the "convenience factor" of our daily lives. So, how do we know that one is not harboring toxins in their body? Because, especially in this day and age they basically are an unavoidable part of our modern lifestyle, and we can be sure that most of the American public have toxins, heavy metals in their body right now!

Eating fast foods in general is one quick way, as is choosing highly processed foods from the grocery store.

Boxed food items, cans, fruit juices, bottled water, cosmetics(make up) and personal hygiene (deodorants), and many other items, are **all laced with trace amounts of arsenic, mercury, cadmium, lead, the top 4** that appear on a **priority list called "The Top Hazardous Substances" from the Agency for Toxic Substances and Disease Registry (ATSDR)** in Atlanta, Georgia, in part of the U.S. Department of Health and Human Services that was established by congressional mandate to perform specific functions concerning adverse human health effects and diminished quality of life associated with exposure to hazardous substances.

There are 35 metals that concern us because of occupational or residential exposure; 23 of these are the heavy elements or "Heavy Metals": *antimony, arsenic, bismuth, cadmium, cerium, chromium, cobalt, copper, gallium, gold, lead, iron, manganese, mercury, nickel, platinum, silver, tellurium, tin, uranium, vanadium,, and zinc (Glanze 1996).* Small amounts of these elements are common in our environment and diet and are actually necessary for good health, but large amounts of any of them may cause acute or chronic toxicity (Poisoning).

Heavy metal toxicity can result in damaged or reduced mental and central nervous system function, lower energy levels, and damage to blood composition, lungs, kidneys, liver, and other vital organs. It is the long term exposure of heavy metal toxicity that may result in a slow progression of physical, muscular, and neurological degenerative process that can mimic Alzheimers disease, Parkinson's disease, muscular dystrophy, and multiple sclerosis. Allergies are also not uncommon, and repeated long term contact with some metals or their compounds have known to cause cancer *(CIS 1999)*.

Possible Symptoms of Heavy Metal Toxicity

The association of symptoms indicative of acute toxicity is not difficult to recognize because they are usually severe, rapid in onset, and associated with a known exposure or ingestion *(Ferner 2001)*. Usually, most people can excrete toxic metals from their body successfully. However, some people – especially those who may suffer from chronic conditions cannot excrete them efficiently enough and a build up occurs. Interestingly, recent research revealed that those who can not excrete heavy metals efficiently appear to be genetically predisposed to this condition.

Over exposure to heavy metals and toxicity can lead to a number of diseases and repercussions at various stages. Some of the symptoms associated with toxicity are problems leading to permanent damage of the nervous system, cardiovascular system, blood production, gastrointestinal system, reproductive system and kidney functioning. Some of the associated prominent symptoms of toxicity are:

- **Muscle and joint pain**
- **Mental confusion**
- **Headaches**
- **Gastrointestinal upsets**
- **Food allergies**
- **Vision problems**
- **Chronic fatigue**
- **Short-term memory loss**
- **Aggression**
- **Irritability**
- **Depression**
- **Speech difficulties**
- **Hypertension**

Cramping
Difficulty breathing
Sweating
 Nausea
Nervousness & emotional instability
Feeling ill

<u>Note</u>**: Symptoms of chronic exposure are very similar to other health conditions and often develop slowly over months or even years. Sometimes symptoms of a chronic exposure subside; thinking that the symptoms are related to something else.**

Chronic exposure may also result from contaminated food, air, water or dust; living near a hazardous waste site; spending time in areas with deteriorating lead paint; maternal transfer in the womb; or from participating hobbies that use lead paint or solder. Chronic exposure may also occur either at home or the work place. And other exposure area's are:

- **Mercury fillings in teeth (amalgams/silver)**
- **Living in a home built prior to 1978 that has lead-based paint**
- **Cigarette smoking and/or inhaling second hand smoke**
- **Living near a land fill**
- **Contaminated water**
- **Consuming fish contaminated with mercury**
- **Mercury contamination from badly fitted dental fillings or silver amalgams**
- **Receiving vaccinations that contain thimerosal (mercury preservative)**
- **Working in an environment where exposure is prevalent, such as a dentist's office where amalgam is used to fill cavities.**
- **. Routes of exposure include inhalation, skin, or eye contact, and ingestion.**

(ATSDR MMGs and ToxFAQs; Anon 1993;Who 1998; CIS 1999; Roberts 1999; Dupler 2001;Ferner 2001)

Natural Chelating Agents For Heavy Metal Toxicity

Without getting into the whole conventional(medical) aspect of heavy metal detoxification, we are going to approach this in a way of detoxifying the body of heavy metal accumulation, and besides its the least cost effective way of removal that has been used by many countries as well. The Liver and Kidneys as well as the Gallbladder and Lymphatic system are the major filters of the blood system, removing toxic wastes and debris.

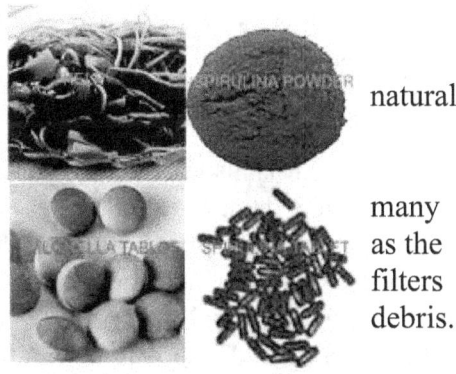

The kidneys especially aid in ridding the body of excess "acids" while rebalancing critical pH levels. The Liver being the supreme organ of metabolism, once burdened with toxic substances can effect many of the body's biological functions, and symptoms of a sluggish liver will show the following signs which include:

- **Heavily coated tongue and bad breathe**
- **Circle under the eyes**
- **Bloated feeling, poor digestion or nausea in the sight of raw meat and after eating fatty foods.**
- **Constipation and flatulence.**
- **Bad breathe.**
- **Weight gain around the abdominal area.**
- **Foggy brain symptoms like short-term memory loss, depression.**
- **Unpleasant mood changes.**
- **Un-explained fatigue.**
- **Skin conditions, and if in a toxic over-load condition, discoloration of the**

skin.
- **Poor liver function that's heavily burdened by the accumulation of toxins can trigger or exacerbate allergic conditions.**
- **Can also impair cholesterol levels.**
- **Can cause unstable blood sugar levels.**

The proper approach first would be to do a short cleanse (see cleansing procedure listed earlier)
get back to a clean recommended diet by omitting all junk foods, processed and refined foods, all sugar by-products, diet should be based on a more alkaline diet (see section on pH) and take on a specific formula (chelating agents) consisting of a blood cleanse to purify and chelate (detox) the heavy metals from organs and blood stream. After you have completed your short cleanse detox, it would benefit your health in an additional, simple detoxifying procedure that can greatly enhance your health and free your liver and the other glands of your body.

Your liver is the largest organ contained within the body weighing nearly 3lbs. Without you could not survive one day. This complex hard working organ performs over 500 biological functions producing over 1,000 essential enzymes and manufactures the cholesterol essential for building healthy cells and hormones. In addition to that, your liver filters more than one quart of blood per minute and produces bile to emulsify fatty foods so they can be absorbed into the bloodstream.

Amazingly, it is also the only organ within the body that can regenerate itself up to 75% if it gets damaged or diseased. And interestingly enough, in typical Chinese medicine the liver and gallbladder are seen as the holding cell for anger and are considered your seat of emotions concerning bitterness, frustration, and happiness. So, it is obvious now on how important it is to keep your liver clean and unburdened from toxic build up and free your emotional hang-ups and a liver cleanse every now and then.

There are many liver and gallbladder flushes that can be found in books and through the internet. Which most of them include variations of utilizing extra virgin olive oil with lemon or grapefruit juice. And usually mixed in various proportions and consumed either all at once or over several evenings in smaller proportions. This particular flush that I have found to be a simple two day flush that comes most highly recommended and effective consists of the following as described below:

Directions for A Two Day Liver Gallbladder Flush

Day 1 : On the night before you start say on a Friday night, take an herbal laxative. The next day (Saturday) drink one gallon or more of pure apple cider juice or freshly squeezed apple juice (juice machine). **Please do not use store bought regular apple juice!**

Consume nothing else, and try not to cheat with anything that has fat or oil in it(important). Then you take another herbal laxative that following evening of day 1.

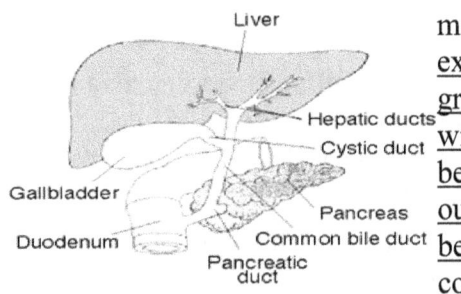

Day2 : upon waking up that following morning, first thing to do is mix eight ounces of extra virgin olive oil with two lemons or half a grapefruit. The lemon or grapefruit is used to mix with the olive oil to make it more palatable. And begin by drinking only between two to three ounces at a time, waiting about 5 to 10 minutes between doses and repeat this until you have consumed all of the mixture. This should take you 20 to 30 minutes or so. After wards, set some time to go and rest and lie down, and try and not to consume any food or beverages for several hours (important). Wait before you have had your first elimination (bowl movement) before eating or drinking anything, and this includes water too! After wards you may begin eating and resume your normal dietary regimen.

This program has worked for so many people with success, and this information is one of the more effective ones that you will find used by many health care practitioners. As mentioned earlier there are many other formulas that you can use for a liver gallbladder flush and you will find that there are many to choose from and many conflicting ideas of how and why it works.

Other natural therapies for liver health, protection, and detoxifying are the amino acid Taurine, which plays a major role in good liver function via the formation of bile acids and detoxification. Abnormally low levels of Taurine have been found in those with chemical sensitivities and allergies. Taurine is the major amino acid required by the liver for removal of toxic chemicals and metabolites from the body. Taurine is also a key componenet in bile acids produced in the liver. As bile synthesis utilizes cholesterol, and disordered bile synthesis may result in elevated cholesterol levels.

Recent findings also suggest that Taurine is one of the major nutrients involved in the body's detoxification process of harmful substances and should be considered in the treatment of all chemical sensitive patients (Fibromyalgia and chronic fatigue). Taurine is also found in high amounts in animal protein, organ meats, invertebrate seafood. Factors that may increase the body's requirements are high stress (CFS and FMS), vegetarianism, fad diets, cortisone therapy, alcohol, and high intake of MSG. The recommended dosage for Taurine is 200 to 500mgs a day.

Kidney function and detoxification can be had with a simple kidney flush by consuming 2 to 3 cups of herbal teas, specifically *"Dandelion root"* known by herbalist as ***Taraxacum officinale.*** One the best herb's used for centuries for liver and biliary complaints. Dandelion root has always been a popular herb as a liver tonic since the 16th century, used by Germans as a blood purifying tonic and liver congestion. Its therapeutic properties are due to in part to its bitter constituents, namely taraxacin and inulin. Other substances in dandelion are fatty acids, vitamins, minerals, especially high in potassium), and flavonoids.

Dandelion 's dual acting action makes it an excellent detoxifying agent for remedies of gout, rheumatism, skin complaints, digestive aid, liver problems (hepatitis), and as a kidney flush. Dandelion leaves can also be consumed and made in a salad for a health treat to the liver and can be made into a tea where it works most easily. One cup a day would do wonders for the health of your liver, digestion and your kidneys.

Natural Heavy Metal Chelating Agents

Now on to some of the best natural blood purifiers and natural chelating agents which include *Cilantro, Chlorella, Spirulina, and Chlorophyl (the green healer)*. Chlorophyll is a chemical formed by the chloroplast cells of green plants. Considered the beginning of the food chain – the plasma of green plants. Without chlorophyll all animal life on earth would become extinct. Chlorophyll is basically the life blood of all plants, structurally similar to hemin, the 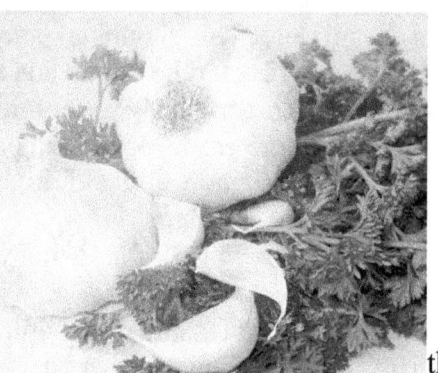 protein portion of hemoglobin that carries oxygen. The only difference is that chlorophyl is bound by an atom of magnesium, while hemin is bound by iron.

Chlorophyll has also been famous for its ability to heal infected and ulcerated wounds. It has been used substantially as an important medicine for heavy metal detoxification, bleeding gums, canker sores, trench mouth, pyorrhea, gingivitis, detoxifying agent of all sorts, and it makes for a great mouth wash to kill bad breathe. Chlorophyl has this unique ability to kill anaerobic bacteria(odor producing) and is the reason it covers up the smell of garlic so easily and fights bad breath, body odor, and acts as a general antiseptic. But our interest lies in its ability to detox heavy metals from our body.

Found in all green plants and algae, especially found in large quantities in Chlorella. In fact its because of its high level of chlorophyll that Chlorella got its name. Chlorella is very good at binding to heavy metals and helping to remove them from your body as well as purifying the blood stream of toxins.

With the ever increasing dangers of unwanted chemicals our body pick ups through the foods we eat, the air we breathe, and the water we drink, it wise to develop a plan of attack to protect ourselves from the many acceptable poisons our government allows through the use of pesticides, hazardous materials in manufacturing and processing of foods tainted with chemical sprays. This damage is just too widespread and pervasive. You have to take it upon yourself to take a subjective measure to protect your family and yourself from harm. And that is to include plant algaes like *Chlorella, Spirulina, Kelp (iodine)*, and several others that we will get to in a moment.

Protecting Yourself From Systemic Pollution – Heavy Metals & Toxins

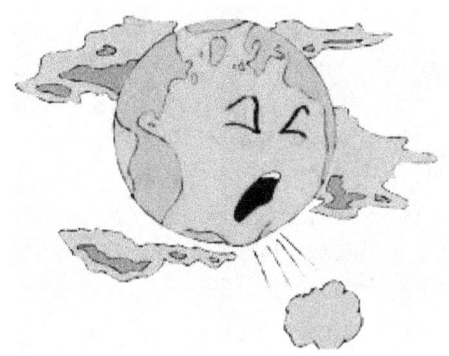

In this 21ˢᵗ century, we're seeing an explosion of growth accumulated toxins, parasites, chemicals, and heavy metals that create diseases like cancer, auto-immune dysfunction, brain disorders like Autism, Alzheimer's and Parkinson's, Chronic Fatigue syndrome, Fibromyalgia, and many more. Many years ago this was not the case, as top soil was fertile and heavily dense with nutrients, our foods were basically all organic and were relatively cheap to buy, and as of now organic foods cost double or even triple the price. Farm lands are not as fertile as they once were with the ever decreasing amount of top soil eroding away due to super storms that appeared once every hundred years or so.

What does this all mean? It means we live in a toxic polluted world! Food supply devoid of nutritional abundance (not years ago when it was rich with nutrients), farm lands not nearly as productive or in numbers, which means our food supply is diminishing in quantity and quality, chemical factories create waste lands with toxic fill that cause cancer and disease, I can go on and on, but the point here is disease is growing and spreading due to pathogens, chemicals and poisons.

We all have to protect ourselves and families by being better aware and watching what we eat, buying organic food as possible, washing our vegetables completely with water and a teaspoon of hydrogen peroxide in a water bath to rid it of pesticides and airborne pollutants. And most importantly adding certain protection like chlorophyll based products that include - *Chlorella, Spirulina, Cilantro, Kelp, and other chelating agents and detoxifiers like: Glutathionine, Cysteine, Magnesium Malate or Malic Acid, NAC(N-acetylcysteine), EDTA, Garlic; and formula's consisting of Milk thistle, ALA's, Vit-C, Selenium, and foods that contain natural chelating agents and exercise.*

We will go through each and everyone describing its effectiveness and application. This list includes many of the most commonly used chelating agents by holistic health care practitioners and some popular formula's that you can use and go back and see which is the most productive one for you.

List Of Natural Chelating Agents For Detoxification
Metals, Toxins, Yeast: Candida

__Chlorella__ – High in natural chlorophyll and one of the most exciting nutritional resources available today to help your body naturally fight off environmental pollution.

Chlorella is also one of the most widely used substances used in Japan, where over 10 million people use it daily, as we Americans use vitamin C as our most popular supplement. Highly prized in Japan for its natural detoxification abilities. Considered a "green food" because of its complete nutritional profile and natural chelating agent. A key component derived from the nuclei of the algae and unique to chlorella is **"Chlorella Growth Factor (CGF)". CGF is named for it's growth stimulating properties. Chlorella Growth Factor is a nucleotide-peptide complex found only in chlorella, which include**; nucleic acids, amino acids, peptides, polysaccharides, and beta glucans.

Chlorella is highly valued for its natural detoxification abilities. Its molecular structure allows it to bond to metals, chemicals, and pesticides found in your digestive tract, your body's pathway to your blood stream where these harmful toxins are delivered and deposited into your cells. Once in your blood stream, chlorella is like unleashing a tiny army inside your body to fight the battle of removing toxins from your tissues and ushering them back outside of your body. There are case reports of patients with dramatic tumor remissions after taking CGF in higher amounts. Chlorella Growth factor will make the detox experience for heavy metal detoxification, much easier, shorter and more effective.

Chlorella is also one of the most widely studied food supplements in the world. A subject of medical research in the USA, USSR, Germany, Japan, France, England, and Israel. Even NASA has studied and considered using it as one of the first whole foods in space on the international space station. Because of its 50% protein and a complete amino acid based food. *Loaded in vitamins, minerals, complete amino acids, RNA and DNA, and enzymes*. Chlorella's benefits include:

- **Aids you in processing more oxygen by purifying your blood stream and cleaning away toxins.**
- **Cleanses key elimination systems like your bowl, liver, and bloodstream. Aids you in promoting optimal blood pressure**
- **Supports the elimination of molds in your body and helps neutralize the bad air you might breathe in**
- **Promotes growth and repair of your tissues**
- **Boosts your immune system**
- **Provides B vitamins**
- **Increases natural energy**
- **Balances your body's pH levels**
- **Normalizes your blood and blood pressure**
- **Reduces your risk of cancer**
- **Freshens your breath**
- **Binds to toxic metals, toxins**

Chlorella can be bought in tablets, powder, and liquid (more expensive and potent) and good sources to buy are from "Sun Chlorella" brand. Can be found online or at any health food store.

A good mobilizing and therapeutic effect is to take 3,000mgs daily taken in 1,000mgs 3 times a day.

Spirulina – Is a micro-algae that is packed with nutrients and many health benefits. Spirulina is another complete food supplement just like chlorella except it lacks the chlorella growth factor. Used in many countries, including in the USA, for its nutritional benefits and its natural cleansing abilities to remove toxins from the blood stream. Those who have enjoyed its energy and vitality effects can testify its wonderful healing qualities. Also sold as a major ingredient in many health drinks and foods, and is considered one of the most popular whole food supplements sold today.

Spirulina is also high in protein, several vitamins and minerals, and in chlorophyll. It includes many B vitamins, such as vitamin B12 that is usually missing from a vegetarian and vegan diets. Vitamin B12 is mainly available from whole foods that are derived from animal sources, such as meat and dairy products, but this micro-algae is a great alternative source of B12 for anyone who does not want to eat meat or dairy products. It is also rich in calcium, potassium and many other minerals. You can also use super food to make sure you are getting enough nutrients from your daily diet.

Spirulina's main health benefit includes its ability to boost energy levels and reduce tiredness by cleansing the blood, stimulate the digestive system and to give a boost to the immune system. Today, many people take it to cleanse their blood of toxins and to make sure their digestive system and elimination works well to get rid of toxins. Some people also take large amounts of spirullina during a detox program and then continue on with smaller daily maintenance doses after finishing the detox. Spirulina can also be used to clean heavy metal toxins from the body. It is often used for this purpose together with chlorella. Spirulina together with chlorella can release these toxins from the body's cells into the blood stream and then purge them out of the body with the normal elimination process. The main detoxifying substance in spirulina is chlorophyll, a powerful blood cleanser.

Spirulina also contains probiotic bacteria that can help help to keep the digestive system healthy, to protect it from a variety of problems, and to make sure the digestive system works properly. Probiotics help to boost the amount of so called healthy bacteria in the digestive system which is needed to keep the digestion balanced. This can also help those who suffer from constipation. Spirulina is available in powder form, tablets, capsules and is added to many natural health drinks and wholefood supplements. The powder is a dark green in color and is easy to digest and is absorbed into the body fast, giving you the instant energy you need. It can be made into a smoothy or juice and can be taken any time instead of that cup of coffee or tea. Spirulina can be taken daily and is very safe to take in large amounts to relieve specific symptoms or for detoxifying, and smaller daily amounts can be used as a nutritional supplement.

A good way to introduce it in your diet is to start out with smaller doses and slowly increase building it up over a few weeks, so as your body gets used to this new wholefood.

Cilantro - A common spice/herb has been found to chelate (remove) heavy metals like mercury, aluminum, and lead from the body. And in fact, it is believed to cross the blood brain barrier and actually remove said metals from the brain. The contention that cilantro is a powerful chelation agent is based on the research from Dr. Yoshiaki Omura, President and Founder of the International College of Acupuncture & Electro-Therapeutics and Director of Medical Research of the Heart Disease research Foundation.

In 1995, Omura observed that subjects had higher than normal levels of mercury in their urine after consuming Vietnamese soup, which has large amounts of cilantro (also called Chinese parsley). He followed up on this accidental finding and discovered that giving cilantro to patients with mercury poisoning for several weeks successfully eliminated the toxin from the body - *[Acupuncture Electro res. 1996 Apr-jun, 21(2):133-60, Omura Y, Shimotsuura Y, Fukuoka A, Fkuoka H, Nomoto T]*

Cilantro: Chelation therapy has been used by conventional medicine to pull lead from people suffering from lead poisoning. Dr. David Williams published in his news letter Alternative *(For the Health Conscious Individual) (Vol. 7, No. 12)* June, 1998 the most interesting piece of information to come down the pike in years – reads, **Cilantro: A common spice/herb** *that can Save Your Life "Let your food be your medicine, and your medicine be your food". "Hippocrates"*

This remarkable discovery which can greatly increase our ability to clear up recurring infections, both viral and bacteria is an inexpensive, easy way to remove (chelate) toxic metals from the nervous system and body tissues. Amazingly enough, how this simple common household spice/herb can remove toxic metals from the body and brain empowers us with a safe and simple alternative.

Cilantro is also an excellent blood cleanser, tonic, and builder, working through increasing the ability of the liver and related organs to strain and purify the blood and lymphatic system. Cilantro achieves it's tonic properties through the astringent purification of the blood supply to the glands and acts as a cleansing herb for the lymphatic system.

This common Mexican and Middle eastern spice must be used fresh with stems and all tossed into a salad is a perfect way to use cilantro, or added it to your favorite salsa dish to really perk it up. You can also use it in a pesto sauce that will also do the trick. **Here is the basic recipe for Cilantro pesto:**

- **1 clove garlic**
- **½ cup almonds, cashews, or other nuts**
- **1 cup packed fresh cilantro leaves (and smaller stems)**
- **2 tablespoons lemon juice**
- **6 table spoons olive oil extra virgin**
- **Celtic Sea Salt to taste (see <u>www.healthfree.com</u> to order salt)**

Blend the cilantro and olive oil in a blender, add other ingredients to make a nice smooth paste, then go ahead and add some nuts and/or seeds: pistachio, cashews, almonds, pumpkin seeds, sun flour seeds. Adding cayenne pepper to anything has a very synergistic effect making all the other ingredients work better.

Note: The recommended "dose" of Cilantro for its detoxifying effect, is ½ a cup a day of chopped fresh cilantro leaves and stems per day for 3 weeks. Or you can easily eat ½ a cup a day by simply adding the fresh leaves to your daily salad.

Recent studies have also shown an unquestionable link between ethyl mercury and Autism, and cilantro with chlorella and garlic has shown considerable improvements in children with autism. **Chlorella: Super Food and Detox Combo makes for a super duo in the removal of toxic metals and common impurities.** Chlorella's detox abilities are already known and have been tested by several great nations in it's effective abilities as far as detoxification and nutritional value. Chlorella and cilantro when used in combination can make a dent in your level of Aluminum, a notoriously difficult metal to remove from the body. Once cilantro binds to the aluminum, the chlorella will then hasten its excretion through your kidneys. Chlorella will also support your liver's detoxification enzymes while supplying plenty of glutathione: a key detox player.

<u>Garlic</u> – I consider this a super food that not only does it add flavor and spice to meals, but it also benefits the body in many healthy ways. Garlic is a natural anti-biotic (natural penicillin) that also acts as a potent anti-fungal, anti-microbial, making it an effective agent against candida albicans and parasites. Garlic also contains an important mineral that protects one against mercury toxicity. It's bio-active Selenium. Garlic selenium is the best form of selenium available. Raw garlic of course would be best in its natural form. But if you don't like raw, the next best thing would be aged garlic extract such as **"Kyolic brand"**. Garlic contains sulphur which oxidizes **mercury, cadmium, and lead** and makes them water soluble. The sulphur found in garlic is the main reason it is able to oxidize heavy metals, and then it might also be helpful to supplement with MSM as it is a form of sulphur.

Garlic has been shown to protect the white and red blood cells from oxidative damage, caused by metals in the blood stream – on their way out – and also has its own valid detoxification functions, including the most valuable sulph-hydryl groups which oxidize mercury, cadmium and lead and makes the metals water soluble. Metal toxic patients almost always suffer from secondary infections, which are often responsible for part of the symptoms.

<u>Selenium</u> - Is now recognized as an important trace mineral. Selenium plays important roles in detoxification and as an anti-oxidant defense mechanism in the body. The most active forms of selenium are sodium selenite, selenomethioine, and high selenium yeast. Excess amounts can be toxic if it were ingested on a regular basis. <u>Selenium helps detoxify heavy metals such as mercury and cadmium.</u>

It also plays a very important part in thyroid function along with iodine and if deficient can affect its production of thyroid hormones. And an interesting aspect of selenium is – it has been found to to specifically counter act the ocular or eye dysfunction of

Grave's disease, called Grave's orbitopathy, characterized by exothalamus (protrusion of the eye ball), and protosis (movement outward of the eye). This is in response to swelling and inflammation of the muscles and structures behind and around the eyeball.

Selenium is also required for the functioning of and development of certain areas of the brain that open up a person to higher emotions and higher thought. Supplementation with selenium is always included in nutritional balancing programs and everyone needs a supplement for it's immune enhancing effect, cancer preventing, thyroid protection and it's heavy metal binding capabilities.

Its involvement in heavy metal detoxification has to do with glutahione production, mainly, although thyroid activity and other functions related to selenium are required for all meta detoxification. It has also been used to reverse cancer in a non-toxic manner by reducing toxic metals and other problems that can lead to cancer. Brazilian nuts are a prime source of selenium: just 3 to 4 Brazilian nuts will supply your body with 200mcgs enough for your days need. Other foods rich in selenium are wheat germ, fresh seafood like tuna, sardines, cod, red snapper, and herring. Beef and poultry and grains. The safe upper limit of selenium is 400mcgs a day in adults.

Selenium is a wonderful aid for general health and is one of the reasons garlic has an ancient and important place among the food kingdom and herbal medicine's history.

N-acetylcysteine (N-A-C) – Is produced in living organisms from the amino acid cysteine. NAC is a natural sulfur containing amino acid derivative found naturally in foods and is a powerful anti-oxidant. Being a powerful anti-oxidant and cell detoxification co-factor, NAC works to eliminate your body of free radicals and heavy metals, which improves your cellular health tremendously. NAC is currently the supplement of choice for building up cysteine or conserving the body's store of Glutathione, Cysteine and other sulfur anti-oxidant resources. This is very crucial for the body's life functions, as NAC helps the body neutralize toxins, heavy metals, such as mercury from dental amalgam fillings, cadmium and lead from paint and cigarette smoke.

NAC is a chelator of heavy metals, binding to toxic metals such as mercury and lead, and remove them from the body. One of the most effective oral chelating agents that if taking regularly over a period of time, will remove many toxic heavy metals from the body. Another interesting aspect of NAC is its ability to be an antidote to acetaminophen (Tylenol) poisoning, and even arsenic poisoning. As a precursor to glutathione, NAC can help strengthen the immune system and has been shown to be a protective agent in many diseases and conditions in which free radicals play a role in. This includes cancer, AIDS, cirrhosis, as well as pollution damage from smoking or other chemicals.

Cancer research has also shown that NAC can dramatically reduce the ability of a tumor to invade surrounding tissue, and decrease the number of metastases by 80% when cancer cells were pretreated with NAC.

A great supplement to include in any nutritional arsenal against health and disease.

NAC is also the standard medical treatment for acetaminophen (tylenol)over dose. And it is prudent to take NAC whenever one uses acetaminophen. Besides its excellent heavy metal detoxification capabilities, NAC is an excellent mucolytic agent, keeping the membranes of the respiratory system moist, thereby lessening the irritation of dry air, dust, and pollutants. **Note:** it is also recommended that when taking NAC to also take plenty of vitamin C. Take 2 to 3 times the amount of vitamin C when taking NAC to prevent the NAC from being oxidized and insoluble, as this form may cause kidney stones.

NAC is one of the good pillars of a good mercury detoxification program, the others being Chlorella, Garlic, MSM, and the herb Cilantro.

Glutathione – Is a very important amino acid that is composed of three amino acids: Glycine, Glutamine, and Cysteine. Glutathione is made by all the cells in the body, and is considered the body's master anti-oxidant and detoxifying agent. In one review, almost 80% of people with chronic ailments were found to be deficient in glutathione. In fact, low levels of glutathione are involved in all disease states. Why? - because the heavier the cumulative toxic burden on the body, the greater this depletes supplies of glutathione. For example, one molecule of mercury will use up one molecule of glutathione.

Glutathione is a major player in detoxifying the body of many toxic pollutants, including toxic metals and chemicals. Glutathione deficiency impairs the body's ability to get rid of toxins whether they are environmental or the by-product of cellular metabolism. If we do have low levels of glutathione we slowly become toxic, storing away poisons in our tissues, organs, muscles, and brain.

WE SIMPLY CANNOT DETOXIFY EFFECTIVELY IF OUR GLUTATHIONE LEVELS ARE TOO LOW, NO MATTER WHAT FORM OF DETOXIFICATION WE UNDERTAKE.

Important: Make sure your supplement of Glutathione is in an absorbable form, as most oral glutathione supplements are extremely difficult to absorb, because the digestive tract destorys the nutrient before it can be absorbed. Other supplements known as Glutathione boosters are - NAC, Alpha Lipoic Acid, Cysteine, Methionine, Selenium, MSM, Melatonin, Glutamine, SAM-e, Astragalus, Garlic, Milk Thistle & Asparagus (herb), Milk Thistle, and two great food sources are 100% Whey protein and Colostrum.

NOTE: The importance of Glutathione (GSH) can not be over stated, being virtually found in every cell of the body, protecting cells from free radicals and oxidative damage. Without this master immune system stimulator, the cells in the body would not be protected from oxidative injury. They would be damaged and killed, setting off an inflammation response.

Your personal level of glutathione directly affects your body's ability to reduce and control chronic inflammation as seen in those with chronic inflammatory conditions like Fibromyalgia, IBS, Rheumatoid Arthritis, and Lyme disease.

Magnesium Malate or Malic Acid – Is a compound of magnesium and malic acid. Malic acid is a natural fruit acid that is present in most cells in the body and is an important component of numerous enzymes key to ATP synthesis and energy production. Preliminary studies suggest that magnesium malate supports the body's own detoxification of aluminum in the brain. As one of the most potent aluminum detoxifiers, it helps reduce the levels of aluminum toxicity of the brain and for that reason could be used to help Alzheimer's disease.

Malic acid has also shown to release fecal and urinary excretion of aluminum. And it can also reduce the amount of aluminum found in the organs. Some research supports magnesium malate for boosting energy and alleviating pain and tenderness in those with Fibromyalgia. Dosage for therapeutic effects are 200mgs of magnesium twice a day, and 600mgs of malic acid three times a day. Dosages with magnesium and malic acid may vary with some people, some may need less and some may need more. It may also take some experimentation to find your optimal dose.(more on this on Natural Therapies for FMS and CFS section).

Milk Thistle – **(Silymarin)** Milk thistle is considered the treatment of choice for liver disease, particularly chronic infection with hepatitis C. It also provides support and protection against liver toxins which can cause free-radical-mediated oxidative damage. Silymarin, milk thistle's active component is as many times more potent than vitamin E in anti-oxidant activity. In addition, it increases liver production of Glutathione and protects red blood cell membranes against lipid peroxidation and hemolysis. Milk thistle helps your liver detoxify and promote the growth of new liver cells, eliminate heavy metals and toxins, plus protecting the liver from inflammation.

Milk thistle is one of the best herbs for liver health and diseases of the liver. Its main ingredient (Silymarin) is the main compound of milk thistle that is both an anti-inflammatory and anti-oxidant. And some of its noted healing effect claims are – provides heart benefits by lowering cholesterol levels, helps diabetes in people who have type-2 diabetes and cirrhosis, helps reduce growth of cancer cells in breast, cervical, and prostate cancers in men. Some other studies have revealed alcohol damage from chronic alcoholics, benefits people whose liver was damaged by industrial toxins, such as toluene and xylene.

Epsom Salt (Magnesium Sulphate)– Taken in a warm to hot bath, Epsom salt can be a great benefit in helping yourself remove heavy metals from your body. It can reduce inflammation to relieve pain and muscle cramps, exfoliates dead skin, improves nerve function through electrolyte regulation, improves heart and circulatory health, helps the body make more efficient use of insulin by reducing the incidence and severity of diabetes.

Plus it can help relieve constipation, improves oxygen, improves the absorption of nutrients, prevents and eases migraine headaches, can be a replacement therapy for a magnesium deficiency/help aid in it, relieves symptoms of Fibromyalgia and Osteoporosis, is used to treat pre-clampsyia, and Epsom salts may be given as a first aid for barium poisoning, eases stress, calms and relaxes, and can be used to flush out the liver and the gallbladder.

An Epsom salt bath can be one of the easiest and very therapeutic in relieving tensed muscles, nervousness by promoting a calm and relaxed feeling, especially for those people who suffer from Fibromyalgia, and chronic Arthritis. Epsom salt baths are simple and very economical, a great cost effective therapy to do two to three times a week. Half a cup of Epsom salt in a hot bath for 20 to 30 minutes utilizing a soft massage type of brush stroking the body lightly as you bath will help you to release the toxins from your body.

Alpha Lipoic Acid (ALA) - Is a fatty acid that naturally occurs in cells, and converts glucose into energy. Our body's natural supply of Alpha Lipoic Acid is replenished by the consumption of green vegetables, and could also be purchased in supplement form as well. New research is creating a great deal of interest showing that alpha lipoic acid can help protect DNA, optimize other anti-oxidants, and even help protect us from mercury and other heavy metals.

Alpha Lipoic Acid is a super nutrient that works in synergy with other anti-oxidants. Research shows that the free alpha lipoic acid in our bodies can even regenerate Vitamins CoQ-10, vitamin C and E, three other essential anti oxidants. ALA also regenerates the potent anti oxidant glutathione which is also found in cells. Further more, because alpha lipoic acid can absorb high energy states, it can also act as a chelator which can bind (or chelate) heavy metal molecules like mercury, lead, and arsenic, so that they can be removed from the body.

Because of its activity as an anti oxidant and heavy metal chelator, alpha lipoic acid is being studied in many areas. Some of the benefits that this powerful nutrient can do is improve insulin sensitivity, improve blood vessel dilation and blood flow in small blood vessels, prevents the formation of blood vessel plaques (heart disease), has a protective effect against nerve damage, improves peripheral neuropathy (diabetes), lowers blood pressure, and promotes rejuvenation via its powerful anti oxidant function by slowing down aging, DNA damage, making it a perfect anti aging therapy for the skin, benefits children with Autism, multiple sclerosis, dementia, age related cognitive disorders, and as a chemotherapy adjunct in the treatment of cancer.

Foods high in alpha lipoic acid are *broccoli, spinach and other dark green vegetables*. Alpha lipoic acid has shown that it to be absorbed quickly into the blood stream, where it "traps" heavy metals, and prevents them from settling in the soft tissue, where they can cause cellular damage. A potent combination for heavy metal evacuation from the body is by using alpha lipoic acid with chlorella and cilantro. *Note: (R-Lipoc Acid is a much better absorbed form of Alpha Lipoic Acid).*

Natural Juice Protocol For Heavy Metal Detoxification - Juicing is an excellent way to rid the body of heavy metals and other toxins. Juicing will supply your body with live natural enzymes, vitamins and minerals and chlorophyll. A home procedure that can be done for 2 to 3 days out of the week can help you to speed up the process of elimination depending on the severity of your symptoms. Juicing can also make you feel instantly energized as live nutrients enter your blood stream.

Juicing can help you normalize thyroid hormones so it is easier to lose weight or recover from any illnesses. Foods like *apples and lemons* can help your body release and excrete heavy metals from our tissues. Their pectin is a natural chelating (binding) agent for *aluminum, lead, mercury, cadmium, nickel, and many other toxins as well.* *Apples* combine very well with *coriander* and other heavy metal detoxifiers such as *Chlorella supplements. Garlic* protects the red and white blood cells while toxins are being released out of the body. At bedtime calcium and magnesium complete the binding process of excretion.

Here is a simple juice recipe that you can do for 2-3 days out of the week. First thing in the morning would be an ideal time to begin: 1 cup fresh coriander leaves, 1 cup of water, 1-2 chopped apples including skin, 1 cup of parsley or celery or wheat grass or a combination thereof, 2 lemon slices with skin. Process the ingredients in an electric blender on high for a bout a minute or two. Strain the mixture through a cloth bag or use a few layers of stocking, stretched over the jug. Squeeze out all of the juice, drink half of it straight away, then eat 1 or 2 apples and take 6-10 chlorella tablets to absorb metal particles as they are loosened and to keep them moving along to the kidneys.

An hour or two later drink the remaining juice with more apples, take 6 – 10 more chlorella tablets, if you get hungry have a snack of cottage cheese mixed with flax seed oil or ground up flax seeds. Eat a lot of garlic will all your food for a few days to protect the blood from suspended heavy metal particles. Eat parsley after wards to protect your friends from your breath!

Later on have a normal lunch and supper, and at bedtime take 1-2 teaspoons of Calcium and Magnesium powder mixed with a little water to help prevent the newly released lead, mercury, nickel, etc., from re-contaminating your brain, soft tissues and skeletal system. Alkaline minerals, especially calcium bind metals and other toxic particles and are then deposited into the toilet instead of back into you. Keep a glass of water next to your night stand by your bed and drink it during the night if you wake up.

Parsley - Is the king when it comes to purging both the liver and urinary system. Rich in chlorophyll natures natural blood cleanser, that also contains good amounts of folate and potassium to help you to quickly alkalize and excrete heavy metals via the kidneys. You can also include dandelions from the garden along with some spinach to the juice for an extra boost.

Green Coriander Leaves(cilantro) : Nature's best heavy Metal Remover – This common spice is one of nature's gift to man kind. When eaten at a meal, coriander automatically stimulates bile, and so aids in the digestion process. As a natural way to help remove heavy metals from our toxic systems, it is invaluable. It even crosses the blood brain barrier helping to repair mecury based damage within the brain cells. And according to one study, it removed aluminum and lead from bone tissue faster than any other detoxifying drugs that were tested.

Garlic Protects the Blood from Heavy Metal: - What can you say about nature's natural penicillin that is also an anti-fungal, anti-microbal, and anti-bacterial. A basic cure all for all the body's needs and sicknesses. Research now indicates that garlic matured in water is a hundred times more potent than fresh cloves. Try this: chop up a few cloves of garlic and cover with water. Keep the mixture in a glass jar for a few days. Add 1 -2 teaspoons of this very pungent garlicky brew to your plate of food. Garlic protects the blood from toxic effects of heavy metals. *(References – Townsend Letter October 2009 page 111, 59-66 (Eliminating neurotoxins). 102-104, Naturopathic perspectives)*

Lemons & Limes – Have an alkalizing affect on the blood stream and the white piths contain pectin that binds up toxic heavy metal particles. It is also rich in vitamin K to control bleeding and is an excellent liver cleanser. Lemons also have anti-bacterial properties and can be used to disinfect cutting boards in food preparation.*(The Food Pharmacy by Jean Carper 1997 ISBN 0-671-71502-X Simon & Schuster Australia)*

Apples – "An apple a day keeps the doctor a way" is a familiar saying to millions that carries good common sense. Apples are one of God's great health giving foods. Apples are a rich source of potassium, vitamin E, biotin, folic acid, vitamin A, C, enzymes, and natural detoxifiers suh as sulphur, iron, iodine, silcon, magnesium, and calcium.. Considered a good old fashioned folk medicine for vibrant health. It is one of the oldest fruits that humans consumed, since the garden of Eden and has stood the test of time. Apples contain pectin that helps to bind and excrete heavy metals via the kidneys and the gut.

An apple detox will revitalize your body and give you a fresh start to change your eating habits for good. Apples help with constipation, lowers cholesterol, and can reduce the risk of colon cancer and is a natural chelator which can take up unwanted heavy metals from tissues. Remember, have an apple a day and keep the doctor away! *(References detox Now by Leslie Kenton 2002 ISBN 0-09-82582-2 Vermillion London)*

Specific Heavy Metal Detox Formula's

You can also purchase ready made natural cleansers, supplements that will help your body to detoxify toxins, heavy metals, chemicals, and parasites that come in an easy to apply kit with instructions, or you can pretty much put together your own formula based on the recommended products listed in the detoxification section.

- **Renew Life – (Heavy Metal Cleanse)** which consists of a 30 day program that combines natural chelating agents with anti-oxidants. Gluten Free.

- **Enzymatic Therapy- (Metal Magnet)** this product is usd for an 8 week periods between cleansings with another Enzymatic Therapy's "Whole Body Cleanse" or Simple Cleanse.

- **Nature's Secret – (Ultimate Cleanse)** excellent product that comes with good reviews and a free wellness CD. This is a two part total body cleanse, delicately balanced for cleansing, detoxifying & elimination. Part is a multi herb digestion

& detox formula. Part two is a multi fiber cleanse. A great formula that combines exactly what you may need Detoxify* Cleanse* and Rebuild*

- **<u>Garden of Life – (Perfect Cleanse)</u>** excellent reviews as well manufactured by a reputable company to where the owner himself suffered a serious illness that did not recover by conventional means, till he discovered Alternative medicine and healed himself from cancer. Perfect cleanse is designed as a gentle internal cleansing system that works in synergy with your own body's detoxification system. It offers a triple benefits of cleansing, capturing and smoothly removing toxins from your body in one convenient 10-day program you can use in the evening. This formula allows you to maintain your daily routine at work or home, without disruption. Great product!

- **<u>Renew Life- (Rapid Cleanse)</u>** A 7 day cleansing program, simple, fast and effective! A 3 part program, 1. to detoxify liver and organ cleanse, 2.captures toxins with natural acacia fiber, 3. Eliminates with colon cleanse. This is also considered a total body cleansing formula with added herbals and vitamins, and anti-oxidant support.

<u>Note:</u> *<u>This is just a quick sample of some of the ready made mixed formula's that are pretty much convenient and easy to use.</u>*

Chapter 16

What You Need To Know About Water

<u>Distilled Water</u> – One of the world's best and purest water, distilled water is excellent for detoxification and fasting programs and for helping to clean out all the cells, organs, and fluids of the body because it can help carry away so many harmful substances. Our normal drinking water from home, the office, work, schools, hospitals, etc., is likely to be overloaded with zinc from old galvanized pipes or with copper and cadmium from copper pipes.

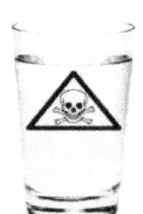

One of the most important functions of water is to flush out toxins and salt from the body. The temperature of the body controlled through water in the human body averages 65%, and water makes up 92% of the blood of your body, and 15 billion brain cells are 70% water. Keeping the body properly hydrated is one of your best natural protections against all kinds of virus infections, such as influenza, pneumonia, measles, and many other infectious diseases. People who drink the right amount of fluids (distilled water, fresh juices of fruit and vegetables have a much better circulatory system which is most important to a super healthy long life.

Water holds the key to our health, our vitality, our youthfulness, and our life Every 90 days we build a brand new blood stream. We can also regain health by the reversal program if we will be careful of the kind of water we drink and the kind of food we eat. Blood is the fluid which carries oxygen and nutrition to all cells of our body and tries to take away poisonous substances. But people are pouring inorganic minerals and toxic poisons into the body so fast

that the blood finds it impossible to purify itself. And that is one of the main reasons we get sick and die long before its our time.

The point here is, that it is important for us to clean and detoxify the body by drinking 100% pure water (distilled) to help our body's to dissolve and eliminate inorganic minerals from your body, and one of the best and healthiest things to do is to go on a 1 week to 10 day fast, eating nothing but Watermelon and watermelon juice, along with distilled water. Distilled water being 100% pure water can actually improve the quality of your complexion and over all skin will radiate with a glow! Regular household water seals the pores of your skin and tends to clog the pores. For a through, healthful cleansing, next time use distilled water and a pure soap (from health food store) on your skin. Distilled water is also excellent as a hair rinse.

Distilled water is almost always recommended and prescribed by doctors for babies for drinking and is also excellent for babies diaper rash and other skin problems. An interesting remedy for Arthritis is a quarter cup of raw apple cider to a gallon of distilled water, flavored with raw natural honey, and drink several glasses daily will help eliminate the inflammation normally associated with it.

Animals can also tell the difference of water, you can place 9 different kinds of water before a goat, for example, and he will amazingly select the glass with distilled water. The 9 different kinds of water are – *hard water, soft, raw, boiled, rain, snow, filtered, de-ionized and distilled water.* Regular tap water contains a variety of poisons such as *chlorine, chloramine, asbestos, pesticides, fluoride, copper, mercury, and lea*d. The best way to remove all of these contaminants is by distilling. Installing a home distilling station is one one the best ways of having pure distilled water. It is the only reliable way of home water purification for taking out the fluoride out of the water.

Distillation provides you with the cleanest water obtainable, distilled water is water which has been turned into vapor, so that all its impurities are left behind. Then, by condensing, it is turned back to pure water free from all of the impurities. Water hardness (inorganic minerals in solution) is the underlying cause of many, if not all, of diseases resulting from poisons in the intestinal tract. These (hard minerals) pass from the intestinal walls and get into the lymphatic system, which delivers all of its products to the blood, which in turn, distributes to all the parts of the body. This is the cause of human disease.

(Reference -Fluoride: The Aging factor, Dr. John Yiamoyuiannis, Ph.D)

As per the American Medical Association - "The greatest damage done by inorganic minerals – plus waxy cholesterol and salt – is to the small arteries ad other blood vessels of the brain (75% water). Hardening of the arteries and calcification of the blood vessels starts on the day you start taking inorganic chemicals and minerals from tap water into your bodies."

In a survey of 79 countries, America came in 79th in health. Heart attacks are the leading cause of death in this world. One cannot get sick unless their immune system is not working properly. This applies to cancer and every chronic disease, such as heart disease and Auto-immune diseases like rheumatoid arthritis. When you're sick, the doctor gives you drugs. Drugs never cure chronic diseases, but only cover up the symptoms while the disease continues to get worse. Doctors learn very little about nutrition and true healing.

Drink plenty of purified water, because water is a "key" element in making sure everything in your system is working right and being flushed out. If you do not drink ample amounts of water in a day your body eventually becomes sluggish like a toilet that has not been flushed for a long time, or like pipes backing up in a septic system. And all those toxins in your body are just sitting there in your gut being very harmful to your body.

This will also put you at risk in developing cancer, bowl disease, and eventually affecting the rest of your organs and tissues in your body. So, get the poisons out and drink plenty of purified distilled water to flush out the toxins and impurities to keep your insides clean from debris. You can look online for distilled water manufacturers that supply the necessary equipment to install a basic water distillation system for your needs.

Sauna Therapy & Exercise – Peer review literature shows that sweating during sauna therapy eliminates high levels of toxic metals, organic compounds, dioxin, and other toxins. Sauna therapy is an ideal way to help your body mobilize toxins from its hiding places. The skin is the body's largest detoxification organs and sweating in a hot sauna can help draw the mercury out from the body. However, during sauna therapy it is important to be on some kind of therapy *(chlorella & garlic)* for heavy metal detoxification, as sauna therapy can also cause toxic metals to be displaced from one body part to another. This means that mercury can be shifted from the connective tissue into the brain. This untoward effect will be prevented completely when one is on *chlorella, cilantro and garlic.*

Exercise - Helps facilitate the detox process and is absolutely needed. There are also many people with chronic illness who are often unable to engage in vigorous exercise e.g. jogging. Finding the right level of exercise for yourself that is appropriate to your level of illness will be of benefit in your detox program. Without exercise, mobilized toxins accumulate in the connective tissue, kidney, lungs, skin and can cause a new set of symptoms. It is recommended that 20 minutes twice a day is the minimum requirement during the active detox phase. And a good exercise program should include 3 components; *a) muscle strength training b) aerobic training c) stretching.*

Exercising for at least 20 minutes or so and immediately following the exercise, sit in a nice hot sauna or under infrared lights (infrared sauna) for up to 30 minutes, then finish off with a cool shower. **Important,** when doing the exercise sauna treatments for body detoxing, consume adequate amounts of water to avoid dehydration.

This is a minimum of two quarts before and after entering a sauna. Learn also to replace the important electrolytes lost to perspiration with grape juice (naturally pure), prune juice, or a sports electrolyte drink like Power-Aide or Gatorade. Vegetable juices are also a great addition to replace the calcium and magnesium lost through the skin.

TESTING PROCEDURES FOR HEAVY METAL TOXICITY

A hair tissue mineral analysis or hair analysis can provide you with a unique reading material of mineral levels in cells over a time period of many months. A hair analysis can help you reveal any toxic metal build up that you may not be aware of toxins that may be stored in the tissues of the body, not in the blood. For instance, you can have normal copper levels in the blood, but high copper levels in tissues.

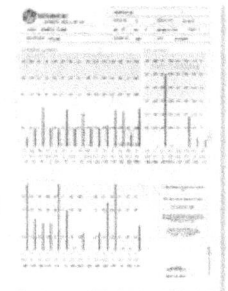

To help you get a better idea of this and of how helpful this can be, think about this: researchers using tissue mineral analysis determined, more than 100 years after Napolean Bonaparte's death, that he had been poisoned by arsenic. Even though his hair sample was tested more than a century ago after his death, it is still revealed pathological amounts of arsenic that had gradually proved fatal.

A hair usually needs to be obtained through a health care professional, such as a holistic health practitioner or any medical office that utilizes and offers hair analysis tests. The technology has been known for at least 75 years or more, and has been improved greatly since then. All commercial hair testing laboratories in America, are licensed and inspected annually by the federal government, as part of the CLIA act. The United States Environmental Protection Agency published a 300 page review, and concluded that hair analysis is a "meaningful and representative tissue for biological monitoring for most of the toxic metals". *("Toxic Trace metals in Humans and Mammalian Hair and Nails", EPA-600 4.79-049, August 1979, US Environmental Protection Agency, Research and Development)*

One reputable hair analysis testing site can be located at ARL, Analytical research Labs, INC., in Arizona and there website is www.arltma.com. They offer a complete individualized testing interpretation in a 15-20 page report that includes information related to one's metabolic rate, energy levels, sugar and carbohydrate tolerance, immune system, autonomic balance, glandular activity and metabolic trends, along with a personal dietary supplement program, basic diet recommendation, menu plans, and a wealth of information covering food preparation, eating habits, changing one's habit, cooking, shopping and other valuable information. I highly recommend this to help you determine your health status.

Chapter 17

ENZYMES THE "KEY" TO HEALING FMS & CFS

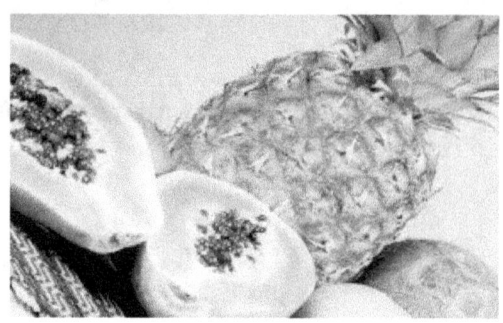

OVERVIEW -   With all the publicity that vitamins and minerals get, its a wonder that know one ever mentions the importance of enzymes, LIFE'S ENERGY SOURCE. Dr. Edward Howell *(author of Enzymes & Enzyme Therapy),* father of enzyme nutrition and therapy. Stated that enzymes are the very substance that makes life possible. Without enzymes, human life as we know it will cease to exist. Without enzymes, there would be no breathing, no digestion, no growth, no blood coagulation, no perception of the senses, and no reproduction. Enzymes are substances that occur naturally in all living things, including the human body. If its an animal or a plant, it has enzymes.

Enzymes are critical for life period! At the present, researchers have identified more than 3,000 different enzymes in the human body. Every millisecond of our lives these enzymes are constantly changing and renewing at an unbelievable fast speed.
Every life process depends on the action of enzymes, each activity that occurs within the body involves enzymes. The beating of the heart, the building and repairing of tissue, the digestion and absorption of food. Nothing can not take place without energy (enzyme activity) and energy cannot be used or produced without enzymes. Our body's ability to ward off disease is directly related to the strength and numbers of our enzymes. That is why an enzyme deficiency can be so devastated to the body's ability to function.

Enzymes complete very, specific jobs and do nothing else. They work on specific molecules and only do specific tasks. The purpose of an enzyme in a cell is to allow the cell to carry out chemical reactions very quickly. These reactions allow the cell to build things or take things apart as needed. This is how a cell grows and reproduces. At the most basic level, a cell is really a little bag full of chemical reactions that are made possible by enzymes. Enzymes are also made from amino acids. Some enzymes break down large nutrient molecules (the proteins, carbohydrates, and fats in our foods) into smaller molecules for digestion and aids the human body incorporating the raw materials from food or supplements. Without enzymes, our bodies cannot process and use the vitamins, minerals, and other nutrients present in our food and supplements. Enzymes can be likened to to the starter in your automobile; they ignite the process into action and the speed is dependent on the amount of power under the hood.

A good example of what an enzyme can do is, people who are lactose intolerance. The problem with lactose intolerance is when the sugar in the milk – lactose – does not get broken down into its glucose components. So therefore it can not be digested. The intestinal cells of lactose-intolerant people do not produce the enzyme lactase, which is needed to break down lactose. This shows how just the lack of one enzyme in the human body can lead to problems. A person who is lactose intolerant can swallow a drop of lactase prior to drinking milk and the problem is solved. There are also many other enzyme deficiencies that are not so easy to fix. The body's ability to function, to repair when injured, and to ward off disease is directly related to the strength and numbers of our enzymes. That's why enzyme deficiency can be so devastating.

Because enzymes are catalysts, their effectiveness can be greatly influenced by their environment. An acid or alkaline environment will affect their activity, as will temperature, concentration of substrate (the substrate upon which they work), coenzymes, and inhibitors. As we grow older our bodies are faced with an array of age related disorders that can correspond to disease rates, a parallel between an increase in age and the occurrence of diseases. Enzymes are one of the most powerful weapons we have against diseases. The benefits of enzymes can be verified by solid scientific data, including clinical studies.

Enzyme therapy has been helpful in supporting the immune system and immune system is affected by every disease. Taking protease enzymes orally may help reduce pain, swelling and over all discomfort of inflammatory conditions such as fibromyalgia, rheumatoid arthritis, lupus, Lyme disease, and injuries as well. Enzymes also help to improve the discomfort of varicose veins, phlebitis, and post-thrombotic syndrome. Enzymes improve blood circulation and therefore reduce the risk of thrombosis.

Chapter 18

ENERGY, ATP, & ENZYMES IN FMS/CFS
"The Road To Sustained Energy production"

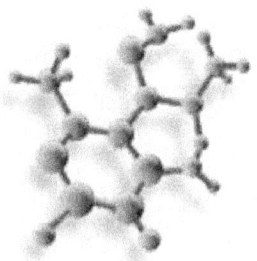

One of the main problems in those with Fibromyalgia and CFS is a lack of energy and weakness. Those with FMS and CFS experience digestive problems early on and eventually will lead to malabsorption. Research shows these people experience the lack of the enzyme amylase. Amylase enzymes are the catalysts that breakdown carbohydrates. Clinically it is also shown that people with FM and CFS have digestive problems with carbohydrates and starches. Many also have lipase deficiency, and lipase enzymes are the catalysts that breakdown fatty foods.

And without the proper lipase enzymes, one can have a fatty acid imbalances and hormonal imbalances as well. All of these deficiencies will lead to a protease deficiency. Since the protein invaders of our body are bacteria, fungal forms, and parasites, it stands to reason why the immune system then becomes compromised.

Dr. Suhadolink professor of biochemistry and member of the University's Institute of Cancer Research and Moleculor Biology, states FM and CFS patients have an inability to control common viruses and an inability to maintain cellular energy. The lack of enzymes control these processes. He feels this explains why FM and CFS patients have a hard time maintaining the energy for cellular growth. All carbohydrates, proteins, and fats contain stored energy that, by biological oxidation in the Kreb's cycle, can be transferred into ATP, Ninety percent or more of all the carbohydrates you eat are used to form ATP in the cells. There are three sources of ATP for muscles to use: *carbohydrates, fats, and amino acid proteins.* Carbohydrates metabolize the most efficiently and therefore used first. If carbohydrates are not available, your body metabolizes fat and amino acid proteins. Adenosine triphosphate (ATP) is the energy molecule for all of the cells in your body. People with FM and CFS tend have low levels of ATP.

This lack of energy so often experienced in those with FM and CFS is suspected to be in the very core defect of energy loss found in each and every cell: the mitochondria, which are (little organelles within cells), which produce energy in the form of ATP, that supplies the whole body with energy.

The one most obvious reason for the symptoms of weakness and fatigue in those with FM and CFS is the failure of the mitochondria which can a major cause of FM and CFS. Possible mitochondria failure could be the result a lack of enzymes due to malabsorption and nutrients for the mitochondria to work.

One of the ways of over coming FM and CFS is to help the mitochondria in supplying more ATP with in the body. And some of these important nutrients that seem help many with FM and CFS are; *D-Ribose, Magnesium and Malic acid, vitamin B3, CoQ-10, and systemic enzyme therapy.* Chronic stress which can block oxidative phosporylation, or blocking translocator protein function, poor anti-oxidant status (so mitochondria are not damaged by biochemical activity), poor hormonal control (poor levels of thyroid and adrenal hormones) and so on.

With CFS, it is suspected that core defect that underlies the disease is a defect in the energy cycle found in each and every cell of the "mitochondria," sited by Dr. Teitlebuam in his book *"Alternative Home Remedies."* According to Dr. Teitlebaum, the mitochondria are microscopic, capsule like structures inside the cells. They produce the energy – in the form of a chemical called **adenosine triphosphate, or ATP** – that powers all the functions of the body.

If the mitochondria are functioning inefficiently, they may generate only one-ninth of the optimal amount of ATP, Dr. Teitlebaum says. The one **"secret"** of overcoming CFS, then, is to help the mitochondria produce more of this energy-giving substance. *(see more on this on The cure and the remedy section of CFS & FM).*

Every century has certain illnesses that stump and baffle physicians, and for at least the last half of the century Fibromyalgia and Chronic Fatigue have been the prime examples. Because of it, ever year, there are up to 10 million people suffering from **Fibromyalgia (FM)** and it's cousin, **Chronic Fatigue syndrome (CFS),** a debilitating and chronic syndrome that has been around for most of the century, but is just now beginning to get recognition and attention in the medical community. In the last 30 years I've been practicing as a Holistic Health Practitioner, no single illness has been more confusing to the health-care system as FM and CFS are. Chances are, you probably know someone with Fibromyalgia & CFS, or either a family member, a friend, or a co-worker, or you could be afflicted with FM/CFS.

Optimize Cell Energy Production By Boosting ATP Levels

Here are some supplements can greatly help boost the production of ATP reserves and finally receive the help you need in reversing FM and CFS:

D-Ribose*** – is a 5 carbon sugar that forms the base of ATP. Supplementing with 3 grams a day may be helpful in boosting ATP production.**(See Life Extension Foundation for D-Ribose Tablest or D-Ribose powder)**

Magnesium & Malic Acid*** – is essential to the healthy muscle function. The enzyme that metabolizes ATP to release energy require <u>magnesium</u> to function. Multiple controlled clinical studies have found that magnesium is effective in relieving the symptoms of fibromylagia. Magnesium and malic acid helps assist cells in turning glucose(sugar) molecules into energy-giving ATP. **(See The Vitamin shoppe)**

CoQ-10 with Shilajit*** – enhances cellular energy by increasing ATP production better than CoQ-10 alone. The combination released brain energy 40% more than CoQ-10 alone and increased energy in the heart 27% more than CoQ-10 alone.**(See Life Extension Foundation for Super Ubiquinol CoQ10 with Enhanced Mitochondrial Support)**

 Potassium Magnesium Aspartate***- enhances energy production and plays a very important role in regenerating and producing ATP, which is the biochemical molecule storing and releasing the energy supply of your body. Potassium Magnesium Aspartate encourages cellular energy production, offers nutrition to support and enhance energy and fight against fatigue and promotes increased stamina.**(For further information see section on other nutritional therapies) (Potasium Magnesium Aspartate can be purchased at the Vitamin Shoppe)**

NADH – **(nicotinamide adenine dinucleotide)** also known as Coenzyme 1, has crucial roles in many cellular process. One of them is acting as a primary enzyme in the production of cellular energy. NADH triggers ATP energy production at the cellular level. The more Coenzyme 1 cells have the more ATP energy is produced.

Everyone needs Coenzyme 1 to fuel your cells so your body can function, so you can move your arm, blink, and breathe!

NADH can also help to increase brain function and cognitive capabilities and is directly involved in cellular immune response. NADH acts quickly to help boost and restore energy and alertness. Clinical studies have demonstrated benefits of Coenzyme 1 and will be a vital part in enhancing energy production so lacking in FM and CFS patients. **(Source Naturals NADH 5mgs for an effective and reliable product)**

Source of Enzymes

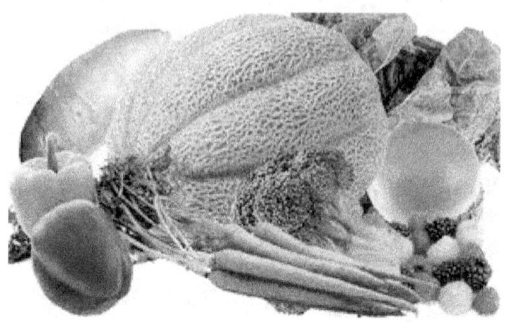

With regular use of enzymes people can enjoy a better quality of life. Traditionally food has been the primary source of enzymes. Uncooked foods (such as fruits and vegetables) are usually high in enzyme activity and, fortunately, taste good, too. However, in practice, with the magnitude of food additives, preservatives, radiation, long term storage, canning, freeze drying, the actual enzymes activity level o foods can be grossly reduced.

Enzymes are also heat sensitive, cooking destroys most of the live enzyme activity found in vegetables. Because of this this there is energy drain, and that is why it is best to consume as much raw vegetables as possible, and if cooking to steam or lightly poached, will be of benefit regarding health. Virtually all fresh, organically grown, uncooked foods are sources of enzymes. Raw vegetables and fruits are nature's rich source of natural enzymes.

While all raw foods contain enzymes, the most powerful enzyme rich food is *"sprouted seeds"*, *grains, and legumes*. Sprouting increases the enzyme content in these foods enormously. A lack of enzymes can also be a factor in common food allergies. *Symptoms of digestive enzyme depletion are bloating, belching, gas, bowel disorders, abdominal cramping, heart burn, and food allergies.* All of us will lose our ability as we get older in life, and in cases where age is a factor, or where a lack of digestive enzymes cause food allergies, supplementation may be helpful. In such , you may want to explore food combining. Below is a list of digestive enzyme supplementation that aid digestion:

- **AMALYASE** – works to breakdown carbohydrates i.e., starches, and sugars.
- **BROMELAIN** – taken from the pineapple plant, helps breakdown proteins.
- **HCL** (hydrochloric acid) – stimulates pancreatic secretion, activates pepsin and sterilizes the stomach from bacteria and parasites.
- **LACTASE** – needed to break down lactose found in milk products.
- **LIPASE** – Works to break down fats into fatty acids and glycerol.
- **OX BILE** – Improves fat digestion, stimulates bile flow, and aids the gallbladder.
- **PANCREATIN** – contains protease, amaylase, and lipase, functions in the

intestines and in the blood.

- **PAPAIN** – breaks down proteins, function depends on availability of HCL.
- **PROTEASE** – works to break down protein into amino acids.
- **CELLULASE** – Is the only enzyme your body cannot produce on its own, and is crucial for the digestion of fiber. It can also be found in alfalfa.

The more raw food you can eat, the better your health will be, digestion will be efficient, and your body will function more smoothly. If you do cook your food, the best way to cook food is to lightly steam, stew, or use a slow crock cooker. Eat as few over-processed and over cooked foods as possible. The body has a difficult time processing and digesting fried, pasteurized, barbecued, dried, and other over processed and over cooked foods which you find in boxed and processed foods.

It would encourage you to consume at least 50% of your food s uncooked as possible. Adding a good vegetable juicing program to your diet will easily put you over the 50% mark and allow you to reap the many health

Super Foods Rich in Natural Enzymes

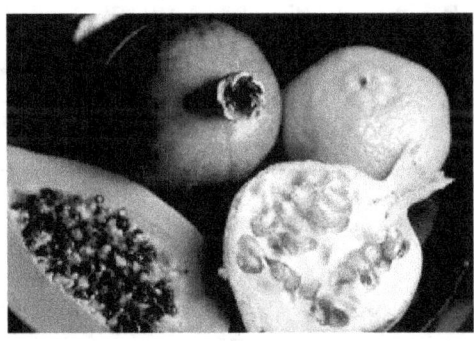

There are two major types of enzymes; synthetases and hydrolases. The *synthetases* are known as *metabolic enzymes* that help to build body structures by making or synthesizing large molecules. The *hydrolases* known as *digestive enzymes* use the process of hydrolysis to break down large molecules into smaller ones by adding water to the larger molecules. The best natural sources of enzymes are *fresh fruits, vegetables, and fresh juice made from them.*

- <u>**Bee Pollen**</u> – One of nature's most dense foods because of its dense nutritional quality. Packed with natural vitamins, minerals, trace elements, enzymes, and amino acids the way nature intended it to be. It contains 18 amino acids, vitamins B1, B2, B6, and B12; niacin; pantothenic acid B5, folic acid; vitamins C, D, E, choline; inositol; rutin; and other bio flavonoids; calcium; magnesium; iron; zinc; ten types of enzymes; coenzymes; and many other nutritional factors.

- <u>**Aloe Vera Juice**</u> – A great healer that has been recognized for its numerous health benefits, both internally and externally. Aloe vera is especially useful in relieving a variety of digestive ailments inside the digestive tract. It provides powerful anti-inflammatory action in the digestive system, it helps to detoxify the bowel, neutralizes stomach acids and relieves constipation and gastric ulcers. The most nutrient dense of all aloes is Aloe Badensis Miller containing 75 nutrients and over 200 active compounds including 20 minerals, 22 necessary amino acids, and 12 vitamins.

- **Sprouts** – one of the most concentrated sources of nutrition. Rich in enzymes, minerals, vitamins, amino acids, and phytonutrients. Some of the most common consumed sprouts are made from beans, lentils, broccoli seeds, alfalfa seeds, and clover seeds. You can also obtain sprout kits from specialty food stores such as www.sproutpeople.com

- **Cereal Grasses** – like wheat grass and barley grass are known for its rich source of chlorophyll, that contain many other nutrients and enzymes including the anti oxidant enzyme "superoxide dismutase" (SOD). Superoxide dismutases are a class of enzymes that provide important anti oxidant defense in nearly all cells exposed to oxygen. Without SOD cells are highly susceptible to damage and inflammation.

- **Microalgae** – spirulina, chlorella, and wild blue green algae contain more chlorophyll than any other foods on the planet. Microalgae are considered by most health experts to be the most healthiest foods on the planet. In addition to its rich chlorophyll factor, it is also a rich source of protein, beta carotene, enzymes, and nucleic acids (RNA and DNA).

- **Green Leafy Vegetables** - They all include chard, collard greens, mustard greens, bok choy, kale, dandelion greens, parsley, broccoli, coriander, and romaine lettuce. They all are a very good source of chlorophyll, enzymes, vitamins, minerals, and phytonutrients.

Natural Food Sources of Natural Enzymes

Pineapple (bromelain) – A *proteolytic* digestive enzyme that has been the study of several important health benefits, most of which is still under investigation. Research has revealed that bromelain is effective in fighting cancerous growth, and has powerful anti-inflammatory properties. 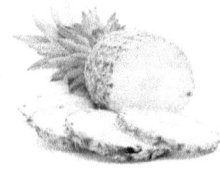 It blocks the growth of a broad range of tumor cells in several types of cancer including breast, lung, colon, ovarian, and melanoma. And Pineapples are a great source of nutrients that include a high content of vitamin C, essential minerals, and fiber.

Papaya (papain) –
Papain is also a proteolytic digestive enzyme extracted from papaya. Papain is normally found as a major ingredient in digestive enzyme supplements, and also used in many of the commercially supplements that are formulated for pain relief such as arthritis, sprains, injuries, etc.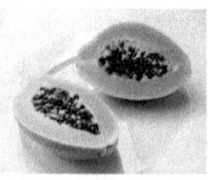
Papain also has anti-inflammatory properties and is an excellent source of other nutrients including vitamins, essential minerals, and zeaxanthin, a bioflavanoid found in almost all herbs, fruits, and vegetables. Zeaxanthin is also one of the two primary

xanthophyll carotenoids contained within the retina of the eye and is used in supplements to treat different disorders of the eyes.

Mangoes

Considered the king of fruits, and besides being delicious, it has immense health benefits with every taken bite. Mangoes are a rich source of digestive enzymes and contain an abundant amount of vitamins, minerals, fiber, and anti-oxidants. Mangoes also have been known for decades of its stomach soothing properties, rich in fiber and if you have at least one mango every day in your diet you are sure to stay miles a way from constipation, piles and spastic colon. Mangoes are also one of the best sources of *Quercertin, betacarotene, and astragalin, powerful anti-oxidants.*

Kiwifruit (actinidin)

Considered as one of the world's most most nutritious foods. The actinidin enzyme in kiwifruit eases digestion due to its proteolytic enzyme qualities. Actinidin is also found in pineapples, mangoes, and papayas.
Aside from being a great source of digestive enzymes, kiwifruit is also a great source of other several nutrients including fiber, high amounts of potassium, manganese, vitamin C (it has twice the amount in an orange), it contains the highest amounts of folate (folic acid) and vitamin K.

One cup of kiwi can supply you with 809% of the daily value of vitamin K. Kiwi also acts as a blood thinner without the adverse effect of aspirin. Still under research and study, scientists have been fascinated for its ability to protect DNA in the nucleus of human cells from oxygen related damage. Kiwi also contains a variety of bioflavonoids and carotenoids that have anti oxidant activity.

Figs (ficin) -

Are one of the prime fruits enjoyed since antiquity in human history. The ficin is another (proteolytic) enzyme that eases digestion, and has been used as a tenderizing agent in meats. Figs are an excellent source of dietary soluble fiber and a good source of concentrated minerals and vitamins, and anti oxidants. Research studies suggest that chlorogenic acid in figs 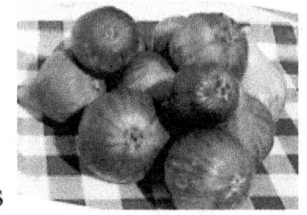 help to lower blood sugar levels and control blood glucose levels in type II diabetes mellitus (adult onset) condition.

The foods we eat are our first line of defense from the negative effects of lifestyle, stress, pollution, radiation, and toxic chemicals. So, wouldn't it make sense to consume the most beneficial health foods as possible? Of course it would! We are what we eat, and know that all disease will manifest in the stomach, meaning, if we eat like crap we will feel and look like crap. Nature has provided us with some of the earth's most nutritious foods, all rich in enzymes, vitamins, minerals, and elements that can prevent sickness and create optimal health so we can live life to its fullest degree. The healthiest foods are you best defense!

Try and make your nutritional meals 50% of raw and live foods rich in enzymes the catalysts of life. Cut back or eliminate foods that really have no nutritional value like sugar and processed foods. All they do is leave us with being vulnerable to poor health and low energy. Consume more water, remember 70% of the body is water, so give it what it needs and it will take care of you. Water will help flush out toxins from your liver and kidneys and help keep your body's pH level neutral, neither too acid or too alkaline.

Avoid the high acid forming foods and drinks, international studies have already shown that populations with little or no history of illness, such as cancer, consume less acid forming foods and drank alkaline waters. Alkaline ionized water "first came to notice in Japan, where researchers noted that people drinking water that came from certain fast moving rocky mountain streams enjoyed extraordinarily good health. It turned out that this naturally occurring water was alkaline and had a different chemical structure and electrical properties. *(Dr. Larry Clapp, Ph.D. In "Prostate Health in 90 Days")*

The Solution For Healthy Digestion

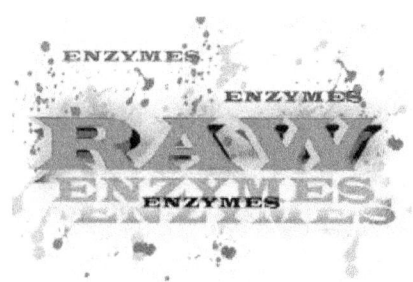

The common solution to this energy drain, is daily supplementation in addition to live foods, fruits and vegetables should be a basic part of your dietary meal plans to ensure an adequate supply of enzymes. We cannot produce energy without catalysts, and enzymes are those catalysts. You cannot start your day and feel young, with energy and vitality, if your body has lost its enzyme punch.

Today, researchers are now able to produce enzymes to treat specific acute and chronic disorders. This technique is called systemic enzyme therapy. Since many chronic disorders involve disturbed enzyme function, it seems logical to take supplemental enzymes. Digestive enzymes provide optimal support for healthy digestion of proteins, carbohydrates and fats. They also help prevent accumulation of undigested foods in the large intestine, which can disrupt the normal healthy bacterial balance in the bowel.

There are three types of enzymes: digestive, metabolic, and food enzymes. The **pancreas** is the organ that produces most of the body's digestive enzymes required for food breakdown and secretes them into the small intestine.

The four general classes of digestive enzymes are: **amylase**, which digests carbohydrates, starches, and sugars found in grains, fruits, and starchy vegetables; **protease**, which breaks down protein found in meat, nuts, and cheese into amino acids;

lipase, which breaks down fats and oils found in dairy and meat products into fatty acids; and **cellulase** which helps digest fibers. The pancreas also secretes **insulin** which we all know, regulates blood sugar metabolism.

Metabolic enzymes are manufactured by the body's own cells to perform highly specific tasks required in regulating the blood, tissues, and organs. They are responsible for the growth of new cells within the body, repair and maintenance of tissues and organs, transportation of blood to the different organs, and the detoxification of the cells, tissues, organs, and blood.

Metabolic enzymes are also responsible for the delivery and absorption of nutrients in various organs. Enzymes that come from food are the vital force naturally found in raw, uncooked foods. There are a lot of well documented cases that attest to the wonderful benefits and healing power of raw food.
They work synergistically with other nutrients like vitamins, minerals, phytochemicals, anti-oxidants, and co-enzymes, allowing your digestive system to take its much needed rest and give your immune system the necessary boost to successfully carry out its search and destroy missions.

Enzymes & Disease Connection

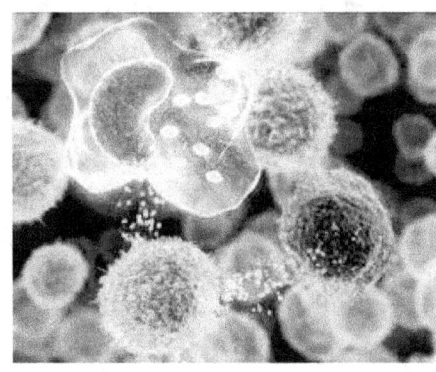

The digestive process begins as soon as you begin to chew the food in your mouth, enzymes in saliva start digesting foods before they leave your mouth, so take your time and chew your food slowly and enjoy your food. Discomfort may result after eating if you consumed your food to fast. Deficiencies of insufficient enzymes may include, feeling of gas and bloating after a normal meal. **Other symptoms of enzyme deficiency include:**

- **Abdominal cramping and pain**
- **Bowl irregularities**
- **Food intolerance**
- **Pale colored stools and foul smelling stools**
- **Muscle cramps**
- **Easy bruising**
- **Bright orange oil droplets in the toilet after bowel movement**

Some of the possible causes of pancreatic enzyme insufficiency may include –

surgeries in which part of the stomach and/or pancreas is removed, a blocked pancreatic duct, or insufficient output, the pancreas may not secrete its juices into the small intestine, or a stomach ulcer. Severe cases of pancreatic enzyme deficiency may lead to malabsorption, meaning the body cannot absorb the nutrients in food. People suffering from malabsorption are normally thin and sickly, and suffer from severe abdominal pain. This is a serious health matter that can create a host of health disorders that must be taken care of immediately.

The leading cause of pancreatitis (inflammation of the pancreas) is alcohol abuse, but causes can also include infections, cancer and the effects of certain medications. Over 80% of of hospital admissions for acute pancreatitis are due to bilarly tract disease and alcoholism.The effects of pancreatitis will come on quickly with mild to severe pain in the upper portion of the abdomen that can radiate to the back and sometimes the chest. The pain will also be constant and can last for hours and often days. And will worsen when the patient eats or drinks alcohol. There can be nausea, vomiting, and fever with a rapid pulse. Its important to be aware that the cause of this pain is not due to a back injury, but rather to a potentially life threatening pancreatic disorder. If you think you have this condition, see your physician immediately!

In some people that may have pancreatitis, they may experience any pain, but most will have the same bouts of discomfort that those with acute pancreatitis go through – nausea, vomiting, and fever. They may have trouble tolerating fatty foods, and may suffer from steatorrhea and/or diabetes. Weight loss normally occurs with those that have pancreatiris even though the person is eating normally, due to the malabsorption of vital nutrients from food. From this you will see oily, foul and smelling stools. Eventually the cells in the pancreas that secretes digestive enzymes are destroyed and abdominal pain may actually subside. In time, pancreatic secretions will be reduced and the patient will develop steatorrhea. And destruction of the islet cells of the pancreas will result in reduced insulin secretion and glucose intolerance. Pancreatitis is something that we must not ignore, as it can lead to serious health complications and even death. The chronic form (usually alcohol related) means that the tissue destruction is irreversible.

Therapy will be limited to dietary measures of , anti-acid administration, and high levels of **_enteric coated pancreatic enzymes_**. A diet low in fatty foods, a vegetarian type of a diet would be ideal, eliminating most dairy products, except yogurt, and low fat milk 1% or skim. Protein that's consumed should always be low in fat. Meats and fish are good if you eat lean cuts such as poultry and baked fish. Your meals should consist of small meals also instead of large meals that may create digestion problems. Healthy carbohydrates are good and should consist of brown rice, pasta, baked potatoes, vegetables, whole grain breads, fruits, and high fiber foods like oatmeal are excellent.

Foods to avoid for pancreatitis are the spicy foods, beans or any type of gas producing foods, pizza, eggs, cheese, all fried foods, bacon, sausage, butter, tea, coffee, sugar, caffeine, alcohol, and all stimulants and tobacco. **Pancreatic supplements** are excellent and should definitely be included with all meals.

A quick and effective way to heal pancreatitis and restore it back to health is to consider buying a juice extractor, this will help you get the vital and necessary live enzymes, vitamins, and minerals in a liquid form – *(for more information on juicing I highly recommend you read "Raw Juices Can Save Your Life: An A-Z Guide to Juicing" by Sandra Cabot) and ("Super Foods: The Food and Medicine of the Future" by David Wolfe)*

Digestion is a vital process in sustaining our body's health status and affecting our rate of aging. And can help with many of the following digestive problems such as the following listed below:

- **Hpyochlorhydria**
- **Achlorhydria**
- **Pancreatic insufficiency**
- **Acute pancreatitis**
- **Chronic pancreatitis**
- **Cystic fibrosis**
- **Celiac disease**
- **Lactose intolerance**
- **Intestinal toxemia**
- **Malabsorption**
- **Steatorrhea**
- **Food allergies**

Stress and Enzymatic Function

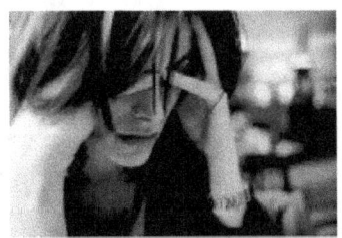

Here we are back to the subject of stress again and its importance pertaining to health related matters. Stress of any kind can interfere with the proper digestion and absorption of foods. And this includes all facets of any stress related situations, such as emotional, physical, anxiety, stress from work, environmental, surgery, injury, and toxins. I'm also sure by now after reading this book we all have become very familiar with how stress can cause a multitude of health problems, and the series of reactions and responses to stress. As explained in the previous chapter of stress and health conditions, the brain's reaction when under stress. The "flight or fight" response will always become a priority first and realizes that digestion is not a priority.

The glands and organs involved in digestion shut down as the body diverts energy to handle the increased needs of respiration, and circulation. And less blood flow to the digestive tract and digestion will virtually stops. Although short term situational stress problems may not be detrimental enough to cause digestive diss-stress, but one condition which does develop from our response to stress is irritable bowel syndrome. This condition appears to be due to an inappropriate response, by the intestinal wall, to stress.

If we are in a constant state of stress, our digestive system will definitely suffer, and impair our ability to properly digest our foods and absorb the nutrients we need to sustain health, and then our nutritional status will set the stage for a variety of health conditions. *(please see the section on managing stress for more helpful information).*

Enzymes and Food Allergies

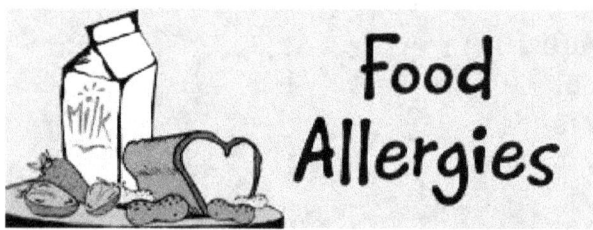

Enzymes can be a great help to those who suffer from food intolerance or sensitivity. The ultimate purpose of eating is to provide each cell in your body with the nutrients it needs. If you can't digest your food well, your cells don't work optimally. Today, one out of every three people believes they have a food allergy or sensitivity. Those with food sensitivities will often experience a wide variety of complaints including – gastrointestinal problems, headaches, low blood sugar, anxieties, skin problems, asthma, arthritis, and rhinitis. Having a food intolerance is also a big clue to a digestive enzyme deficiency.

And throughout my practice I have found enzymes to be an effective tool in relieving people from food sensitivity. Having one digestive enzyme deficiency may be an indicator that you may have another one as well. And <u>in this case its best to include a broad spectrum digestive enzyme or a multi-enzyme formula.</u> There are so many people that have enzyme deficiencies, making them unable to adequately digest specific foods or food groups. When left unresolved, enzyme deficiencies prevent complete digestion of specific compounds in foods and can lead to symptoms of food intolerance. Because enzymes are specific, we need to have a lot of different types to digest specific food components.

Adding the use of digestive enzyme supplements and enzyme dense foods, can help you support your body so that you have fewer sensitivity reactions. Enzymes also will help reduce a leaky gut and food sensitivities because there is less irritation in the small intestines. Some excellent digestive supplement that can be purchased through the *"Life Extension Foundation" called "Enhanced Super Digestive Enzyme" a*nd one of the best enzyme formula's *"Wobenzym-N".*

Essential Fatty Acid Deficiency & FMS / CFS

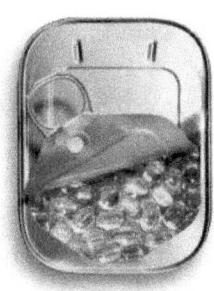

"Every Case of Fibromyalgia is Found To Have a Deficiency in EFA's"

Essential fatty acids **(EFA's)** have been a hot research topic because of it's impact on the functioning of the human body and disease. When you see the term *"essential"* whether it be in front of particular vitamin, mineral, amino acid, nutrients, or *"good fats"*, it means that humans cannot synthesize a particular nutrient, and must be obtained through the diet. In the average American diet most people are now becoming deficient in essential fatty acids which include – Omega 3 & Omega 6 fatty acids.

Omega 9 is also including but is not necessarily essential because the human body can manufacture a modest amount on its own, providing Omega 3 and Omega 6 are present within the human body. **EFA's** are considered long chain polyunsaturated fatty acids and super unsaturated acids derived from **linolenic, linoleic, and oleic acids**. There are actually two kinds of **EFA's: Omega** 3 are derived from Linolenic Acid & **Omega 6** from Linoleic Acid, , and the second being **Omega 9** from Oleic Acid.

Deficiency of **EFA's** are common in United States at an estimated 40% of the population suffers from some amounts of EFA deficiency. Particularly Omega 3/6 deficiency, this imbalance is linked with serious health conditions, such as - *heart attacks, cancer, accelerated aging, insulin resistance, asthma, lupus, schizophrenia, depression, insomnia, anxiety, GI disorders, muscle pain, poor mental function, postpartum depression, stroke, obesity, diabetes, arthritis, ADHD, ADD, and Alzheimer's disease, among many others*. When EFA's are deficient, cell membranes are weakened in their abilities, and the wrong substances are allowed to enter into the cell. A deficiency in EFA's can cause some of the very symptoms associated with CFS and FM as noted above.

Many people fear that by consuming too many fats will make them fat and obese, but by not realizing that the fat they consume is of the wrong type deter them from making the correct choice in choosing the healthy fats from their diet. Just by the word itself "fatty acids" make them wonder that it's a fatty food and omit it from their diets. Its time to let go of your fears and be sure that your getting the "essential fats" you need in your diet to remain healthy. It is too much of the nonessential fatty acids, especially the "hydrogenated fats" (fried) like margarine and shortening, that can cause high cholesterol and heart disease.

What Do EFA's Do In The Body?

It is important for the average consumer to realize that "good fats" (essential) compete with bad fats, so its important to minimize the intake of trans fatty acids and cholesterol(animal fat) while consuming enough of the essentially good fats. Good fats help to raise your "HDL" (good cholesterol) levels and lower the bad fatty acids(LDL) levels.

One of the jobs of HDL (high density lipoprotein) or "good cholesterol" is to grab your bad cholesterol, LDL (low density lipoprotein), and escort it to the liver where it is broken down and excreted. In other words, these good fats attack some of the damage already done by the bad fats. This is very important in an age when so Americans are struggling to get their cholesterol down, and fight heart disease.

EFA's support the cardiovascular system, reproductive system, immune system, and the nervous system. The human body needs these EFA's to manufacture and repair cell membranes, enabling the cells to obtain optimum nutrition and expel harmful waste products. The primary function of EFA's is the production of series of *"Prostaglandins (PGE1, PGE2, PGE3)"*, hormone like-chemicals that have a high turn over rate and play a large part in managing the daily housekeeping of cells, which regulate body functions as *heart rate, blood pressure, blood clotting, fertility, conception, and play a role in immune function by regulating "inflammation" (FMS) and encouraging the body to fight infections*. The PGE series of prostaglandins 1, 2, and 3 are all needed by the body in proper balance:

- **PGE 1** – keeps the blood mobile, helps remove excess sodium and fluid from the body, relaxes blood vessels, decreases inflammatory symptoms(FMS), regulates calcium functions, and supports the immune system and nervous systems.
- **PGE 2** – constricts blood vessels, promotes inflammation, fluid retention, and stcky imobile blood.
- **PGEs** 1 & 3 – keeps PGE2 production under tight control.

Problems occur when an over consumption of cholesterol and trans-fatty acids encourage the production of PGE2, leading to a systematic imbalance of the worst kind. When EFA's are digested in a healthy person, they will enter the cell by means of protein transporters, where they will convert to GLA (from Omega6) and EPA from (Omega3) the important precursors to PGE1's and 3. EFA's are also involved in, systemic metabolism, cellular energy production (FMS/CFS), manufacturer of hemoglobin, removal of lactic acid from the system, and proper brain development in infants and children.

Omega 3 and Omega 6 must be taken in proper proportions, 2:1, in order for them to be fully effective. A person who cannot digest their food (FM people) will also be unable to utilize their EFA's. And even if digestion does improve, other factors can and will prevent the conversion of EFA's to GLA and EPA, (such as diabetes, viral & bacterial infections, FMS, and poor diet.

When this happens the symptoms of EFA's deficiency will begin to occur and systemic imbalance is upset, and eventually leading to a disease. It is for this reason that Omega 6 oils should always be supplemented with a source of GLA, such as Borage oil, to make sure PGE1 production occurs.

The conversion of omega 3 EFA's to EPA is easily taking care of by the regular consumption of cold water fish (once a week is sufficient) or seaweed, both sources of EPA. Fish oil capsules are generally recommended as well, but be aware that some fish oil capsules can become rancid and post the prevalence of toxins such as *"polychlorinated bihenyls"* which will create extra problems for the immune system. So, when purchasing fish oil capsules make sure that their made from a reliable manufacturer that takes the necessary steps in removal of rancidity.

The Importance of EFA Supplementation

There are several interesting interrelationships between EFA metabolism and viral infections commonly chronic in those with FMS and CF. EFA's do have a direct anti-viral effects and are lethal at surprisingly low concentrations to many viruses. Interferon, a modulator of the immune system in fighting off viruses and bacteria is dependent on EFA's and in their absence will be compromised. Viral infections lower the blood levels of EFA's and has been confirmed in cases of Epstein Barr Virus (EBV).

In a Scottish trial, patients with CFS were given EFA supplementation with great success. Placebo controlled trials were held for 70 patients with persistent CFS giving them Linoleic acid (flax seed oil) and eicosapentaenoic acid (fish oils), after 6 months, an astonishing 84% of the patients in the group receiving EFA supplements, and only 22% of those in the placebo group rated themselves as better or much better.

And in another successful study, 63 adults with CFS were enrolled in a double blind placebo controlled study with essential fatty acid therapy. The patient's were ill for an average of 1 to 3 years after a viral infection. They all suffered fatigue, mylagia (muscle pain), and a variety of psychological symptoms. After one month, 74% of the patients taking EFA supplements, and 23% of those on placebo, assessed themselves as improved. [*Ref' – Artical; Fish Oil For Fibromyalgia and Chronic Fatigue Syndrome; Dr. Roger Murphee, Feb. 24, 2012]*

As you can see from the above studies done with CFS and EFA's supplements, the importance of including EFA's in your diet and from supplements are very important in the recovery and relief of the symptoms associated with both FM and CFS.

Essential fatty acids work to keep us mentally and emotionally strong in three ways:

1. **Omega 3 fats acts as precursors for the body's production of pre-prostaglandins and neurotransmitters (specific hormones).**

2. **Omega 3 fats provide the substrate for B vitamins and co-enzymes to produce compounds that regulate many vital functions, including**

neurotransmitterss.

3.   Omega fats provide energy and nourishment to our nerves and brain cells.

Fat Facts

- Every cell in our body is made up of a fat(lipid) coating. The fat acts as a barrier to keep out harmful microbes.
- Our endocrine glands (pituitary, hypothalamus, pineal, adrenals, thyroid, parathyroid, thymus, pancreas, testes, ovaries, all requires fats in order to construct hormones like estrogen and testosterone.
- The human brain, the most complex organization of matter we know is compromised of 60% fat.
- Fats maintain the integrity of neuron connections – the brains vital communication system.
- Nerve, brain, eye, heart,, and adrenal and thyroid cells must have essential fats to function.
- Essential fats are necessary for normal reproduction and growth. They are converted into prostaglandins, which regulate all body functions at the cellular level. Prostaglandins control blood pressure, clotting, inflammation, allergies, sodium,, and water excretion, tumor growth, among other functions.
- Fat is required for the production of <u>Serotonin</u>, which elevates mood and promotes good sleep.

[Reference & Resources - from "The Diet Cure" -8 step program to rebalance your body's chemistry and end food cravings, weight problems, and mood swings -now; Julia Ross, M.A.]

"Handbook of Essential Fatty Acid Biology: Biochemistry, Physiology, and Behaioral Neurobiology" by Shlomo Yehuda (Nov 5, 2010.

European Journal of Medical Research, (2003; 8(8); 355-7)

Journal of Nutrition, (2005; 135(3): 562-6)

Journal of the American Pharmaceutical Association (40(2): 234-242, 2000)

Supplementing EFA's In Your Diet

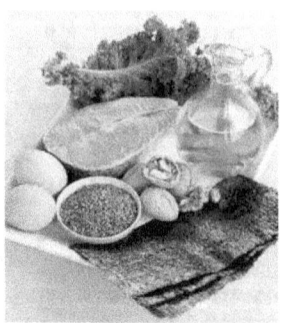

One of the simple ways in determining essential fatty acid deficiencies are fat cravings. Many people who crave fatty foods and tend to over eat them are essentially deficient in EFA's and are basically eating the wrong type of fats and eventually become fat addicts. They are so deficient in certain essential, healthy fats that their body continually calls for oily, creamy foods, hoping that they will eventually swallow the particular kind of fat that it really needs. According to Artemis Simopoulos, MD, distinguished researcher and author of "The Omega Plan", states that Americans are getting one tenth of the EFA's we really need, and 20% of us have levels so low that they are undetectable.

Most people that tend to over eat fats soon start to develop health problems. And that is also one of the health problems today in America. You have to realize that when you start to crave and over eat fatty foods, especially when you are trying not to is a signal that something is wrong. The solution is to cut out all the bad fats and start to eat the correct fats. The Omega 3 fats, sometimes called Vitamin F2, and Omega 6 which is equally important must be consumed regularly in your foods, or other wise we cannot protect our selves.

Important Facts About Fat Sources

Cholesterol, a word that many people have learned to fear, is made from fatty foods. All of our necessary hormones are made from cholesterol – our sex hormones – estrogen, progesterone and testosterone, and our stress hormones – pregnenolone, DHEA, adrenaline, and cortisol. Fats like saturated fats are the "solid fats" like high fat cheeses; high fat cuts of meats, whole-fat milk and cream, butter, ice cream and ice cream products, and the fats in shellfish, and poultry are all high in cholesterol.

With animal fats being the primary source of saturated fat. Certain plant oils are also another source of saturated fats: palm oils, coconut oils, and cocoa butter that are often added to commercially prepared foods, such as cookies, cakes, doughnuts, and pies. Solid vegetable shortening often contains palm oils and some whipped dessert toppings contain coconut oil as well. But if they are not hydrogenated (to prolong shelf life), they don't cause harm and can help lower triglyccrides. If we eat fats like these in excess, these oils will block the benefits of the essential Omega 3 and Omega 6 oils that we do take in.

A low cholesterol diet does not usually help much either. We actually do better by increasing our vitamin and mineral intake from vegetables and fruits, and take special supplements, including essential fats. So, the question is, how do we control our saturated fat intake? The answer is we do need both types of fats to stay in balance, red meat actually contains some beneficial fats, as well as important vitamins and minerals (iron and zinc). Lamb even contains some Omega 3 fat.

We can balance our saturated fat intake by trimming some of the fat off of the meat, as well as in poultry is a good idea. Choose leaner cuts of meats that do not have a marble appearance (where the fat appears imbedded in the meat). Leaner cuts include round cuts and sirloin cuts. Trim all visible fat off the meats before eating. Remove the skin from the poultry (turkey & chicken) before cooking.

When cooking soups or stews, skim the solid fats from the top before serving. Drink low fat milk (1%) or fat free (skim) milk rather than whole or 2% milk. Buy low fat or non fat versions of your favorite cheeses and other milk or dairy products. Pay attention to snacks and sandwhich crackers contain saturated fats. Stay away from margarines that are high in trans fatty acids, and always read the nutrition label. Most of the fat that you eat should come from unsaturated sources: polyunsaturated and monounsaturated fats. In general, nuts, vegetable oils, and fish are sources of unsaturated fats.

- **Good sources of Omega 3 polyunsaturated fats** are from – fish (trout, salmon, mackerel, sardines, anchovies, herring), soybean oil, canola oil, walnuts, flax seeds, walnuts, Brazil nuts, sesame seeds, avocados, wheat germ, hemp seeds, dark green leafy vegetables (kale, spinach, purslane, mustard greens, collard greens).

- **Omega 6 sources are** – soybean oil, corn oil, safflower, flax seed oil, grape seed oil, pumpkin seeds, pistachio nuts, chestnut oil, chicken, borage oil, evening primrose oil, black current seed oil, sun flower oil, cotton seed oil, and pine nuts.

- **Excellent sources of Monounsaturated (Omega 9) fats** are – nuts, vegetable oils, canola oil, high oleic safflower oil, sunflower oil, Olive oil (extra virgin or virgin), olives, peanuts, almonds, sesame oil, pecans, pistachio nuts, cashews, hazelnuts, macadamia nuts, and avocados.

- One to two tablespoons of extra virgin olive oil per day should provide sufficient oleic acid for adults. However, the "time released "effects of these nutrients from nuts and other whole foods is thought to be more beneficial than consuming the entire daily amount via a single dose.

Important Tips & Facts

- Remember, animal fat is only junk fat if you consume it in excess, and always remember to trim the excess fat as well.
- Animal and dairy fat also harbor pesticides and anti-biotics, so buy the organically produced versions whenever possible.
- Blood types also seem to play a part in the digestion of animal fats. People who have blood type – O, seem to digest animal fat quite well, and seem to need meat, poultry, eggs and fish. But do not seem to do well with cow's milk products. Blood-type A people have a difficult time with the utilization of saturated animal fats and are best adapted to a vegetarian type of a diet based on legumes, corn, rice, nuts, seeds, and leafy green sources of fat (*Ref- Dr. Peter JD. D'Adamo; "Eat Right For Your Blood Type"*). Both blood types O & A need to get enough Omega 3 oils. And vegetarians tend to get too much Omega 6 and meat eaters can be deficient in both Omega 3 & 6.
- Malabsorption problems not being able to digest healthy fats due insufficient

enzymes specifically "lipase" as a result of illness and health conditions (FMS, IBS, Leaky Gut syndrome), and/or Liver and gallbladder problems can have a severe essential fatty acid deficiency.

- Signs of an improper fat digestion include – feeling full, heavy, or nauseous after a high fat meal, have oily skin or experience burping or belching after eating fatty foods. By supplementing with the fat digesting enzyme "Lipase" can help. Having insufficient amounts of Lipase will not allow you to obtain the full nutritional value of digesting the fatty acids your body needs.

- A sluggish liver and gallbladder will also lead to improper breakdown of fatty foods consumed, bile a powerful acid made by your liver and stored in your gallbladder breaks down fat into little pieces so that lipase can easily dissolve it for your body to utilize it it, rather than just store it.

- By not correcting a sluggish liver problem can lead to an overload of fats to process and turn into a vicious cycle as the liver gets more inefficient and congested in the breakdown of fats and cause significant health problems like hepatitis.

- Symptoms of liver problems include yellowing of the skin and eyes, intolerance to greasy foods, and unusual bowel movements. **(See section on liver detoxification for liver health and supplementation).**

- Tiny intestinal parasites, called "blastocystis hominis or blasto" can also increase your appetite for fatty foods. These little microbial parasites actually will feed on the fat you consume until it gorges itself and explodes. They can also invade your liver and gallbladder too. If you increase your omega 3 fats and improve the function of your liver and gallbladder, and you still have strong cravings for fatty foods, get yourself checked with your doctor and ask for a complete parasitic panel and/or follow the recommendations on the section of detoxification and whole body cleanse.

(Note) the normal medical treatment for parasitic infestation is anti-biotics which does not kill them off and just grow back with more eggs). Natural Holistic treatment is what kills them completely! The herb <u>Ginger</u> is a good staple to keep in your diet, it has a long history in India and Africa in treating parasitic infestations, use it in foods and drink it as a tea 2 to 3 times a day. Also see the herb "<u>wormwood bark</u>" to treat common parasites.

- A sluggish or congested liver can also give you some of the symptoms of CFS and FM that include weakness, fatigue, lack of energy, indigestion problems, nausea, constipation, moodiness, etc. *(see liver specific herbs and detoxification section)*

Good Quality Essential Fatty Acid Blends To Take

<u>A Flax/Borage Oil blend</u> is good to take, that provides you with an optimal ratio of 2:1 Omega 3 to Omega 6 oils, with 23% of GLA for the conversion purposes and vitamin E for optimal absorption seems to work the best. The flax/borage oil combination consistently has worked well for people experiencing a variety of EFA's deficiency symptoms, including various arthritic symptoms, gastrointestinal symptoms, hormonal imbalances, FMS/CFS, Crohn's disease and auto-immune dysfunction. Flax seed oil is the highest Omega 3 food known, with only one tablespoon per day providing enough Omega 3 acids for the whole day.

Also, in order for EFA's conversion into PGs (prostaglandins)to occur you must have protein available in the body to carry EFA's into the cells. Because if you are protein deficient you will not digest the oils and you will not get them into the proper location for the manufacturer of prostaglandins.

Recommended EFA's are –Udo's Choice - Udo's Ultimate Blend, Spectrum Naturals "Organic Flax Borage Oil". Second choice "Enzymatic Therapy" Eskimo-3 Fish Oil.

Recommended reading – **"Omega-3 Oils; A Practicle Guide", by Donald Rudin, MD and Carla Felix and "The Omega-3 Connection" by Andrew L Stoll, M**

Hypoglycemia and FM/CFS Connection

It is estimated that over 40% of FM patients are hypogylcemics that suffer from carbohydrate intolerance. This is expressed by the body's inability to use certain carbohydrate loads effectively without adverse consequences. With symptoms occurring 3 to 4 hours after eating, including fatigue, irritability, nervousness, depression, insomnia, flushing, dizziness and fainting, anxieties, headaches, blurred vision problems, numbness and tingling of the hands, excessive gas, abdominal cramps, loose stools, and diarrhea. In fact, individuals with FM are likely than individuals who do not have FM to have this condition.

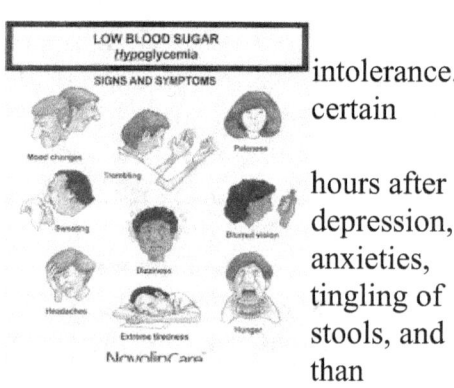

What is Hypogylcemia & How is it Linked To FM/CFS

Hypogylcemia is a condition most often associated with diabetes, however, it can also occur in individuals who do not have diabetes. The following reasons are causes of hypoglycemia in individuals who do not have hypoglycemia:

- certain medications
- alcohol
- certain types of cancer
- heart, kidney or liver failure
- hormonal imbalanced disorders that cause the over production of insulin

As such, hypoglycemia is not considered an illness in and of itself, but an indicator or a more serious health problem.

Diagnosis

- **Symptoms of hypoglycemia:** are checked for after the individual under goes either an overnight fast or an extended fast in a hospital setting, or symptoms may also be checked after a meal.

- **Documentations of symptoms**: a blood sample is then taken to analyze blood sugar levels
- **Reduction of symptoms**: symptoms are then monitored to see if they disappear after blood sugar levels are raised.

Treatment of Hypoglycemia

A healthy diet is the main tool through which hypoglycemia is treated. Individuals with hypoglycemia should not consume sugar in any form, including: corn syrup, honey, sucrose, glucose, dextrose, maltrose, and table sugar. In addition, heavy starches, including rice, pasta, and potatoes, should also be avoided, as should be caffeine products. Only a single piece of fruit should be consumed within a 4 hour period.

The biggest problem FM/CFS people have is the carbohydrate consumption that increases insulin, decreasing blood sugar levels, this high glycemic load breakdown into tremendous amounts of sugar within your body and should be avoided as they make your FM/CFS worse. Foods to eat for FM/CFS are light complex carbohydrates with healthy proteins and healthy fats will keep insulin levels from rising and keep FM symptoms from getting worse. Carbohydrates, proteins and fats form the three main macronutrients that are essential in every diet your body basically needs in proper amounts.

When you eat carbohydrates, they get converted into glycogen and are either used immediately for energy, providing you with a steady dose of blood sugar, or they are stored in the muscles and liver for energy at a later time. Simple carbs by contrast, cause a spike in blood sugar that quickly dissipates, complex carbohydrates consist of a chemical structure that is made up of three or more sugars, which are usually linked together to form a chain. These sugars are mostly rich in fiber, vitamins, and minerals. Due to their complexity they take a little longer to digest, and don't raise the sugar levels in the body as quickly as simple carbohydrates do. Complex carbohydrates act as the body's fuel, and they contribute significantly to energy production.

Without getting into the complexity of complex carbohydrates and simple carbohydrates, it is basically important to know that complex carbs have a higher nutritional value than simple carbohydrates. Their chemical structure are different, and therefore, they can be distinguished by their nutritional properties. The consumption of simple carbohydrates are not recommended, especially for diabetics. The simple refined carbohydrates, found in many processed foods tend to be devoid of important nutrients and pose a greater risk that some of the energy will be converted into fat and stored. Natural complex carbohydrates are often devoid of additives and preservatives and therefore the recommended choice for your carbohydrate needs. Foods that are high in complex carbohydrates are:

- **wheatgerm, oat bran, barley, maize, cornmeal, buckwheat, oatmeal, brown rice, rye bread, yams, shredded wheat, beans, peas, lentils, chick peas, bananas,** nuts, root vegetables, wholemeal pasta, parsnips, potatoes, sweet corn, wholegrain cereals, wholemeal breads, broccoli, cabbage, eggplant, spinach, string beans, apples.

Complex carbohydrates will help provide a slower and more sustained release of energy tha carbohydrates. In their natural form they contribute to long term good health, appetite control and sustained energy levels. Hypoglycemia contributes to FM/CFS, particularly with muscle tightness, fatigue and brain fog. Changing your diet to exclude all of the simple sugars that you have been consuming will be a big advantage in reducing the severity of your symptoms. There is no reason to suffer anymore when you can eliminate the foods that aggravate your condition. The results from a simple diet change will be very gratifying and you will be on your way towards a healthy and speedy recovery!

In his book *"What Your Doctor may Not Be Telling You About Fibromyalgia"* by Dr. R. Paul St. Armand, recommends the following advice:

- **Meats: ensure sugar is not added, especially to low fat cold cuts.**
- **Dairy: as long as it is unsweetened(e.g. Unsweetened yogurt)**
- **Vegetables: most vegetables, except potatoes**
- **Nuts: all nuts.**
- **Fruit: maximum of one piece every 4 hours, avoid bananas. 1 cup of unsweetened orange, grapefruit or tomato juice is allowed as a serving of fruit.**
- **Grains: wholegrain wheat, corn or rye is acceptable. Rice must be wild rice, only consume a small portion. Bread: sugar free whole grain wheat, corn or rye. Consume a maximum of one piece per 4 hours. Eliminate bread temporarily if symptoms persist.**
- **Desserts: artificially sweetened dairy based desserts. Cheesecakes may be made with ground nut base or crust. Avoid chocolate.**
- **Drinks: artificially sweetened drinks, soda water. Avoid all caffeine products. An occasional drink of spirits and dry wine is allowed.**
- **Herbs, spices, dressings, oil and vinegar: all herbs, spices and imitation flavorings are allowed. Use sugar free sauces, salad dressings, mayonnaise, oil and vinegar.**
- **Sweeteners: splenda made using sucralose a natural sugar is a good sweetener to use. It is available in tablets (one tablet is equal to one teaspoon) or in powder form (as an equivalent to sugar). Some chemical sweeteners such as aspartame have negative side effects such as headaches and should be avoided.**
- **Other:**
- **Low carb and sugar free protein bars, shakes and bake mixes**
- **All fats**
- **Carob powder**
- **Gluten, soy or nut flours(high protein, low carbohydrate).**
- **Tofu**
- **Popcorn, maximum 1 cup of popped popcorn**

- **Pork rinds**
- **Tacos**
- **Xanthan gum(used as a thickener in gravy and baking.**

This is considered the basic caveman or paleolithic diet our ancestors have followed for million of years ago and bears no relationship to the modern food pyramid. Atkins, South Beach, Mediterranean and low carbohydrate/glycemic index (GI) diet cook books are an excellent source of recipes.

You may crave sugar initially as your body begins to adjust to the diet; this is normal and will pass after several days. Once you have been on this FM diet cure for after about a month you can treat yourself to an occasional treat, but don't get carried away, because that's how you got to to this condition in the first place, so be careful!

Some people after following the FM diet for at least a month might still have some symptoms of FM/CFS due to food particular intolerances. This may be due to a common dairy and/or wheat gluten which are common food allergens for some people. If that's the case, simply remove all dairy and wheat from your diet for at least one month; if symptoms seem to improve reintroduce one at a time to determine if one or both are responsible for your symptoms. If elimination of dairy and wheat fail to give an improvement in symptoms it may be necessary to get a food allergy test completed or begin an elimination diet by keeping a food diary with the associated symptoms.

According to Dr. Donald J. Lepore, ND, DN, NMD a nutritional research pioneer and director of the "Life Extension Research Center in Jersey City, N.J., has utilized bio-kinesiology in nutritional therapy, believes that all food allergies (Metabolic Antagonist) have a nutritional antidote. He points out in his book *"The Ultimate Healing System:The Illustrated Guide To Muscle Testing & Nutrition"* based on his experience in treating clients, states that "many illnesses are cause by the body's inability to absorb nutrients because the source of these nutrients are hostile to the body, referring this hostility to Metabolic Antagonism" which is another way of saying "Allergies".

Dr. Lepore attributes this condition to each substance that is a metabolic Antagonist (or allergic substance) is caused by or attributed to a certain nutrient, or combination of nutrient deficiencies. And furthermore, it has also been found that specific vitamins, minerals, and amino acid combinations are necessary for the complete absorption of particular foods.

For example, in the absorption of yeast, which is a source of B complex vitamins, the mineral important for the *absorption of yeast is Zinc*. Therefore an allergy to yeast can be corrected by just taking *Zinc*. Other vitamins that could also be lacking and could subsequently cause a yeast allergy, would be the vitamin *B1(thiamine) and B6 (pyrdoxine). Herbs* which can be used to correct a yeast allergy are; *Pau D'Arco, red Clover(rich in zinc) and Comfrey.* And the amino acid necessary to alleviate a yeast allergy is *Lysine, also found in Comfrey.*

The common allergy that we're concerned with "Wheat". Vitamins such as *vitamin E* are often made from wheat germ and are not absorbed properly by the person with a "wheat allergy" have found the antidotes to wheat allergy to be *"Magnesium"*, the *amino acid "Histidine"*, and *vitamin "F" (Linoleic Acid)* which exists in poly unsaturated fats such as *olive oil(also contains vitamin E), safflower oil, castor bean oil, and peanut oil.* The *herbs Black Walnut and kelp* are also helpful in correcting wheat allergies, as they are naturally rich in *Magnesium and other essential minerals.* A *lack of Sodium* and the *amino acid Histidine* will also cause an allergy to wheat.

Dairy allergies can be corrected by the administration of *"Potassium"*. Dairy products like milk and cheese can be allergic if there is a deficiency in potassium in the body. Once the potassium deficiency level is brought back up, the person will tolerate milk more readily. The milk or dairy allergy is also corrected by the amino acid *Aspartic Acid and vitamin D*. It is also interesting to note that when a person's sodium and potassium levels have been depleted, they have been found to be allergic in everything. And this may also be a reason why more people tend to eat more salads in the summer.

The salads have the natural sodium that is needed to correct the allergic condition that arises when heat and temperature is excessive. When there is a sodium deficiency, greens are very important as they contain the vital organic sodium that is needed to help correct the allergic condition. That is also why many times in the summer when people go to the beach for the day and return home feeling exhausted. Usually due to the loss of **Sodium and Potassium** and the loss the **vitamin F(EFA's)** burned up from the sun.

Another likely common cause of food intolerance that more than half of the FM/CFS patients is *"Leaky Gut Syndrome"* that research has been conducted on was proteins, particularly dairy and wheat (gluten), not being fully digested and via leaky gut passing into the bloodstream where they shouldn't be and causing disruption/blocking biochemical and neurological processes. Leaky Gut Syndrome is one of the many concepts in medicine that cuts across the boundary lines of specific diseases. It is a major example of an important medical phenomenon that causes distress in one organ to cause disease in another. Leaky Gut syndrome is not generally recognized by conventional physicians, but evidence is accumulating that it is a real condition that affects the lining of the intestines.

Chapter 20

What Is Leaky Gut Syndrome?

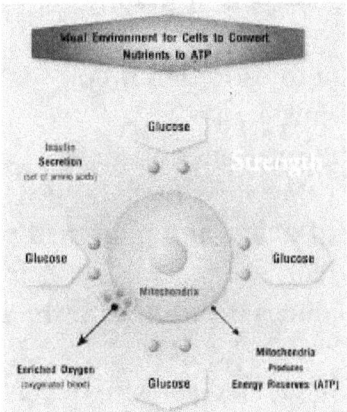

Leaky Gut Syndrome (LGS) is a name given to a condition in which the ability of the intestinal wall to keep out large and undesirable molecules is reduced. Hence the name, substances that are normally kept outside of the body and within the intestines, are "leaking" across the intestinal wall and into the body as a whole. This happens when the spaces between the cells of the intestinal wall become enlarged for various reasons.

Leaky Gut Syndrome is ever hardly tested for a diagnosed by doctors in general practice but there are vast amounts of research implicating altered permeability of the intestinal wall in a large number of illnesses. Indicators that might reveal a diagnosis of Leaky Gut syndrome are normally of the inflammatory bowel conditions which include – Crohn's disease, celiac disease, IBS(irritable bowel syndrome), rheumatoid arthritis, or asthma.

Dr. Sandy Newmark, who deals with leaky gut syndrome in children, states that it isn't clear how many people have this disorder or exactly what problems can be attributed to it, but states also that a significant percentage of children with autism have <u>increased intestinal permeability</u>, but it isn't known whether this is a cause or an effect of food sensitivities and an underlying metabolic problem.

What Causes Leaky Gut Syndrome?

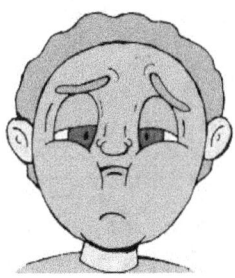

There are quite a number of factors that can increase the permeability of the intestinal wall, and according to reports from the [***Lancet 341:49:1993, American Journal of Physiology, 258; 603: 1990, and the Annals of Allergy, 1990***], The following agents can damage gastrointestinal mucosal integrity which can set the stage for "***Leaky Gut Syndrome***", which can be an important source of chronic inflammation, systemic toxicity, and a key factor in food hypersensitivities.

- **Bacterial infections of an intestinal matter.**
- **Ethanol (beer, liquor, wine, etc.)**
- **Food allergy (insufficient nutrient anti-dotes)**
- **Drugs and Xenobiotics (the worst include NSAIDs -non-steroidal anti-inflammatory drugs, anti-acids, and pain med's-aspirin & ibuprofen)**
- **Toxic Heavy Metals**
- **Stress (chronic stress reduces blood flow to the gut leaving it unable to repair itself)**
- **Poor quality diet (high in refined carbohydrates, high sugar diet, food additives, preservatives, etc.)**
- **Parasite infestation.**
- **Mycotoxins (candida, caused by anti-biotic use and endotoxemia)**
- **Viral infections(deficient immunoglobulins)**
- **Alcohol and caffeine (these irritate the gut wall)**
- **Insufficient digestive enzymes(caused by maldigestion)**
- **Poor liver functions resulting in inflammatory toxins being excreted into the intestines in bile.**

Due to the above attributed affects in "Leaky Gut Syndrome", the immune system starts making anti-bodies against the larger protein molecules because it perceives them as a being foreign, invading substances. Anti-bodies are produced against the "invading proteins" and previously well tolerated foods. It is then that these antibodies can get into various tissues and trigger an inflammatory reaction when the corresponding food is consumed.

This will occur because the bodies tissues have antigenic sites very similar to those on the foods, bacteria, parasites, candida, or fungi. Which then auto anti-bodies are thus created and inflammation can become chronic. If this inflammation occurs in a joint, auto-immune arthritis develops.

If it occurs in the blood vessels, vasculitis (inflammation of the blood vessels) is the resulting auto-immune problem. If it occurs in the muscles and multiple organ systems, the result may very well be Fibromyalgia or ME.

<u>Note:</u> it is possible to measure the permeability or "leakiness" of the gut wall be a simple test called the "Indicans Test". You are also likely to have a leaky gut if you suffer with one of the ""Clinical Conditions with Altered Intestinal Permeability" Listed above. The Indican test is an efficient aid used by many naturopathic practitioners in screening for bacterial links to digestive issues. The Indican test can be a valuable and useful tool for monitoring degeneration or improvement in digestion efficiency of your system in dealing with protein. Indican is formed by an abnormal metabolism of tryptophan (which is normally associated with FM/CFS patients).

Indican is a by-product of putrefacation (protein degradation), usually in the intestine, but possibly in other locations as well. Putrefaction is the anaerobic bacterial decomposition of proteins. When the product of this putrefaction is absorbed into the blood stream, an increase in urinary indican is seen. This increase can also be seen if bacterial decomposition of body tissues or fluids occurs, as in gangrene, abscesses, etc.

Among the pathological conditions in which urinary indican is likely to be elevated are hypochlorhydria (low stomach acid production), inhibited peristaltic movement (the involuntary muscular "waves" that move food through your bowels), and the poor production of digestive bile secretions from the gallbladder and liver. Elevated indican levels are often high in cases of diarrhea, and it is also a good indicator for the breakdown of proteins accompanied by gastrointestinal permeability (the leaky gut). To perform this test, urine is collected and treated with "Obermeyer reagent "(ferric chloride dissolved in hydrochloric acid) and chloroform. The color of the solution is then observed. A clear solution indicates a negative test while an opaque or indingo color indicates a positive result. The conditions normally associated with increased Indican are:

- **Inflammatory bowel disease**
- **Celiac Disease**
- **Hypochlorhydia**
- **Gastric Ulcer**
- **Biliary and intestinal obstruction**
- **Sclerodema**
- **Diminished peristalsis**
- **Increased protein or tryptophan consumption**

(Additional Resources "Indican Test"- "Pizzorno, J., Murray, M. textbook of Natural Medicine. 2nd ed. New York, Churchhill. 1999; p 245-246) -(Todd J. Clinical diagnosis and management by laboratory methods. Philadelphia, PA: WB Saunders. 1979: p 592-593)

A high lectin diet also typically increases indican levels. Foods high in lectins include grains, beans, and night shades. To reduce your intake of lectins, avoid all types of grains, especially wheat, corn, barley, oats, rye and rice, according to a paper published in 1999 in "World Review of Nutrition and Dietetics", which includes *breads, crackers, buns, pizza dough, breakfast cereals, tortillas, muffins, cakes and cookies.* Avoid the beans found in "hummus", soups, and bean salad as well as peanut butter and soy based foods. Limit night shades, vegetables and fruits, such as tomatoes, eggplants, potatoes, bell peppers, hot peppers and goji berries.

Your lectin diet should consist of low lectin foods. All vegetables and fruits contain some lectins, but most vegetables contain low levels compared to some night shades, vegetables and fruits. For example, *you can eat onions, garlic, mushrooms, broccoli, bok choy, cauliflower, leafy greens, pumpkin, squash, sweet potato, carrots and asparagus as well as berries, citrus fruits, pineapple, cherries and apples.* You can also eat *animal proteins, from fish, seafood, eggs, meat and poultry, as well as fats from olive oil, avocado, butter, cream and lard, which all have low levels of lectins.*

(References- "Worls Review of Nutrition and Dietetics"; Cereal Grains: Humanity's Double Edged Sword; Loren Cordain;199(PDF) (Vitamin Research Product: Lectins; Carolyn Pierini)(Weston A. Price Foundation: Be Kind To Your Grains; Sally Fallon and Mary G. Enig; Jan. 2000)

Treatment For Leaky Gut Syndrome

A Leaky Gut Syndrome is basically caused by inflammation of the gut lining. This inflammation causes the spaces between the cells to enlarge, allowing the absorption of large protein molecules. These protein molecules are normally broken down into much smaller pieces before being absorbed through the normally small spaces between the gut lining cells. Treatment involves avoiding inflammatory agents, involves avoiding alcohol, NSAIDs, allergic foods. One of the best treatments for leaky gut syndrome is **"Bovine Colostrum."** *Findings published in the March issue of the "American Journal of Physiology-Gastrointestinal and Liver Physiology,"* stated bovine colostrum can massively reduce gut permeability – otherwise known as 'leaky gut syndrome.' *(http://ajpgi.physiology.org/)*

Among the list of findings caused by leaky gut syndrome it was attributed to the following – Leaky Gut syndrome causes most food allergies; A Leaky gut causes a weakened ability to resist infectious organisms; Leaky gut syndrome creates a long list of mineral deficiencies; Leaky gut syndrome is almost always associated with auto-immune disease.

(Sources – Immune-Tree; "Colostrum Heals Leaky Gut Syndrome"; by Thomas E. Stone, ND, CNHP)

In addition, make sure you include eating an anti-inflammatory diet that includes *essential fatty acids like fish oils (see EFA's diet & supplements), and GLA.* In addition, try supplementing with *L-Glutamine*, an amino acid that helps maintain intestinal metabolism and function and seems to benefit patients who have had intestinal injury from chemotherapy and radiation. Leaky gut syndrome also creates a host of nutritional deficiencies, including minerals, essential fats, vitamins and proteins. Leaky gut syndrome can also create a host of nutritional deficiencies, including minerals, essential fats, vitamins and proteins, if left uncorrected.

This inflammation process damages the various carrier proteins present in the gastro-intestinal tract, needed to transport vital nutrients from the intestines to the blood. For example magnesium deficiency is quite common in conditions such as FM and CFS, despite a high magnesium intake through diet and supplementation.

If the carrier protein for magnesium is damaged that is required for magnesium to be transported, a magnesium deficiency thus develops as a result of this malabsorption. Muscle pain and spasms can occur as a result of this. Similarly, other mineral deficiencies result due to malabsorption. For example, a Zinc deficiency can result in hair loss or baldness as occurs in alopecia areata, another auto-immune disease.

A leaky gut syndrome does not absorb nutrients properly. Nutrients are vital to bodily functions and glandular functions, without the required nutrients that our cells depend on, situations or conditions such as bloating, gas, alternating diarrhea with constipation, and cramps occur, leading to irritable bowel syndrome. Eventually, systemic complaints such as fatigue, headaches, memory loss, poor concentration, or irritability develop. ***Leaky Gut Syndrome can be resolved, you have before you the necessary information to reverse this condition.***

(References and Resources)
(Leaky Gut Syndrome, Professor Keith Scott Murphy)
(Leaky Gut Syndrome: A Modern Epidemic Part I & II, Jake Paul Fratkin, OMD)
(Leaky Gut Syndrome: The Internal Terrorist – Gloria Gilbere)
(Leaky Gut Syndrome: Breaking The Vicious Cycle – Dr. Leo Gallard)

How You Can Improve the Intestinal Integrity

Having a proper and healthy digestive system is very important to your overall health and quality of life. We are what we eat, scientifically speaking and it is necessary that we do our best to take care of one of the most important systems in our body - "the digestive system". Foods we eat on a daily basis nutritionally, effect every aspect of bodily function. From our brain to overall organ and glandular function, digestion and absorption of nutrients are important in preventing disease and maintaining health.

Correcting a malfunctioning digestive system can have an immediate impact on the relief of symptoms and a gradual improvement in the underlying condition. Maintaining a healthy population of bacterial flora(good bacteria) by consuming proper amounts of probiotic cultures
That can help you maintain the natural balance of other organisms in the digestive tract and intestines. The human digestive tract ranges from 25 to 35 feet and houses over 400 species of bacteria. And in total there are over 100 billion organisms in our digestive tract. Disrupting this balance can easily be obtained by an over use of anti-biotics which is equivalent to pouring bleach into a fish tank to kill an overgrowth of algae.

 It is necessary for people taking antibiotics to alternate with Probiotics because antibiotics kill beneficial bacteria along with the bacteria causing the illness. In addition to supplements, probiotics can be found in such foods as yogurt, fermented and unfermented milk, some juices and soy drinks. ***Dannon's Activia Yogurt***, for instance, is an example of a probiotic food.

Today most people are starting to use probiotic supplements to support their digestive system and help them to fight off any infections and to maintain regular bowel movements and cleanse the digestive systems. Researchers are also studying whether probiotics taken as foods or supplements can help treat or prevent illness. There is encouraging evidence that probiotics may help in:

- **Treating diarrhea problems.**
- **Preventing and treating vaginal yeast infections and urinary tract infections.**

- **Treat IBS**
- **Reduce bladder cancer recurrence.**
- **Shorten the duration of intestinal infections.**
- **Prevent and treat inflammation follow**ing colon surgery (pouchitis)
- **Prevent eczema in children.**

To maintain a healthy digestive system it is also important to avoid the unnecessary foods and substances that can contribute to a malfunction digestive tract, which include the following items:

- **Avoid refined sugars and carbohydrates, as this is what feeds unhealthy organisms, especially yeast.**
- **Avoid preservatives, additives, food chemicals, as in processed and can goods, etc.**
- **Avoid moldy or pickled foods such as old peanuts, green tomatoes, dried fruits that are moldy or bitter and yeast extracts.**
- **Avoid long term use of anti-biotics and steroid drugs**

Instead try and do:

- **Eat plenty of fiber in the form of vegetables and fruits, ground seeds and hemp seeds.**
- **Use gluten free fiber powder daily to cleanse the colon.**
- **Follow good hygeine practices.**
- **Use natural *anti-biotics to kill* intestinal yeasts, bacteria and parasites.**

Natural anti-biotic foods include, herbs, garlic, cabbage juice, cruciferous vegetables, cauliflower, brussels sprouts, broccoli, onions, leeks, radishes, fenugreek, ginger, hot chili, lemon juice, tumeric, mustard, rosemary. *Colostrum, Bee Propolis, Kyolic Garlic extract, Olive Leaf Oil extract, Oregano Oil extract are all very good and helpful natural anti-biotics that have a broad spectrum of killing microorganisms and preventing infections.*

- **In many instances it may be necessary to follow a gluten free diet. To see if you are gluten intolerant, have a blood test to check your HLA DQ HLA DR genotype.**
- **Take a good probiotic supplement.**
- **Some people find that by eating fermented foods brings great relief.**

Raw garlic is the most powerful natural anti-biotic for the digestive system. And eating several cloves of garlic every day for several weeks can help you eradicate and expel from your bowels parasites, yeasts, and kill bacteria that could be infecting your digestive tract. For an even more powerful and natural anti-biotic adding rosemary, oregano can also be an affective means of killing bacteria instead of using prescription antibiotics. They can also be used for those who cannot tolerate garlic.

Chapter 21

Establishing The Ultimate Diet For FM/CFS

"The Doctor of the future will give no medicine but will interest his patient in human frame, in diet and the cause and prevention of disease." **Thomas Edison**

"Eat Your Vegetables"
---Your Mother

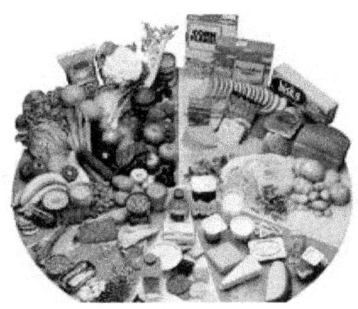

Once your whole body <u>detoxification</u> is complete, you liver, kidneys, your bowels and blood supply is cleansed, and free from toxins, heavy metals, parasites, yeast over growth, your ready to begin your diet. Nutritional support through supplementation will help speed up the healing process and can be looked up in the nutritional healing protocol. The foods that will be listed here will help you to win the battle against FM and CFS.

When dealing with a diet change, especially when one has been so accustomed to eating incorrectly for years and have destroyed their health unknowingly, can sometimes be one of the hardest in making a change. This, I have found out to be very difficult with most people, many just like to eat what they have been so accustomed to, such as the popular junk fast foods and sweets. Avoiding them has been a major problem for many, but if we want to stay and be healthy free from disease and illness, we must make this change! If you want to be free from FM and CFS.

<u>Know that statistics show that by just changing your diet to healthy and nutritious foods, over 90% of those that have, recovered from the illnesses 100% of the time.</u> And many of those patients that have recovered from FM and CFS after treatment and recommendations, have improved their quality of life. Remember, your body in general always strives to heal itself, nature and "God" has designed us in that way. Healthy foods provide the nourishment we need to sustain life and function correctly to fight off disease. It is imperative that you get in the right frame of mind in order to establish a healthy diet regimen.

 Supplements are derived from foods, plants, and herbs and are of a natural order that are bodies are able to distinguish and utilize for healing, drugs are not and are made of synthetic chemicals that do not agree with the body.

That's why every prescription drug has a given side effect, and in supplemental herbs, nutrients, vitamins, and minerals, side effects are a beneficial thing that normally corrects the main healing objective and creates an additional side effect that's normally beneficial by correcting other area's of the body.

It is important for you to keep a list of foods to avoid while on your FM/CFS diet and post where you can see it on a daily basis on the refrigerator or office area, or anywhere where you'll likely see it the most. This way it will remind you and embed itself in your thoughts. So, before we list the healing and most nutritious foods, we list the most harmful and nutrient devoid foods that do nothing but create illness and side effects.

Foods To Avoid: The Link To Illness & Disease

- Commercialized, heavily processed and packages foods designed for long shelf life have artificial preservatives (Nitrates, BHT, BHA), additives (Olestra, MSG)) and chemicals (potassium bromate). They contain hidden toxins, metals and contaminants that get processed and stored in your liver.

- Foods that contain **Trans Fatty Acids** -found in cookies, crackers, icing, potato chips, margarine and micro-wave pop corn. 80% of trans fats in the American diet comes from factory produced partially hydrogenated vegetable oils, and is sometimes added to packaged hamburger meats. Trans fats pose a higher risk for heart disease than saturated fats, which were once believed to be the worst kind of fats. Trans fats raise total cholesterol levels and deplete the good cholesterol (HDL) which helps protect against heart disease.

- **Aspartame** – this artificial sugar substitute in ***Equal and Nutrasweet*** is added to 9,000 food products, and is not fit for human consumption. This toxic poison changes to "formaldehyde" in the body and has been linked to *migraines, seizures, vision loss and symptoms relating to Lupus, Parkinson's disease, Multiple Sclerosis, and other health destroying health conditions.* Aspartame/Nutrasweet breaks down to poisons in the body, and besides that it cause carbohydrate cravings leading to unnecessary weight gain. There is also evidence that the *"Burning Mouth Syndrome"* experienced by desert storm troops was actually Methanol poisoning from the diet coke they drank lots of, after exposed to desert temperatures. Why the FDA allows this poison to be used by the American public remains a mystery and is beyond me. To find out more about the deadly health risks posed by this toxic sweetener go to www.aspartamekills.com (stay away from this harmful substance)

- **Propyl gallate** – this preservative used to prevent fats and oils from spoiling, might cause cancer. It is used in vegetable oil, meat products, potato sticks, chicken soup base and chewing gum, and is often found with BHA and BHT.

- **(MSG) Monosodium Glutamate** – is actually an amino acid used widely as a flavoring agent in frozen food dinners, salad dressings, chips and restaurant food. This additive is also found in Asian foods, like egg rolls, wontons, and is so ubiquitous in or food chain that you would go very hard pressed to go MSG free. Junk foods and instant foods and other mixes contain MSG. Prepared foods in grocery stores and fast food outlets like Kentucky fried Chicken skin is massively loaded with MSG and also fine dinning restaurants. So, when you see the word "citric acid" in prepared food ingredient lists, think MSG. In rats, from early studies in the 1950's reported significant issues with MSG killing the inner layer of their retina, and injuring certain parts of the brain (hypothalamus). Human beings are 5-6 times more sensitive to MSG than rats are. MSG is also a chemo-inducer of obesity, type ll diabetes and metabolic syndrome X.

- **Potassium bromate** – is an oxidizing agent that has been used as a food additive, mainly in the bread making process. It is considered carcinogenic in rats and nephrotoxic in man and in experimental animals. It has been demonstrated to cause renal cell tumors, follicular cell tumors of the thyroid. In addition, experiments were shown that it possesses carcinogen actions.

- **Food Colorings (Blue, Red, Green, Yellow)** – research on animals suggests that these additives may cause cancer, ADHD, ODD(oppositional defiant disorder), and OCD (obsessive compulsive disorder). It also causes thyroid tumors in rats, and may cause them in humans as well. Artificial food colorings are made from coal tar and petrochemicals. Now, who knowingly would eat that? Among other things food colorings are shown to increase hyperactivity in a wide range of children.

- **Sodium Chloride** – known as salt, large doses can lead to heart and blood pressure problems, as well as strokes and kidney failure.

- **Acesulfame-K** – this is a new sweetener used in soft drinks and some baked goods, approved by the FDA in 1998 for use in soft drinks. It is 200 times more sweeter than sugar. Testing on this sweetener has been thus far scant, but some studies do show that it may cause cancer in rats, wow, do you think? Approved by the FDA, what does that supposed to mean? The FDA was set up to protect our health, not to destroy it!

- **Sodium Nitrate** – is a food additive in mostly processed meats, such as, hot dogs, regular bacon, turkey bacon, bologna and many other lunch meats. Used as a preservative to extend the life of meats, and to prevent the growth of bacteria. When eating products that contain sodium nitrates it forms nitrosamines in the human body which are dangerous compounds that are highly carcinogenic. In fact, cancer risk is thought to be higher in meat than other foods, not simply because of the higher saturated fat content, but because of the sodium nitrate content.

- **BHA & BHT** – these are food additives used as preservatives to keep food from spoiling. BHA and BHT can be found in butter, meats, chewing gum, snack foods, dehydrated potatoes, and beer. These additives are approved by the FDA as safe for human consumption. However, they are proven carcinogenic There is proof that some people have difficulty metabolizing BHA and this can result in health and behavioral changes. When ingested by humans, BHA and BHT form a compound that reacts in the body.

- **Olestra** – is a fake fat used to make non-fat potato chips and other type of non fat foods or snacks. Olestra has been show to bind with fat soluble vitamins A, E, D and K and carotenoids, substances thought to keep the immune system healthy and prevent some cancers, and to eliminate them from your system. Proctor and Gamble, the company that produces olestra, has acknowledged the problem with vitamins A, E, D, and K and is now fortifying it with them. Olestra has also caused digestive disturbances in some people, especially when they eat a lot of it.

- **White Sugar** - The white crystalline substance we know as sugar is an unnatural substance produced by industrial processes (from sugar cane or sugar beets) by refining it down to pure sucrose, after stripping away all the vitamins, minerals, proteins, enzymes and other beneficial nutrients. What is left after all the stripping is a concentrated unnatural substance the human body is not able to handle, and consists of the large quantities that is ingested in today's lifestyle. Sugar is very addictive, and in that sense can also be classified as a drug. The average American is known to consume over a 150 pounds of sugar per year. The damage that sugar does is a sow and insidious one. It takes years before it ruins your pancreas, adrenal glands, throws your whole endocrine system out of balance and produces a huge list of damage. It is the main cause of diabetes, hyperglycemia, and hypoglycemia. It is a contributor of heart disease, arteriosclerosis, mental illness, depression, senility, hypertension, and cancer.

NOTE: These additives are some of the main reasons for health issues and disorders that cause many people to become afflicted with serious health problems, and also one the other reasons to turn to organic foods. But by being informed of the potential hidden dangers that lie in our food supply, it can help you make better choices to shop healthier.

Reasons Your Health May Fail

- Consumption of processed and refined foods.(see the list above)
- Accumulation of toxins, poisons, and waste materials.
- Lack of the correct combination of nutrients that all humans need in order to be healthy.
- Lack of oxygen at a cellular level
- Lowered vitality (energy) due to stress, shock, injury, emotional upsets, losses, relationship or financial worries, being unhealthy, etc.

Your healthy depends on you! It's nature's law of the survival of the fittest. Take charge of your health, cause no one can do that for you, not your doctor, your mother, not your spouse, and certainly not the government (FDA). Only you can make that decision.

Avoiding Illness If You Do The Following

- Give your body the nutrients it needs to heal and maintain health – food is medicine!
(see the list of super foods in previous chapters)
- Increase your body's oxygen levels, and it's ability to utilize and transport

oxygen.

(see the list of super foods)

- Improve your digestion and your body's ability to eliminate toxins, <u>by introducing live raw foods rich in enzymes, nutrients, and natural anti-oxidants to help the body rid itself of wastes and toxins naturally.</u>
- Eliminate as many sources of toxins and poisons as possible.

By doing these listed suggestions, you will be better able to withstand the negative influences of stress, shock, injury, emotional upsets, relationship or financial worries and concerns, etc. And you can ensure yourself of a long and healthy life. The body will always try to heal itself, as if having a self built mechanism to adjust itself if need be, but by providing yourself a little assurance it can do a much better job of helping it to speed up the process.

When your body lacks the nutrients and oxygen it needs to heal and maintain health it results in the diseases that are so prevalent today, including cancer, diabetes, auto-immune diseases, fungal diseases (yeast/over growth), degenerative diseases, FM/CFS, malfunctioning organs and systems throughout the body, etc. Some foods, processed foods, sugars, and man made vegetable fats and oils, can all contribute tremendously to diseases and malfunctioning of organ and glandular systems. In the case of cancer, Dr. Otto Warburg who won a Noble Prize for his discovery of the cause of cancer, stated - "Cancer has only one prime cause, the re[placement of normal oxygen respiration of the body's cells by an anaerobic [oxygen-deficient] cell respiration."

<u>Cancer cannot survive in a highly oxygenated state,</u> and <u>its favorite food is sugar in all forms</u> of it, <u>including blood pH that is of an acidic state.</u> That is because man-made vegetable fats and oils (except olive oil), sugars and high carb foods cuts off oxygen from the body's cells. They make your cells weak and lack the necessary oxygen it needs which is a perfect environment for cancer, auto-immune disease, and candida/fungal over growth to occur. On the hand, with the proper nutrition it is possible to reverse cancer, diabetes, and heart disease (the 3 leading causes of death today), along with other diseases and malfunctions, i. e. asthma, CFS, FM, obesity, etc...

Compromising the cells structural integrity with sugar and unnatural fats causes the body to incorporate them into the cell membranes which weakens them until they lack oxygen. This is a perfect scenario for the growth of cancer cells, and candida(yeast over growth). When the body is in a diseased state, such as:

- When cells are not able to utilize and transport oxygen and nutrients.
- Allow toxins and waste material into them.
- Not capable of getting rid of wastes and toxins.
- Blood pH is below 5.0 pH (overly acid state)

Sets the stage for a perfect environment for diseases like cancer, multiple sclerosis, amyotrophic lateral sclerosis, auto-immune disease, lupus, etc. Most of the foods today in grocery stores are laced with chemical additives that contain dangerous toxins and chemicals that disrupt the natural flow and integrity of the human body. Processed foods should be eliminated from your diet, particularly – sugars, and genetically modified foods.

 Industrialization has created foods that aren't really considered "real foods" , because of the many additives and preservatives that doesn't really support or create good health as it did many years ago. Making today's standard American diet unhealthy mainly because the food industry is driven by the food processing and agricultural businesses whose only motivation is for making profits, and not healthy foods.

Foods today are loaded with sugars, damaging man made oils and fats, white flour products, chemicals, food additives and colorings, preservatives, pesticides, and heavy metals, all which are very damaging to health. In fact today we are living in a toxic polluted world. Chemical compounds that are found everywhere in our food supply, water, and air are also found in every person. It is the accumulation of these compounds in people that cause a variety of dysfunctions and diseases affecting our immune system, neurological, and endocrine systems leading to the diseases we have today – auto-immunity, cancer, asthma, neurological illnesses(Alzheimer's, and Parkinson's disease), reproductive dysfunction, diabetes, obesity, etc., etc.

Our food sources are seriously becoming a source of toxin laden compounds that have been approved by the FDA only because the food industry and agricultural businesses spend millions of dollars lobbying for laws that will save them time and money, having been so successful in getting laws passed that allow these poisons in our foods, i.e. preservatives, additives, coloring agents, dyes, binders, stabilizers, emulsifiers, thickening agents, MSG, Nitrates, BHT &BHA, trans fatty acids, Aspartame, potassium bromide, etc.

These laws are passed to only benefit them, and damage our health. The two most significant common ingredients in today's foods that totally disrupt the body's balance and creates illness are sugar and regular table salt (sodium & potassium chloride). Sugar can be classified as a drug, because of it's addictive nature it has on the brain, the brain's primary fuel is glucose (sugar) and chronic use of can lead to over a hundred health problems and diseases. Here are some examples that long term use of sugar can cause:

- Too much sugar can suppress and destroy the immune system which scientists have proven.
- Can upset the mineral balance of the body, interferes with the absorption of calcium and magnesium (vital for healing CFS & FM)
- Produces a low oxygen state which can induce serious diseases, like cancer and yeast over growths (Candida albicans)
- Sugar can cause eye sight problems and cataracts.
- Contributes to diabetes and obesity.
- Can impair the structure of DNA genes.
- Sugar is the #1 enemy of bowel movements.

- Sugar can cause depression, indigestion, constipation, headaches, migraines. Sugar feeds bacterial infections, cancer, fungal diseases, candida/yeast over growth.
- Can cause high blood pressure in obese individuals.
- Sugar can addicting and intoxicating similar to alcohol.
- Sugar can cause or lead to diabetes, candida albicans (yeast over growth), atherosclerosis, cancer, eczema, gallstones, hyperglycemia, hypoglycemia, periodontal disease, osteoporosis, arthritis, asthma, MLS, heart disease, varicose veins, emphysema, gall stones, appendicitis, and many others.

New research confirms that sugar (glucose) competes with vitamin C for insulin mediated uptake into the cells, because of it's similar chemical structure, as was revealed by Dr. John Ely's 30 year study and theory on sugar metabolism.
So, by consuming more sugar or sugar by-products, less vitamin C will be allowed into the cells, and vice-versa. It is also interesting to see that the intake of vitamin C also helps to lessen the carving for sugar, alcohol, and carbohydrates. So does the amino acid *Glutamine* and the herb *Gymnestra Sylvestra* also help to stop or reduce the craving for sugar products and carbohydrates. An excellent book to read about sugar and the physical and psychological disorders it can create is *"The Sugar Blues"* by **Bill Duffy**.

Sugar is one of the most easiest and deadliest substances to become addicted to, because it is literally put in so many food products. **Table salt** is another widely used poison, and know that there is a big difference between regular table salt and natural salt. *Sally Fallon,* author of *"Nourishing Traditions",* sates that salt contains two very important macronutrients that are critical to health, which are sodium and chloride, that all bodily fluids contain sodium and it is essential to life. Needed for many of the biological functions that include water balance regulation, fluid distribution on either side of the cell walls. Muscle contractions and expansions, nerve stimulation, and acid alkaline balance.

The adrenal glands also require sodium for the proper functioning as well. Chloride on the other hand is necessary for the production of hydrochloric acid and for protein digestion, plus chloride helps to activate the production of amylase produced by the pancreas which is needed for carbohydrate digestion. Chloride is also required for the growth and functioning of the brain. The most important source of chloride is salt, and only trace amounts are found in most foods that include celery and coconuts. Fermented beverages, and bone broths also provide easily assimilated chloride.

And contrary to popular belief, natural salt doe not cause high blood pressure like what most people are led to believe, it is actually essential for the regulation of of blood pressure in conjunction with water. Most people do not realize that there are differences between the standard table salt and healthy natural salt. Most common table salt is poison and does not even compare with natural salt, table salt is made up of chemicals that pollute your body and wreck havoc on your health. Healthy natural salt is composed of natural elements and have over 84 minerals necessary for your health. We can not live without salt

- Salt is an essential nutrient required for blood pressure regulation, transport of nutrients into and out of our cells, ion exchange, and brain muscle communication.
- Low salt diets are associated with higher cardiac risks.
- Natural salt is 84% sodium chloride, 16% naturally occurring trace minerals, including silicon, phosphorus and vanadium.
- Natural salt (sodium chloride) is a major component of blood plasma, lymphatic fluid, and even amniotic fluid.
- Supports the function of your adrenal glands, which produce dozens of vital hormones.

While natural unrefined salt has many health benefits and is essential to life, that does not mean you should ingest it with impunity. Another factor to consider is the potassium to sodium ratio of your diet.
As an imbalance in this ratio can lead hypertension and can contribute to a number of diseases, including: heart disease, kidney stones, dementia, osteoporosis, cataracts, erectile dysfunction, ulcers and cancer of the stomach, and rheumatoid arthritis. And the easiest way to achieve this imbalance is to consume a diet of processed foods, which are notoriously low in potassium while high in sodium.

If you eat a diet of processed foods, you van be virtually guaranteed that your potassium-sodium ratio is upside down. To ensure yourself of getting these two important nutrients in more appropriate ratios, stop eating processed foods, which are high in processed salt and low in potassium and other essential nutrients, and eat a diet of whole unprocessed foods, ideally organically grown to ensure optimal nutrient content. This type of diet will naturally provide much larger amounts of potassium in relation to sodium. Interesting books to read are *"Water: Rx for a Healthier Pain-Free Life" by Dr. Batamanghelidj.*

By being aware of the hidden potential of sugar and refined salt, two of the hidden poison ingredients in today's processed foods, among the other listed toxins that are also added will be the first step and the correct path towards wellness.

The **basic specific food rules** for people with FM and CFS to consider avoiding to improve your recovery towards optimal health are:

- **Aspartame (NutraSweet)** this artificial sweetener can exacerbate pain. Other artificial sweeteners such as splendida, saccharin, and stevia do not appear to have the same effect as aspartame.
- **All food additives** including MSG can intensify pain.
- **Sugar, fructose, and simple carbohydrate**s like sugar, cake, or white bread can also have an impact and should be avoided. They can contribute to infections, such as yeast over growth and impair the function of your immune system and vitamin absorption.
- **Caffeine** including coffee, tea, colas, and chocolates are also false sources of energy that quickly exacerbate fatigue. Avoid them also all together along with

beer and alcohol products.

- **Yeast and gluten** – yeast can foster overgrowth of yeast fungus which may cause or exacerbate joint and muscle pain. Gluten intolerance results in a variety of stoma ch ailments and digestive problems and is also associated with fatigue in patients with Fibromyalgia.
- **Dairy products** do contain calcium to build bones and protein to build muscle but for some people with FM and CFS may experience an increase in symptoms from consuming dairy products. You can avoid them completely or limit use but make sure their of organic sources.

Take charge of your diet and learn to discover your own food sensitivity by experimenting with an elimination diet. Keep track in a food diary by tracking your intolerance to foods that may cause symptoms and eliminate the foods that trigger any pain or discomfort.

List any associated trigger that brings on a reaction and learn to replace that food with another food source of the same nutrients. For example, if you think corn is causing you a problem, you can replace corn with another carbohydrate such as rice.

If allergy symptoms go away after the food is taken out of your diet, and then they come back when the food is eaten again, a diagnosis may be made. Educating yourself about how your body reacts to different foods so you can practice good nutrition and create a diet that works for you is the best thing you can do yourself to treat Fibromyalgia. Sticking to a diet that's best for you is the hard part. But if you don't succeed, try, try again!

A study published in the Journal Rheumatology International showed that free radicals and inflammation may play a role in the development of Fibromyalgia., so adding more of the rich anti-oxidant type foods to your diet may help relieve some of the symptoms. More than 60% of FM and CFS patients diagnosed with chronic digestive disorders, such as, food allergies, irritable bowel syndrome and leaky gut syndrome, which can be triggered by certain foods. That's why diet is a potentially powerful weapon for controlling FM and CFS symptoms, AND can be reversed by making appropriate nutritional healthy lifestyle choices. Even many doctors, who have traditionally been long on drugs and short on proper nutrition in their practices, now recommend whole foods to their patients. Because of the continuing increase in cancers and diseases that have been linked to junk food diets have finally gotten the attention of people and the medical community it deserves.

People are finding that they are feeling much better when they eat natural foods, and that they actually taste better as well. School systems are also replacing their vending machines with fresh fruits instead of the junk foods normally found. Consumer awareness is increasing and people are starting to realize that old fashioned natural foods are much healthier for them. Making the transition from the addictive junk foods to whole natural healthy foods can be difficult for some people, so, therefore the best way in doing this is to make substitutions from dead junk foods to live wholesome foods.

Making Transitional Changes From Junk Food To Live Healthy Foods

Junk food is in my view characterized as being dead, refined, and adulterated. It can be summarized simply by saying – junk food is just that "junk food", it produces deficiencies, toxicities, and eventually sickness. Food manufactures know that sugar and salt are addicting and take advantage on millions of people to become addicted, with the average American consuming over 150 pounds of sugar a year. Nearly all commercially processed foods, condiments, including vegetables, fruits, cereals, and meats, contain some kind of sugar either as a flavoring agent or preservative. And it almost seems impossible to buy anything in the supermarket that does not contain sugar or a sugar substitute that may be even worse. We have become a society of "Sugarholica".

It's become so bad now that the Senate Select Committee on Nutrition and Human Needs received testimony that if sugar were being proposed as a new additive today its "metabolic behavior" would undoubtedly lead to it being banned. Sugar causes the blood sugar to rise rapidly and in this process the pancreas is over stimulated resulting in too much insulin going into the blood stream to control the sugar.

This cause the blood sugar level to plummet only to result in the sugar addict needing another sugar fix to raise the blood sugar levels again, by having another doughnut and a cup of coffee. When sugar becomes like a drug its called "hypoglycemia"

Completely changing one's diet overnight often results in withdrawal symptoms and as a holistic health practitioner, I have noticed it is sometimes the hardest thing to do for most individuals. The change for some leads to feelings of deprivation, nervousness, and anxiety. By using this simple withdrawal program that follows you can get unhooked from junk food and make this transition the same way you got hooked, gradually. You didn't get to become a junk food addict over night, and neither will you get unhooked overnight, but you will get unhooked!

Fibromyalgia pain relief will always begin with what you put into your stomach. A diet for Fibromyalgia. which includes lean meats, poultry, fresh vegetables, and fruits should be what your eating. And if you think that a healthy diet change will make no difference think again!

"We are at a point now where we know that diet plays a role in this disease." Kent Holtorf, MD, medical director of the Holtrof Medical Group Center in Torrance, California.

Step 1 – adopt the correct attitude and withdrawal can succeed, know that it is for your benefit, and only you can make that change for the betterment of your health. Keep

FM/CFS food diary will help you eliminate personal triggers for pain and also let you know which foods make you feel good. It may be a trial and error process, but rest assured it will be worth it. By eating healthy, you will be working toward a better quality of life because you'll be healthier overall.

Step 2 – **choose *power foods like vegetables and fruits that are listed in the super***

food section of this book. They are _low in calories, high in live enzymes, high in fiber, and rich in anti-oxidants and phytochemicals._ This will be especially helpful for those battling obesity, digestive problems, or auto-immune disease, all of which is common with FM and CFS. Plus natural foods lack the additives that we want to avoid that can aggravate the symptoms of FM/CFS.

Step 3 - choose lean high qulaity protein foods _(not processed),_ and reducing your carb intake can help you to avoid blood glucose levels from fluctuating, which can trigger unnecessary fatigue. Choosing _lean beef, eggs, fish, pork, chicken, turkey, and whey protein isolates, as in a powdered shake,_ are important to FM sufferers. Proteins should be the essential part of your FM diet. Because they will help repair the damaged muscle tissues and fibers that FM and CFS patients suffer from.

Step 4 – Include the "good fats" (**EFA's**) found in cold water fish and in nuts (walnuts) to help with anti-inflammatory support. Omega 3 fatty acids can give some much needed Fibromyalgia pain relief. Natural fats like avocados, guacamole, organic butter, coconut, seeds, nuts, olives/olive oil, helps produce hormones that promote cell repair and brain function. You need essential fats to help digest and metabolize proteins.(see section on essential fatty acids for specific foods)

Step 5 – _Avoid caffeine, sugar, white flour, and simple carbs_ that can cause hypersensitivity to blood sugar highs and lows. _Cutting back on starches, which are also carbs in bread, pasta, candy, baked goods, regular soda, and rice, should be avoid as well._ Some of the carbs from fruits and vegetables (fibrous starches) are OK, and will be about choices and discipline. Example, if you find a food contains more than 20 grams of carbs per serving just skip it. As a general guide line, you should be only consuming between 75 to 90 grams of carbs a day.

Refined Carbohydrates: White sugar and corn syrup is in everything, it seems. And fructose and high fructose corn syrup is no better, corn products that are highly refined carbohydrates that drastically depress the immune system. Something that FM and CFS patients do not need, and according to the _"Linus Pauling Institute"_ high glycemic load diets have been associated with increased serum levels of C-reactive protein (CRP), a marker of systemic inflammation that is also a sensitive predictor of cardiovascular disease risk." If you eat something that is high in sugar, it stimulates the

inflamation response and taxes the immune system. The more processed the food, the higher the glycemic level, the more chemicals, and the less food value.

Step 6 – Avoid artificial sweeteners and chemical additives as exposed in **recent list of specific food rules to follow and avoid. Basically items that you should not be consuming are:**

- White sugar and white flour products
- High fat dairy foods
- Fried foods or greasy foods
- Preservatives, junk foods, and salt

- Red meat, cured bacon, smoked foods, or nitrate cured.
- Coffee and caffeinated beverages
- Colas, soda pop, carbonated beverages
- Alcoholic beverages
- Liquid with your meals
- All forms of tobacco
- Nutrasweet and saccharine

Conclusion:

A diet for FM/CFS which is all natural is the "key" and one of the best ways to achieve pain relief quickly. Just mix and match from the recommended foods till you find the ones that sit well with you, we are all different and what may work for you may not work for another person. If submitting to your FM diet correctly, you should start to seeing a notable difference in your appearance and your FM pain relief.

Books that I highly recommend are *"The Fibromyalgia Cookbook" Mary L. Moeller, and "The Fibromyalgia Nutrition Guide" Mary L. Moeller.* The rewards and benefits of changing dietary habits far outweigh any detriment. At first it may seem like a tall order, so it is important to realize that no one expects perfection.
 A minor indulgence on limited occasions will not cause any significant harm. The key is to make major changes in dietary habits over the long term haul. Once you begin to experience the benefits, the motivation to continue eating well will not wane. I hope this helps to shed some light on what constitutes the best diet for FM and CFS.

The best diet for Fibromyalgia is the one that best suits your needs, that is easy to digest and breaks down the foods and absorbs the nutrients the food has to offer you. Your pain relief begins with what you put in your stomach. You are at a point now where you know that diet will play a big role in this dreaded disease. Your goal is to get you headed towards a natural and safe treatment plan without any side-effects.

Chapter 22

PUTTING IT ALL TOGETHER: THE ESSENTIAL STEPS IN HEALING FMS/CFS

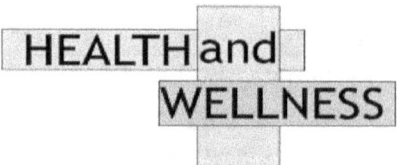

"Every Case of FMS & CFS Is Said To Have a Deficiency"

To Fully understand the treatments given for FMS and CFS it is best to restate the findings in these cases, in which many are complications or associated conditions found progressively among the many and each symptoms governing the multiple causes of affliction concerning FMS and CFS. We will break down each one at time, so you can further get a better understanding of each possible area of the body that could be affected by FM and CFS.

The Digestive System *** – Malabsorption of foods consumed > can create Protein (amino acids) deficiency resulting in enzyme loss, essential fatty acids (EFA's), vitamins, and mineral deficiencies. **Which can create a multitude of deficiencies – hormonal & neurotransmitters.**

Toxicity Syndrome* ** – of heavy metals, toxins, parasites, yeast over growths, toxic bowels (ileocecal valve malfunction), liver malfunction, sluggish gallbladder and bile secretion. Infected and toxic kidney function. **Prelude to disease manifestations.**

Chronic Viral Infection *** – particularly Candida albicans, Epstein Barr virus = CFS and FMS. **Can cause the destruction of the immune system to malfunction (auto-immune illness)**

Tissues *** – including bones (calcium/phosphorus) low levels from lack of protein transport due to malfunctioning digestive system.

Lack of Neurotransmitters & Hormonal Output of Imbalanced levels *** – insulin, thyroid, cortisol, adrenal, glutathione, serotonin, dopamine, acetylcholine, DHEA, and sex hormones, testosterone, estrogen, progesterone, from improper amino acid metabolism and absorption from digested food intake. **(Leaky Gut Syndrome)**

Lymphatic Slow down *** – improper functioning of the immune system. Improper function of the immune cells. **(auto-immune disease)**

Sinus Infections ** – viral, bacterial, yeast, and fungus. Resulting from improper dietary habits (too much sugary products and poor lifestyle habits) can also be the cause of a widespread infectious problem.

Other infections bacterial ** – Possible Lymes disease, parasite infestation, yeast over growths.
(same as sinus infections)

Lack of Detoxification Mechanisms in the Liver *** – allowing heavy metals (mecury is the only one) to remain in the body. This is where the lack of sulfur results in removal failure and Glutathione's inadequate production. Liver unable to function and retain body's natural detoxification mechanisms **due to impurities and toxins imbedded in deep tissue cells. Resulting from very bad dietary habits that include too much staturated fats, sugar, and chemical residues from contaminated food products and preservatives.** Most important organ in the body for preserving whole body detoxification and proper functioning of liver health in creating a healthy body and state of mind.

Immune Deficiency* - Possible combination of several things, malabsorption problem, leaky gut syndrome, food allergies, improper protein & vitamin-mineral absorption, or combination of. Can create an auto-immune disease.**

Mercury or Other Heavy Metal Poisoning ***– Years of accumulated heavy metal build up, possibly due to mercury fillings, or mercury tainted fish contamination, and possible improper food packaging and processing. Can also create an auto-immune problem leading to the start of auto-immune disease. **(Common problem in our society today that goes by unrecognized)**

Sulfur Deficiency** – Malabsorption problem due to leaky gut syndrome, lack of proper protein digestion, and enzymes. Improper mineral absorption from foods eaten. (Leaky Gut Syndrome) **Can also create an immune system disorder.**

Vitamin/Mineral Deficiencies*** - (same as sulfur deficiency) **Resulting from Leaky Gut syndrome, malabsorption and improper supply of vital enzymes.**

Essential Fatty Acid deficiencies*** -(same as above)

Anti-oxidant Deficiencies ***– (same as above plus not consuming high anti-oxidant foods raw foods or supplements)

Note: *This information has not been reviewed by the FDA. It is general and is not meant to diagnose, prevent, treat or cure any condition, illness, or disease. It is very important that you make no change in your healthcare plan or health support regimen without researching and discussing it in collaboration with your professional healthcare team.*

Natural Therapies For Fibromyalgia & CFS
"That Work"

"Our studies at Harvard suggest that the average physician knows a little more about nutrition than the average secretary --- unless the secretary has a weight problem. Then she probably knows more than the average physician."
------**Jean Mayer (1920-93), Nutrition expert and president of Tufts University in Medford, Massachusetts (1976-92)**

Please note that – *Foods, herbs, and drugs can all interact, sometimes in unexpected ways. Always be alert in what you are taking, as in medications or herbs, vitamins, amino acids, etc., they can all interact and should not be taken together, except your standard vitamins, minerals, and amino acids which are basically derived from food.*

It is sad that the average medical schools in the US receives just 2 ½ hours of training in nutrition over four years, and that's from over 125 medical schools in the US, and 30 of these schools have a required course work in nutrition. As a result of this, most physicians often disregard diet, and nutritional supplementation as an effective means of treating and preventing disease.

Fortunately for those who do find a physician who truly understands the importance of optimum nutrition and who dispenses meaningful advice on diet and nutritional supplementation, are lucky enough to be had. Such physicians are now becoming a rare breed, but let's thank God for Alternative and Holistic Medicine which undermines the whole concept of healing and treating the root cause of disease. You are about to learn some of nature's most powerful substances known to man that have <u>incredible curative healing powers</u>. I have also used many of these, which I call *"Miracle Nutrients"*, in my own personal use, which I have recommended to many of my clients, family members and friends.

"Know that FMS and CFS are Now Treatable"

The nutrients listed below are some of nature's most powerful healing agents that have cured and eliminated many diseases. They are mentioned here to give you an idea of which ones can be best applied to your current given circumstances. ***<u>The ones listed with an asterick* mark are the ones which I feel will give you the most healing benefit</u>. The number of <u>Asterisk marks</u>*-*-* will indicate the importance of the recommended supplements, ranging from one mark (*) being <u>important</u>, to two marks (**) being <u>very</u> important</u>, and three marks (***) <u>most important.</u>***

The first order of requirement is to include a broad spectrum *Multi-Vitamin & Mineral* supplement to use as a solid foundation for nutritional support with extra *B Complex vitamins* taken 2 to 3 times a day for the first two months and then reduce down to one time a day taken with your main meal of the day.

<u>Note:</u> *At the end of the chapter will be a list of examples and combinations of supplements pertaining to your required protocol. The supplements listed in this chapter/book were the ones that dispensed the most healing results. And should be addressed accordingly to your specific illness and symptoms.*

<u>**All One Green Phyto Base Multiple Vitamin and Mineral Powder*** – (by Nutritech)**</u> – This is a very good formula that contains all the necessary vitamins and minerals, amino acids, complemented by a unique blend of organic greens that are rich in catalytic enzymes, chlorophyll, and trace minerals. One scoop of the powder replaces 15 to 20 pills a day, it mixes very easily with any juice and provides you with a potent source of easily assimilated vitamins, minerals, and phytonutrients. All One vitamin and mineral powders come in many different formulas that may be of interest to you, they are highly regarded by many professional and Olympic athletes because they work and you can feel the difference once taken.

<u>**B Complex Vitamins**</u>** - Supplying your body with extra B complex (50 to 100mgs) vitamins will enable you to better handle stress and support vital bodily functions. Even though you are getting plenty from your dietary meals and in your All One Multi-Vitamin supplement it wouldn't hurt by taking a little more for extra added insurance due to the given circumstances as in FMS/CFS. Reputable sources are *Solgar, Solary, Twin Labs, and Country Life.*

<u>**Bovine Colostrum**</u>*** – Produced by pregnant lactating cows. This food/supplement called or referred to as *"the first food for life"* has existed since the first mammals roamed the planet and used by humans of various cultures for thousands of years. In

my opinion, Colostrum should be on every Fibromyalgia/Chronic Fatigue and Auto-Immune patients list of supplements.

Colostrum's potent anti-inflammatory action make it an ideal substance for the healing of many auto-immune system disorders, and that includes especially Fibromyalgia and CFS. Colostrum is a type of milk made by mammals just before and after pregnancy.

Classified as a "high octane milk" colostrum is loaded with nutrients and growth factors supplied by nature to sustain the new born infants initial stages of adolescents. It's full of immunoglobins, which help protect newborns as they come into our world of bacteria and viruses.

Colostrum appears as a clear fluid, golden in color, manufactured by nature to provide a new born with perfect nutrition tailored specifically to their needs, giving them large amounts of living cells which will defend their early years of life against harmful bacterial agents. It is like giving your new born it's first natural 100% safe vaccination.

Bovine colostrum is more potent than human colostrum. The biologically active components are either identical or functionally identical regardless of the species of origin or use. The biologically active components in colostrum can be divided into four basic categories.

(1). **Immune Factors**: Active components that have very significant effects on the immune system, promoting a stronger, more efficient immune response and providing anti-bodies which fight specific infections.

- **Colostrum contains over 95 Immune Factors** to provide protection against bacteria, toxins, viruses and disease. They activate numerous process that are critical to the healthy function of the immune system.

- **Proline-rich Polypeptides (PRP)** are hormones that regulate the thymus gland, stimulating an under active immune system or subduing an over active immune system in cases where it has begun to attack the tissues of the body (auto-immune disorder). An over active immune system has been linked to auto-immune diseases such as multiple sclerosis, rheumatoid arthritis, lupus, scleroderma, chronic fatigue syndrome, fibroblast, and allergies. An under active system is associated with an increased risk for infectious conditions, cancer and bacterially related heart disease.

- **Colostrum** contains all 5 Immunoglobulins (known as antibodies) that support the human immune system.

- **IgA:** neutralizes toxins and microbes in the lymphatic and circulatory system.

- **IgM**: destroys bacteria.

- **IgE and IgD**: highly antiviral

- *IgG*: helps against invading pathogens.

Lactoferrin, has been shown to contain antiviral, anti bacterial, and anti-inflammatory properties. It is also an iron-binding protein with therapeutic actions in cancer, HIV, cytomegalovirus, herpes, chronic fatigue syndromes, fibromyalgia, candid albicans, and other infections. Lactoferrin helps to deprive bacteria of the iron they require to reproduce, and releases iron into the red blood cells enhancing oxygenation of tissues.

Interestingly, many drug manufacturers have tried to isolate and synthesize the individual immune factors found in colostrum, includin interferon and gamma globulin. There is no question that the significantly elevated concentrations of the immune factors, essential factors, and growth factors, and the basics found naturally in colostrum are far superior to medical drugs for many people.

(2). ***Natural Growth Factors: Effective in reducing the symptoms of aging.***
Rejuvenating the body's levels of human growth hormone (HGH) is one of the hottest therapies for helping aging men and women maintain a more youthful vitality. Studies show that an aging person exhibits lower levels of growth hormone than a younger one. With all 87 naturally ocurring anti-aging growth factors found in colostrum, many of the diseases and conditions of aging can be improved.

The biologically active growth factors found in colostrum protect the body against disease and assist the body in the following processes:

- **Stimulates cellular and tissue growth.**
- **Repairs and helps reverse the damage done by disease and the natural aging process.**
- **Increases metabolism.**
- **Reduces fat and increases muscle mass.**
- **Involved in regeneration of the heart, lung and liver tissue, plus other organs and tissues throughout the body.**
- **Stimulates protein synthesis, which is critical for the renewal of the skin and bones.**
- **Affects neurotransmitters in the brain, improving moods and mental acuity.**

These regenerative effects of colostrum extend to nearly all of the body's structural cells, making colostrum invaluable in the quest to prevent premature aging.

(3). **Metabolic Factors:** Influence the restoration and maintenance of the body's proper metabolic levels. One key benefit of colostrum is a rich source of *human growth hormone*, one of the master growth factors that assists the body to efficiently burn fat. This is also supported by research from the Medical Endocrinological Department of the University Clinic of Internal Medicine, Aahus Dommune-hospital, Denmark.

It covers such a broad range of healing effects that target most of the related causes of diseases. Research has shown that colostrum is the one supplement that can bring help to everyone that uses it, largely because of its ability to perform many of the functions of human growth hormone (HGH) in the body. Many scientists believe that colostrum may also be the most important preventative that can be consumed by a mammal.

(4).Essential Factors contained in Colostrum. Compounds whose primary effects are to; promote healing by building, maintaining and repairing bone, muscle, nerves, and cartilage; stimulate fat metabolism, regulate protein metabolism during fasting; maintain balanced blood sugar levels; help to regulate the brain chemicals that control mood; and promote wound healing. Colostrum also contains:

- ***All essential amino acid**s*, the building blocks of the body

- ***Essential fatty acids****.*
- ***All essential glyconutrients*** that facilitate cell to cell communication, support the immune system, and promote proper functions of the nervous and endocrine system. They also are important factors in keeping the cardiovascular system functioning at optimum level.

- ***Epithelial Growth Factors (EGF)*** - are instrumental in protecting and maintaining the skin, and can stimulate normal skin growth. It does this by the combination of IGF-1 and TGF A&B.

- ***Insulin-Like Growth Factors 1 & 2*** – insulin growth factor 1 & 2 are the most abundant growth factors in bovine colostrum. They affect how the body uses fat, protein and sugar; stimulates the immune system; and promotes cell repair and growth. Because every cell in the body has a receptor for IGF-2, it can help every cell actively heal or reproduce. IGF-1 is one of the few substances known that can stimulate growth and repair the important nucleic acids RNA and DNA.

These healing properties make IGF-1 a powerful anti-aging substance. IGF-1 has become a big interest in athletes, bodybuilders and weight management programs because it can help burn fat and stimulate growth of lean muscle tissues. As its name indicates, IGF-1 has properties similar to insulin and has improved blood sugar profiles in type II diabetics. And there is also evidence that IGF-1 helps to lower cholesterol levels LDL and raise HDL cholesterol levelsm, which can help prevent heart disease.

- ***Fibroblast Growth Factor (FBG)*** performs a helper function by increasing the binding ability of IGF-1 by 60% -70%.

- ***Transforming Growth Factors A & B (TGF- A&B)*** stimulate proliferation of cells in connective tissue, assist in formation of bone and cartilage, help repair tissue and , according to one study, support the growth of the gut lining, which is very important in leaky gut syndrome (Fibromyalgia/CFS).

Colostrums many health benefiting values have been documented in clinical observations and is supported by a large data base. Interestingly, a team of scientists in London has now found that colostrum can prevent the death of human neurons and effectively treat Alzheimer's patients. In addition, another team of research scientists was documenting that colostrum can eliminate intestinal inflammation. Colostrums various growth factors have anti-inflammatory actions and help repair damaged cells lining the gastro-intestinal tract, which decreases cellular spacing and prevents further leakage of toxins into the body. Colostrum naturally contains EGF-Epithelial growth factors, which research shows can actually help grow and repair intestinal tissue.

Also, there have been many drug manufacturers that have tried to isolate and synthesize individual immune factors found naturally in colostrum, including **interferon and gamma globin.** But there is no question that for most people, the whole intact immune complement found in colostrum is the far superior source.

As it was also reported in the March 1998 issue of the "American Journal of Natural Medicine", by Dr. Zoltan P. Rona, M.D., M.Sc., in which he stated: *Historically, Ayurvedic physicians have used bovine colostrum therapeutically in India for a thousand years. In the US and throughout the world, conventional doctors used it for its anti-biotic purposes prior to the introduction of sulfa drugs and penicillin. In the early, 1950's colostrum was prescribed extensively for the treatment of rheumatoid arthritis. In 1950, Dr. Albert Sabin, the polio vaccine developer, discovered colostrum contained anti-bodies against polio and recommended it for children susceptible to catching polio."*

Several studies have also shown that by taking pain relievers, also known as NSAIDs, over a short term 1-7 days increases gut permeability (leaky-gut) by approximately three fold. Leaky gut syndromes can lead to auto-immune disease. This can obviously contribute indirectly to many of the symptoms from those who suffer from CFS and Fibromyalgia, who have taken NSAID's for pain associated from FM and CFS. This has been shown in a clinical study conducted in London Raymond Playford and his team of researchers at the Imperial College of Medicine showing that colostrum keeps the gastro-intestinal tract from becoming more permeable, even while taking NSAIDs. They attributed this anti-inflammatory response to the numerous growth factors that occur naturally in colostrum. Unlike other known therapies, colostrum is the only natural substance that has the capability of healing the gastro-intestinal tract and preventing it from becoming too permeable. Thus colostrum may have the potential to slow or stop the progression of an auto-immune disease that progresses as a result of a **_leaky gut syndrome._**

Conclusion – Through studies and research, colostrum has proven to be truly one of nature's wonder substances that can provide a wealth of healing capabilities for individuals who suffer from many health related illnesses and injury. It's healing response can be a great and effective substance in potentially slowing or stopping auto-immune disorders by healing injury in the gastro-intestinal tract and eliminating the leaky gut connection to the disease. Scientific research and clinical studies show the evidence of the powerful immune and growth components in colostrum which can regulate the over active immune response as well as heal tissue damage caused by auto-immune disease.

Reliable resources of "100% pure certified true first-milking colostrum" are – Health

Direct (www.healthdirectusa.com), Immune-tree (www.immunetree.com), Garden of Life (www.gardenoflifeusa.com) which also makes the only goat's milk protein colostrum formula on the market today, called **"Goatein-IG "**. Colostrum also comes in a powder, capsules, and liquid.

(Sources & References – CNR, Center for Nutritional Research; Colostrum & Auto-Immune Disorders; John Balmier, MS; www.icnr.org)

("The Colostrum Miracle" and "Colostrum Life's First Food" by Daniel G. Clark, M.D.)

(Henderson D. (2000) Colostrum: Nature's Healing Miracle. CNR Publications, Sedona, Arizona)

[References – Henderson D., Mitchell D., Colostrum – Nature's Healing Miracle, CNR Publications, Salt Lake City, UT. 1999.]
[Walker M, "The Benefits of Bovine Colostrum", Health Products Business, April, 1999.]

[Rona Z., "Bovine Colostrum emerges as immunity modulator". Alternative Health Directory, Vancouver, BC.,Canada.]

[Burke E, "Athletes; Have You Heard About Colostrum?", health Journal, Vol. II, No. 13: July 21,1999]

[Klatz R., Kahn C., Grow Young with HGH, Harper Collins, New york, NY, 1997.]

Magnesium/Malic Acid*** – Studies show that 90 to 95% of the US population is deficient in magnesium. Most Americans do not obtain the recommended daily allowance of 400 to 500mgs. Additionally, a large majority of Americans consume a diet of processed and cooked foods, which increases the body's demand for magnesium. A very vital element our body needs in order to properly function. It is a co-factor in over 300 enzymatic biochemical functions and is required for energy production, stress management, adrenal gland health, bone formation, nervous system function and relaxation of muscles, and protein synthesis.

Magnesium is also involved in specific enzymatic functions which turn sugar and fat into ATP, an important energy source and it is commonly found in low levels in those with FM and CFS *(Sendur 2008;Bagis 2012)*. A magnesium deficiency worsens the symptoms of Fibromyalgia due to the breakdown in the body's energy production. The brain also relies on ATP for numerous functions as well for sending certain signals along specific brain pathways. Approximately 20% of the body's ATP is locate in the brain. And low levels of ATP can diminish brain cognitive functions, a common problem in people with FM and CFS. Insufficient levels of magnesium causes an increase in a body chemical called substance P, which is responsible for pain perception. In other words, you will experience more pain if you are deficient in magnesium. Fibromyalgia patients have 3 times more **(substance P)** than normal.

Diet and digestion plays a big role in magnesium deficiency due to malabsorption. Often times people with FM have other conditions such as irritable bowel syndrome, leaky gut syndrome, or gluten intolerance, which limits nutrient absorption. Excess amounts of fructose (sugar from fruits and honey) may interfere with magnesium absorption.

Phosphates, which are found in soft drinks, chocolates, ice cream, processed meats and hot dogs, can bind magnesium in the gut and create a magnesium phosphate, a salt that can't be used by the body. Insufficient levels of magnesium experienced in those with FM and CFS affects the nervous system by causing nerves to fire too easily. Noises sound excessively loud, light sensitivity that seems too bright, emotional reactions are exaggerated, and the brain is over stimulated, often times resulting in insomnia which is a big issue with FM and CFS. And most migraine headache victims will also demonstrate a magnesium deficiency as well.

Also most of the B complex vitamins are essential for the electron transport in the respiratory system, and for the utilization of magnesium. Current research has definitely confirmed that a deficiency of magnesium for optimal synthesis of ATP can very clearly lead to the symptoms of fatigue and depression in FM and CFS people. The Kreb's cycle) is a magnesium dependent mechanism and even a slight deficiency of the element will severely impair its function. It is now known that magnesium is needed to help body block toxic effects of aluminum; therefore, aluminum toxicity may play a role in symptoms experienced by magnesium deficient fibromyalgia patients *(Weintraub, 1997).*

Magnesium is also involved in thyroid production and protein synthesis and is necessary in the production of stomach acid and digestive enzymes, which are deficient in people with auto-immune disease and Fibromyalgia. Unfortunately, a magnesium deficiency is not easily detected and is often over looked by doctors. While this mineral is no cure all by any means, but it has been shown to relieve muscle pain and fatigue in individuals with FM and CFS. Magnesium is often given in combination with **Malic acid**.

Magnesium and malic acid has been used quite successfully in people with FM and CFS for quite some time now and the results have been promising. Malic acid in itself can act as a most potent aluminum detoxifier and is especially effective at decreasing aluminum toxicity in the vital organs of the body, especially the brain. It has been shown to significantly increase the fecal and urinary secretion of aluminum, reducing the concentration of the metal found in the internal organs, tissues, and the brain *(Weintraub, 1997)*. A most interesting study revealed that 15 patients between the ages of 32 and 60 were used in an open clinical setting where 600mgs of magnesium and 1,200-2,400 mgs of malic acid were used. The results reported significant relief within just 48 hours of treatment. Results such as this gives us continuous hope that FM and CFS can be remedied effectively and even reversed completely.

Magnesium is the main element in the magnesium malic acid formula as a dietary supplement. The combination of magnesium and malic acid is a form of chelated magnesium that is highly absorbable in the body. Magnesium malic acid or malate is one of the better choices when it comes to choosing a mineral magnesium supplement that is effective.

Magnesium and malic acid can also be purchased in specific fibromyalgia formulas such as
"Fibro-Care" which also include the necessary nutritional factors like *vitamin B6, B1, vitamin C, and manganese*, all of which are necessary for energy production.

The recommended intake of *Fibro-Care* is 6 tablets a day, however, with some people may get diarrhea at this dose of 6 tablets because of the magnesium. If that should happen, reduce the dose by 2 tablets till the diarrhea stops and then slowly increase back up to 6.

Foods rich in magnesium include dark green leafy vegetables, salads, nuts (almonds, cashews, brazil nuts), seeds, cocoa, dark chocolate, brown rice, green vegetables, seafood, baked beans, molasses, kidney and lima beans. **Important**: *Do not take extra magnesium if you have kidney disease, because it is the kidneys that process the magnesium*.
Note: People with FMS and CFS should consider having *a red blood cell magnesium test* to ensure that they are not deficient in magnesium.

Manganese *(The FMS & CFS Connection) - A critical mineral involved in the Hypothalamic-Pituitary-Thyroid-Axis (HPTA). The link between CFS and FMS, and specifically why fatigue is one of the most prominent features in both syndromes. The HTPA function is dependent on manganese for the neuro-endocrine changes that begin with the production of thyrotropin-releasing hormone hormones (TRH). Thyrotropin-releasing hormone is stimulated by the pituitary gland to produce thyroid stimulating hormone (TSH) which in turn stimulates thyroid production of thyroxin. *(Sources – www.ithyroid.com)*

Since fatigue is one of the primary conditions of both FM and CFS patients, hypothyroidism is a distinct possibility. Manganese directly influences the metabolic rate through its involvement in the hypothalamus-pituitary-axis and may therefore be a very critical trace mineral for both CFS and FM. Manganese is also required for normal functioning of the adrenal glands. Especially, this can also be a mineral deficiency due to the malabsorption of dietary nutrients from people with CFS and FMS that is so frequent with both of he syndromes.

Supplementing with a digestive multi-enzyme and a multi-mineral supplement may be a good idea in assuring yourself of getting adequate amounts of manganese and other trace minerals. The top foods rich in manganese are – *blueberries, spices (ginger, cloves and saffron), wheat germ, bran, rice bran, oat bran, hazelnuts, pine nuts, pecans, mussels, oysters, clams, roasted pumpkin seeds, squash seeds, cocoa powder and dark chocolate, flax seeds, sesame seeds, sesame butter, chili powder, roasted soybeans, and sunflower seeds.*

SAM-e* – (400-1200mgs daily in dived dosages)** SAME-e is must have supplement in your arsenal for the therapy of FMS and CFS, and should be included most definitely. It is literally involved in numerous life-sustaining metabolic processes.

Low levels of SAM-e have been connected with FMS and can be a very effective treatment for the variety of symptoms FMS/CFS often experience. **SAM-e** donates methyl groups to other chemical compounds, assisting in the synthesis of important neurotransmitters including ***serotonin and dopamine***, hormones and more. SAM-e is also the most active methyl donor in your body.

(Important) when purchasing SAM-e, make sure your product is a full-strength SAM-e, and tablets must be **enteric coated**, meaning the tablets pass through the acidic environment of the stomach intact, and can be absorbed most efficiently by the body. The amounts used in various studies may vary widely, but for the many patients who have taken SAM-e for Fibromyalgia relief reported that SAM-e has helped them more than anything else. **Dosages** for them that used SAM-e were 200mgs to 800mgs a day, and in some cases even more. Because of the no side-effects dosages can be increased when necessary, and consider that this is something that normally you couldn't do with prescription drugs (increasing the dosage without side effects).

SAM-e works through a process called transulferation, helping the body's cell produce Glutathione, an essential compound necessary to protect the liver from oxidative damage. And is the human body's major source of Glutathione, which is sometimes referred to as the ***"master anti-oxidant."*** Maintaining proper glutathione levels is also vital for immune system protection and is beneficial for many liver conditions including alcoholic liver disease, and is good for overall liver health. **Reputable and reliable manufacturers are by Jarrow Formulas, Life Extension (very good), Source Naturals, and Natrol.**

(Important) – FMS and CFS are difficult syndromes which now medical science is beginning to grasp on it being better understood. We are lucky to have something (SAM-e) as natural and effective from nature to be made available for those of us that suffer from crippling and annoying diseases. SAM-e seems to be very safe and is free of any side effects, even after taking for long periods of time. **Contraindications** - *While there are no confirmed drug interactions with SAM-e, individuals using prescription medications such as anti-depressants, including SRRI's and MAO inhibitors, should consult a physician before using. Individuals with Parkinson's disease, bipolar disorder or manic depression should not take SAM-e. The safety of SAM-e in pregnant or nursing women or children has not also been established.* **(References- Jacobsen S, Danneskiold-Samsoe B, Anderson RB. Oral SAM-e (S-adenosylmethionine) in primary fibromyalgia. Double blind clinical evaluation. Scand J Rheumatol. 20.4 (1991): 294-302 – Tavoni A, Vitali C, Bombardi S, Pasero G. Evaluation of S-adenosylmethionine in primary fibroblast. A double-blind cross-over study. Am J med. 83.5A (1987)(: 107-110)**

- **5-HTP***** - **5-hydroxytryptophan** is naturally produced in the body from tryptophan, an essential amino acid. 5-HTP can increase the level of serotonin the brain produces and reverse serotonin deficiency. Although there has been no established safe dose regimen yet, anything from 50 to 300mgs has been used in clinical trials shown to be effective. Dosages may vary among individuals taking 5-HTP, finding your optimal dose is recommended. Start off with a low dose of 50mgs and judge as you go along increasing the amount slowly. Also make sure you include vitamin B6 that will aid and speed up, in the conversion of serotonin.

Along with helping people manage depression, sleep and eating disorders, 5-HTP also appears to offer relief from various symptoms associated with CFS and FMS. According to fibromyalgia researchers **H. Moldofsky and J.J. Warsh** theorize that primary FMS may arise from a deficiency of circulating tryptophan. In a study published in pain; *(1978;5:65 71;Moldofsky and Warsh)* reported that the higher the concentration of unbound tryptophan in the plasma of FMS patients, the more profound the symptoms.

Many fibromyalgia people may be interested to know that clinical studies published in peer reviewed medical journals report that 5 HTP can be effective in relieving musculoskeletal and other symptoms in those diagnosed with FMS and CFS. Also the (***The Journal of International Medical Research;1992; 20:182 – 1189)*** concluded that "good" or fair" clinical improvement occurred in 50% of fibromyalgia patients.

5-HTP effectively improved the symptoms of FMS/CFS by helping to mediate slow-wave sleep as well as influence how pain is perceived by the body/mind *(1978; 5:65 71 Modoldofsky and Warsh). Some studies also show it to work as well or better than – SSRI's antidepressants, such as Prozac, Zoloft, Paxil, and Celexa.*

Tryptophan ***– In peer reviewed scientific studies tryptophan had been repeatedly proven to – *reduce or eliminate depression, relieve insomnia, reduce the tendency to over eat, reduce pain (FMS/CFS) reduce the compulsion to commit suicide, and reduce the tendency towards angry or violent outbursts*. Tryptophan may be a better choice for fibromyalgia patients than 5-HTP, as 5-HTP lacks the many of tryptophan's beneficial actions on pain control and muscular relaxation which are very important in reducing many of the complaints fibromyalgia patients have.

As a patient deals with the myraid of concerns that FMS/CFS produces, tryptophan can clear and calm the mind/body and also allow for a more restful period of sleep at night. Tryptophan helps to control muscle stiffness and spasms, the twitches that tend to wake up a person at night are greatly reduced. When used in lower doses during the day, tryptophan can smooth out the rough spots, lower tempers, frustrations, calm stress levels, and provide for a better sense of well being.

Fibromylagia patients not finding relief from medication or support from family and friends tend to over eat comfort foods which are high in carbohydrates and therefore fattening. By combining the over consumption of carbohydrates with the sedentary nature of fibromyalgia, one will have the recipe for creating obesity.

By raising serotonin levels through tryptophan use, you can increase the sense of comfort and well being and decrease the appetite. Pure pharmaceutical tryptophan (the purest form) has no side-effects and is essential to proper brain function and to life! Dosage is usually one 500mg capsule for each 50lbs of body weight when taken before bed time, taken always on an empty stomach or at least one hour away from food. You can also freely experiment in taking less than that amount and work your way up to the full dose if needed. During the day you may try one to two capsules in-between meals to maintain a higher production of serotonin during your waking hours. Try adding vitamin B6 and vitamin C to help with the metabolism and conversion of serotonin.

Reputable manufacturers are Jarrow Formulas, Life Extension (very good), Source Naturals, and Natrol.

Tryptophan will provide all of the benefits a higher level of serotonin brings, however when combined to a comprehensive program or protocol to over come FMS/CFS, such as outlined in this book, your road towards wellness and healing will add a fuller more pain free life.

(References -*Liberman, J., et al; Mood, performance & pain sensitivity: changes induced by food constituents. J. Psychiat. Res., 17(2): 135-145, 11982-83), (Braverman, E., R, Pfeiffer, C., C. :Suicide and biochemistry. Biol. Psych., 20: 123124, 1985.)*

Natural Food sources - The highest dietary food source of **Tryptophan** are protein foods that include – chicken, turkey, tuna, soybeans, beef, lamb, halibut, salmon, shrimp,snapper, dairy products, nuts, seeds, and bananas.

Natural Homemade Serotonin Boost (Recipe) - This is a simple recipe that you can make at home with ingredients that are normally found in the kitchen of the average American home: Get one whole banana, one cup of warm to hot milk, 2 tablespoons of pure un-refined honey, a pinch of nutmeg, and blend all together in a blender, let it cool down so it is warm but not too hot and then drink and enjoy! This drink/recipe will provide you with a nice calmness (serotonin induced) to help relive stress or anxiety, or take it before bed for a nice deep relaxing sleep!

Royal Jelly** - Absolutely, one of nature's most amazing natural health products that doesn't get the publicity it deserves. Pure royal jelly, and not the type that you see put in capsules or tablets, but the actual real thick milky, creamy type of paste that has to be refrigerated is loaded with nutrients that can help you fight off sickness and speed the healing of disease and illness. Royal jelly is made by the glands of nurse bees. They synthesize it from bee pollen, propolis, and other things and produce it with their enzymes. Then they secrete it into the comb and give it to the queen bee as an exclusive food to help make her fertile to produce more worker bees.

Queen bees live exclusively on royal jelly and it accounts for their incredible size and longevity. The queen is 4 times larger than worker bees and amazingly live 40 times longer than worker bees, 7 years as compared to 7 weeks. Queen bees ail also produce over 2,000 eggs per day with each day's brood equal to 2 ½ times her own weight. Biochemically, royal jelly is very complex, a very rich source of proteins, contains 8 essential amino acids, important fatty acids, sugars, sterols, minerals(calcium, copper, iron, phosphorus, potassium, silcon, sulfur), vitamins A, C, D, E, folic acid, biotin, inositol, B vitamins, and especially high in vitamin B5 (pantothenic acid).

Royal jelly is also noted for its rich source of vitamin B5 (pantothenic acid), recognized for its ability to reduce stress levels. There is also nothing richer in pantothenic acid, bar none than Royal jelly, the top source. Royal jelly is also extremely rich in nucleic acids, RNA and DNA. The main active ingredient in royal jelly is a very special hydroxy acid called – 10-HDA, which helps to boost the immune system. German and French researchers have shown that 10-HDA helps the body kill off viruses by getting into the white blood cells and stimulates them to kill them off. Royal jelly is one of the best natural ingredients to give some one who has a low white blood cell count.

Royal jelly is also a great natural source of natural steroid hormones that are safe, and absolutely non-toxic. One of those natural hormones is DHEA which can help you to boost adrenal gland health or adrenal insufficiency. Adrenal weakness rapidly responds to royal jelly treatment, and addresses the case of steroid hormone insufficiency precisely. It is also helpful for those going into menopause, hot flashes, and menopausal symptoms. For problems of a sexual disorder that's caused by FMS and CFS, it can be of great value in restoring your own hormones back to health.

Royal jelly is beneficial for hundreds of illnesses, because it works by strengthening cells, and increasing their resistance to disease. Plus, it also regenerates cells, bringing new life to the tissues. Thus royal jelly is one of those supportive nutrients that at a maximum can help the body in its recovery process. Royal jelly is a regenerative substance because of its nutrient dense profile that can be used as a supportive therapy for numerous conditions. It should also be touted as a miraculous curative tonic to aid the body's natural healing processes. Royal jelly can be a great addition to your nutritional protocol in healing FMS and CFS. To purchase real 100% royal jelly please the recommended sites, see - www.beeroyalproducts.com or www.beealive.com for pure royal jelly. Recommended reading - *"Health From The Hive: Honey, Bee Pollen, Bee Propolis, Royal Jelly" by Carlson Wade, and "The Miracle of Royal Jelly" by Raymond Dubois.*

Note: Royal jelly is a food and is considered as such, so when purchasing it in it's natural creamy thick-like paste, it has to be kept cold and refrigerated to preserve it's natural state or else it will spoil(keep that in mind), also it can be bought in a freeze dried form that is also effective and does not lose any of it's nutritional potency. Freeze dried costs a bit more and has no preservatives added to it with just the water removed. It still contains it's 100% of the original nutrients.

Note: Other beneficial and healthy bee products are – Natural Honey -unheated and filtered, Bee pollen and Propolis.

Bee Pollen-** Considered one of natures super foods, bee pollen comes from the male reproductive part of flowering plants and is collected by worker bees and taken back to the hive where they add enzymes and nectar to it. Bee pollen is the only food in the world that contains all the vitamins, minerals, amino acids and enzymes that we need to live on. So good, that you can live on 20 grams of bee pollen plus water. It also has an immediate effect on diabetics, coeliac disease and people recovering from serious illness, injury or stress or people wishing to achieve maximum quality of life.

Pure bee pollen has been know to promote a youthful feeling, builds resistance to disease and boosts the immune system. And one thing that is almost certain, people who consume bee pollen almost always experience an increase in energy, zest, and physical endurance. This is also precisely what world class athletes supplement their diets with.

Bee pollen contains; an incredible array of vitamins, minerals, amino acids, co-enzymes, and hormones; especially rich in B vitamins and anti-oxidants, including lycopene, selenium, beta carotene, vitamin C, vitamin E, and several flavanoids. Its composed of 55% carbohydrates; 40% protein(more protein & amino acids than a pound of steak or eggs have), 3% vitamins and minerals, 2% of fatty acids and 5% other substances. Overall its one of the most nutritionally complete natural substances found on earth. *(Schmalzel, 1980)*

When you first start to take bee pollen you may feel a significant energy increase right away, or definitely within a week or so. Over time the consistent use of bee pollen will improve stamina, and endurance. Over long-term use, you will probably also note a general feeling of well being, and the alleviation of many different health problems, slow down the effects of aging, and improve the quality of life.

The Institute of Apiculture, Taranov in Russia, declares that bee pollen has one of the highest sources of "rutin", a powerful anti-oxidant and circulatory enhancer found in nature, as well as packed with both RNA and DNA the building blocks of our biological body. Because of its complex nature, science cannot even duplicate bee pollen in laboratories.

Bee pollen comes in granules, powdered form, capsules, tablets, or mixed with pure honey. Look for bee pollen that comes from multiple sources, as it will contain more nutrients than just a plain single source. The best way to consume bee pollen is in its original form of granules, just make sure its from a reputable manufacturer that specializes in bee products, tablets will contain fillers and binders and other un-neccessary ingredients that will hinder its nutritional effect. Bee pollen can found in many health food stores and online as well. Look for certified sellers for quality. Good sites online are www.maxalife.com, and another good bee pollen source is New Zealand-Bee-Pollen, considered one of the best in the world.

Dosage; Always start off with a quarter teaspoon and chew it slowly to mix with your saliva and wash it down with water. Later on as you get accustomed increase it to half a teaspoon and then to a whole teaspoon. You can also use it sprinkled on your cereal, add it to protein shakes or smoothies for a great nutritional boost.

Important: ***If on prescription medications for FMS and CFS, do not take any nutritional supplements at the same time with your medications.***

Bee Propolis* – This is a substance made by the honey bees that provides protection against harmful bacteria, viruses and fungi. Propolis is a plant resin collected by bees for use in and around the hive. In plants it is usually the sticky substance or coating around the buds that serve to protect the plant from natural elements of weather plus bacteria, fungi, molds, and viruses. Like bee pollen propolis (bee glue) is a product that cannot be duplicated or clearly defined. Hundreds of chemicals compounds have been identified from bee propolis extract. The main chemical classes present in propolis are flavanoids, phenolics, and various aromatic compounds.

Scientific studies that have been taken on bee propolis have been promising and are still in their preliminary findings. However, propolis does have proven anti-biotic, anti-septic, anti-viral and anti-inflammatory properties. And is considered safe and useful as a home remedy. It has been recommended by many health care practitioners as a good topical treatment for uncomplicated wounds, and when used as a gargle or in spray form, as a remedy for sores and irritations in the mouth.

Flavanoids are well known plant compounds that have anti-oxidants, anti-bacterial, anti-fungal, anti-viral, and anti-inflammatory properties. Bee propolis has been used as a local anesthetic, reducing spasms, healing gastric ulcers, and strengthen capillaries. If you are allergic to bee stings that does not mean you cannot take bee propolis. However, any bee product can produce an allergic reaction in susceptible individuals. Bee propolis is relatively very safe and has been used by thousands of people as form of immune stimulating protection. Good sites online are www.maxalife.com.

Velvet Deer Antler*** - This is one the top 5 products that are listed in FMS and CFS protocol that is a must try product for healing FMS and CFS. Velvet Deer Antler has been highly prized in traditional Chinese and Korean medicine for over 2,000 years now. Derived from the antlers of Elk which grow each spring, are among the fastest growing soft tissue in any mammal, growing as much as an inch a day.

When harvested, the Elk are not killed or harmed in any way in the collection of the soft tissue cartilage. The tissue contains the essential building blocks for a variety of cells, nerves, blood, cartilage, bone, and tissue. Velvet Deer Antler is believed to work by stimulating our own immune systems and internal growth mechanisms, allowing the body to heal itself.

Velvet Antler contains: *Growth hormones, Growth factors like IGF-1(insulin-like growth factor), and Epidermal Growth Factor (EGF); proteins (including essential amino acids); Collagen; Lipids (fatty acids omega 3 and 6); Glycosaminoglycans including Chondroitin Sulfate, Glucosamine Sulfate, Hyaluronic Acid, Erythropoeitin, Prostaglandins, Phospholipids, and Glycosphingolipids, Minerals and Trace Elements are Calcium, Copper, Iron, Manganese, Phosphorus, Magnesium, Selenium, Sufur, and Zinc.*

It appears that the ancients had it right all along, It's use for supporting the body range from joint support, anti-inflammatory, building kidney energy and strength (adrenal glands), nourishes the blood and circulation, enhances oxygen uptake and number of red blood cells, sharpens the mind, strengthens the cardiovascular system, increases sexual vitality and health, balances the endocrine system making it a new old remedy for the millennium. It's other interesting aspect is it's ability to help increase natural growth hormone levels and IGF-1 response. This is where it can be of a great benefit with those who suffer from FM and CFS. Patients with FM and CFS may be one of the largest populations of growth hormone deficient individuals.

New evidence suggests that FM patients are deficient in growth hormone secretion. And growth hormone therapy may be warranted in theses patients. Research also has revealed that a possible FM connection and growth hormone deficiency syndrome share many of the same clinical features. Which include muscle weakness, reduced exercise capacity, and chronic fatigue. It was also assessed that more than half of those patients with FM had low levels of insulin-like growth factor levels (IGF-1). Fibromyalgia affects about 4% of the United States women and about one-half percent of the men. It is also believed to be the number two reason for office visits to rheumatologists, second to rheumatoid arthritis. IGF-1 (Velvet Deer Antler) may, in fact, be a miracle medicine for FMS and CFS patients in that it can return strength, increase energy and endurance, and improve the immune response simultaneously.

"A recent clinical study on 40 patients lasting 8 months was conducted by V. James de Franco, M.D., at the Toledo Center for Clinical Research, with the following results: 90 – 95% of participants overcame fatigue with better work performance. Five participants with Fibromyalgia had less pain, better sleep patterns and much more energy"

<u>The best Velvet Deer Antler product can be purchased</u> from www.nutronicslabs.com. Not all deer antler products are the same, and some have no nutritional value at all, so it pays to research when purchasing difficult products that work and are copied because of it. Recommended reading on this amazing product is from ***"The Remarkable Healing Powers of Velvet Antler" by Betty Kamen Ph.D and "Velvet Antler, Nature's Super Tonic" by Alison Davidson***

<u>**Noni Juice**</u>** – Made from the fruit of Morinda Citrifolia (Noni juice), a popular Polynesian fruit that has been under extensive scientific scrutiny for its amazing pain relieving qualities. Traditionally it has been used for thousands of years to heal the body, mind and spirit. Dr. Neil Soloman, a professional and health physician trained at John Hopkins University of Medicine has written quite a few books outlining the benefits of noni juice and its active pain relieving component, Xeronine.

His studies show definite improvement for a quantity of ailments and diseases including: allergies, arthritis, asthma, fibromyalgia, depression, digestion, heart disease, HIV, immune system, kidney disease, menstruation, multiple sclerosis, obesity, Parkinson's disease, respiratory problems, skin and hair problems, sleeping, smoking, stress, stroke, well being, blood pressure, diabetes, coughs, and colds, flu's, pain, and yes even cancer!

Noni juice has been used to ease the intense and persistent pain of Arthritis and Fibromyalgia. Noni juice works by blocking the pain enzyme while encouraging the healing enzymes of the body. This is achieved without any related side effects.

One study reports that noni juice is 75% as effective as morphine at relieving pain. Since arthritis and fibroblast are inflammatory conditions caused by immune system malfunction, anything that decreases the inflammation and modulates the immune system can be helpful. There are also two theories on why Noni helps with pain:

1.   **Noni Juice contains powerful anti-inflammatory nutritional elements that reduce the inflammation and the associated pain.**
2.   **Noni Juice's ability to stimulate the immune system helps correct your**

body's attack on your joints, ligaments, tendons, and muscles.

The reviews on noni juice have been excellent concerning its pain relieving affect and in general well being. Researcher Mian-ying Wang, MD says she first became interested in the study of noni juice in 1999 after being convinced that it helped reduce her pain from wrist fracture. In a study performed at the University of Hawaii, administration of noni-ppt significantly enhanced the duration of survival of mice with lung tumor. The researchers concluded that were possible clinical applications of noni-ppt as a supplemental agent in cancer treatment. Make sure when buying <u>Noni juice it's 100% certified true Noni Juice from Hawaii</u>.

(Ref- Dr. Ralph Heinicke, Xeronine and Cell Regeneration; Noni Juice, Xeronine, Damnacanthal & Scientific Studies), (Fairchild, Diana, Noni: Aspirin of The Ancients, Hawaii: Flyana Rhyme, 1998)

<u>*Recommended reading*</u> *- "Superfoods:The Food and Medicine of The Future" by David Wolfe and "A Physician's Guide To Natural Health Products That Work" by James A. Howenstine.*

Note: Noni has many other interesting health attributes that I thought you would be interested in that may be helpful for some people and that includes – Noni has been reported to be a good therapy for tobacco addiction. Take 4 ounces of noni juice twice a day for three days, which seems to be a long enough to break the cigarette habit with noni. *(Ref- "A Physician's Guide To Natural Health Products That Work", James A. Howenstine, MD: 2002)*

Noni's seems to be nature's universal antidote for almost all illnesses, French researchers confirmed that noni is a non toxic and exhibits consistent (central brain) pain relieving activity. Dr. Heineke, Ph.D in biochemistry from the University of Minnesota has showed much interest in the healing effects of noni, especially its pain relieving affects. He believes that much of noni's healing effects come from the alkaloid called proxeronine that becomes converted in the body to the enzyme Xeronie.

<u>He also states that xeronine is depleted under any kind of stress, and the proneronine from noni was readily converted to xeronine by intestinal cells full of serotonin.</u> *We have also discussed serotonin's effect on pain in the previous section on serotonin and Fibromyalgia, and so this connection is of interest to us concerning xeronine.*

He has also discovered that a lack of xeronine disrupts the body's resistance to illness, infections, and chronic degenerative diseases. The quantity of xeronine produced in the body declines with aging and also with all forms of stress, be it viral illness, injury, surgery, difficult occupations, worry, anxiety, and anger. This may also explain why high stress persons are vulnerable to more illnesses and chronic degenerative illnesses. In this regard, noni can help you to avoid depletion of xeronine that would ordinarily ensue from a stressful lifestyle. Low xeronine levels may cause proteins and enzymes to fail or not function properly which results in every cell, tissue, and organ needing that protein or enzyme may fail and cause heart disease, kidney disease, and diabetes. Restoring correct levels of xeronine may help to alleviate those illnesses.

One other area of interest that's worth noting, is its effect on reversing hard-core drug addiction. Dr. Heineke believes that xeronine may possibly be the best treatment for drug addictions. He states that, "by flooding the brain with xeronine, the proteins in the brain are changed. Within a matter of days, brand new receptor sites are created due to xeronine's work on proteins. Now you have a normal receptor sites in the brain that respond to xeronine instead of drugs." And nicotine addiction can be cured in three days by the same mechanism.

Without proper xeronine levels in the body, vitamins do not work and serious illness may result, including cancer, premature aging, viral illness, and immune system malfunction.

(Ref - "A Physician's Guide to Natural Health Products That Work"- 2009, Dr.Ralph Heineke)

D-Ribose*** – Is a naturally occurring simple sugar found in all living cells. It is the fuel that the mitochondria use to produce adenosine tri-phosphate (ATP), which provides the body's cellular energy. Studies show that patients with FMS, CFS, and congestive heart failure are low in D-Ribose. It is also clear that people who have FM and CFS are low in levels of ATP and have a reduced capacity to make ATP in their muscles. Recent studies show that ribose supplementation can reduce muscle pain and enhance quality of life for those suffering from FM and CFS.

According to Tori Hudson, ND, "As cellular energy is depleted, fatigue and muscle pain become more and more severe, and the muscles require additional energy in their recovery efforts. Energy is used faster than fuel is made available to renew it, and the fatigue, soreness, pain, and stiffness continue to progress. Energy depletion reaches a critical point, and CFS/FMS becomes a state in which the mechanisms are overwhelmed." *(References, Oz, M, MD & Roizen, M, MD, Authors of You:Being Beautiful, "Call Ribose One of the Decade's 'real Nutritional Heroes'. "PR Newswire. 2009. HighBeam research.(Dec. 14, 2009)*

A 2006 study published by Dr. Jacob Teitelbaum, M.D., in the Journal of Alternative and Complementary Medicine showed that D-Ribose significantly reduced clinical symptoms in patients suffering from FM and CFS. Forty one patients with a diagnosis of FM and/or CFS were given D-Ribose, at a dose of 5 grams a day, 3 times a day. The study found that two thirds of the patients reported significant improvement of their symptoms in 12 days of using D-Ribose as a treatment. The average rate of improvement was an average of 45% and quality of life improved by 30%. patients reported less muscle pain and soreness and stiffness, and were better able to overcome fatigue, as well as simply feeling better.

(Teitelbaum JE, Johnson C, St Cyr J. The use of D-Ribose in chronic fatigue syndrome and Fibromyalgia: a pilot study, J Altern Complementary Med. 2006 Nov. 12 (9):857-62).

Ubiquinol CoQ10 with Shilajit *** **(for energy support)** has been also shown to enhance cellular energy by increasing ATP production better than CoQ10 alone. The combination increased barin energy by 40% more than CoQ10 alone and increased energy in the heart by 27% more than CoQ10 alone. *(Ref- Dr. Michael A. Smith, MD; Living With Fibromyalgia? These Nutrients can help; Life Extension Foundation Magazine)*. <u>*Recommended supplement by Life Extension "Super Ubiquinol CoQ10 with Enhanced Mitochondrial Support". Dosage: Take one soft gel once or twice a day, or as recommended by your health care physician.*</u>

<u>**Important Facts about Shilajit:**</u> Shilajit has been used for centuries by Traditional Ayurvedic Indian Medicine to strengthen the body and treat many ailments. In ancient Sanskrit, Shilajit means *"conqueror of mountains and destroyer of weakness". Shilajit is composed of humus and organic plant material that has been compressed by layers of rock in the high mountains of India. It is a rich source of 84 different naturally occurring raw minerals in ionic form which are vital for maintaining the equilibrium of energy metabolism in our body. Ionic form of minerals are easily and fully absorbed more readily than regular minerals.*

One of it's benefits has been in treating anemia as it helps in retaining iron and other minerals in the body which can be of great help in people with FM and CFS. It's other benefits are in helping to improve liver function, blood circulation, oxygen uptake by cells, stress protector, anti-allergen, provides strength and stamina to the body, boosts the immune system, restore functioning of the digestive system, mental fatigue, hormonal imbalance, libido restorer, and is highly effective in recovering from weakness and general disability. Effects usually take 3 to 6 weeks to start seeing results. Shilajit has also been a favorite in professional athletes in providing the strength and resistance in coping with physical strenuous activity. Shilajit has been well researched by Russian scientist for its amazing adaptogenic qualities. It also goes by the name of Mooyimo.

(Suraj P Agarwal, Phytotherapy Research, Volume 21, Issue 5, pages 401-405, May 2007)

NOTE:
Shilajit may also help those who suffer with sexual dysfunction problems and may be an alternative in helping to restore sexual function with those that have FMS and CFS. Also when looking to purchase Shilajit or Mooyimo, make sure its the extract and its from a reputable manufacturer that specializes in the sales of the two products.

<u>Note:</u> *D-Ribose can be taken by itself or in combination with the "CoQ10" formula for an even more potent synergistic effect.*

<u>Important:</u> *Look for a brand of D-Ribose that is pure, and the normal dosage in the pilot studies were 5 grams 3 times per day. You also need to take it for an average of 12 days to start feeling better.* <u>*See The Life Extension* Company Brand (D-Ribose powder) or Solgar, Cardiovascular Research, and Solary.*</u>

<u>**Probiotics*****</u> - Are live microorganisms or good bacteria with Lactobacillus Acidophilus and bifidobacterium being the two predominant beneficial bacteria in our

intestinal tract that we need to have in a healthy digestive system. These friendly bacteria are called intestinal flora, probitics, or eubiotics with the last term meaning *"healthful to life"*. Probiotics are also becoming one of the fastest growing dietary supplements, and are now very prominent on drugstore and health food store shelves. U.S. Sales of probiotic supplements have totaled nearly $770 million dollars last year, and are steadily increasing. Why? Because they work and are vital to our health, and 77% of our immune system is located within your digestive tract. As it is known that disease manifests in the stomach, it is important that we keep the friendly bacteria flowing.

Friendly bacteria keep the immune system strong and the digestive system functioning smoothly. The wrong bacteria or harmful variety can set the stage for disease. Most of American diets have the inverse ratio of bad bacteria to good bacteria which can seriously compromise the immune and digestive system, leading to a number of chronic conditions and disorders like Fibromyalgia and chronic fatigue syndrome.

In addition, many FM and CFS suffers have compromised gastrointestinal problems from the many drugs that are often prescribed for them. These drugs alter the levels of beneficial bacteria in the gut.

For this reason it is very important for those who suffer from FM and CFS to take probiotics, including the lactobacillus group of beneficial bacteria, to restore intestinal health and function. Lactobacillus is particularly helpful in treating Candida albicans, It is also thought that Candida albicans yeast over growth is prevalent in many Fibromyalgia suffers. It is important to keep our gastrointestinal tract in good working order and our friendly flora in an abundant supply and the way we do that is our nutrition and diets.

We can also supplement with probiotics which may also be necessary since many people have had several doses of anti-biotics throughout their lives. It's been said that our stomach is our second brain and when we fully appreciate that 77% of our immune system is located there, it's no wonder. Beneficial bacteria or friendly flora is responsible for manufacturing many vitamins including the B complex vitamins.

The B complex vitamins are our stress fighting vitamins and we can only make them by eating the right foods. Foods that enhance beneficial flora that contain either lactobacillus acidophilus or Bifidobacterium, or both are: *yogurt, sauerkraut, cottage cheese, tofu, miso, natto, tamari, shoyu, tempeh, and kimchee*. Chinese Green tea and Ginseng also help to increase friendly flora. Green tea contains polyphenols which are believed to be the enhancing substance while ginseng extract was found to increase beneficial flora. Introducing probiotic supplements is a very important step in healing FMS and CFS. Adhering to the health protocol as listed with the addition of probiotic supplements will help you recover that much more rapidly. ***Recommended choice of supplements are – Udo'S Choice Probiotic Super 8, Enzymedica -Digestive Gold + Probiotic, and Enzymatic Therapy – Acidopilus Pearls.***

Digestive Enzymes* – With the average American diet being high in refined carbohydrates and processed foods, its no wonder that many suffer from malabsorption problems and the consequential illnesses that may result from it. Digestive enzyme therapy can be used as an effective treatment for digestive problems (malabsorption), illness, pain relief, and restore some of the nutritional losses that are caused by improper food digestion. Enzyme supplements and a proper diet recommended in this protocol can help FMS/CFS patients maintain energy for cell growth and as well as strengthen their immune system. Plus provide the necessary enzymes that they may be lacking due to intestinal disorders to help breakdown carbohydrates, proteins, starch, and fats.

Systemic Enzymes ***– *("meaning "body wide")* are metabolic enzymes that operate not just in digestion but throughout the body and all organs and systems. Most of the systemic enzymes are your "proteases" (or protolytic enzymes), regulating protein function and ailing the digestion of those proteins that are no longer needed or are even harmful in the body *[e.g., cellular debris, plaque, scar tissue]*.

The inability to break down dietary proteins into amino acids plays a very important part in FM, lupus and auto-immune diseases. Studies have shown that CFS/FMS patients and auto-immune disorders have significant reduced levels of amino acids from protein break down from defects of malabsorption of amino acids. Thus affecting many of the body's neurological functions of serotonin metabolism, sleep disorders, and hormonal production. Most CFS patients were found deficient in amino acid absorption, specifically tryptophan, methionine, phenylaline, with the highest deficiency being Tryptophan(80%) and Phenylaline(72%). This was published in the "Journal of Applied Nutrition" *(Lord, 1994).*

Other essential amino acids were also found to be lacking as well. This amino acid deficiency is typical of the symptoms FM and CFS patients normally suffer from, such as weakness, fatigue*(tyrosine)*, lack of energy*(carnitine)*, and inability to have restful sleep *(lack of growth hormone)*, *(serotonin/melatonin)*. Amino acids are involved in every aspect of bodily function from neurotransmitter production, energy production and hormonal production, thyroid, adrenal, and enzymatic functions. And it is this lack of amino acids that is found in FM and CFS that is the result of inability to digest and metabolize dietary proteins and other vital nutrients that contribute to this syndromes multi dimensional complaints. If we don't do not digest and absorb nutrients from the foods we eat we sets the stage for many illnesses to begin.

Systemic Enzymes - have a unique features which make them very valuable in healing many diseases and disorders. The systemic effect of enzymes can be used to prevent and resolve many diseases. In Europe, therapies of malignancies usually includes enzymes in large dosages which has lengthened survival. Enzyme preparations are carefully formulated so the are able to avoid dissolving in the stomach acid and thus are available to get into the blood without being destroyed. Enzymes also allow the immune system to function more efficiently and assist the immune system in fighting off and eliminating diseased conditions.

For example, in cancer, the cancer cells are surrounded by a layer of fibrin which may be up to 15 times thicker than the layer of fibrin that surround normal cells. This fibrin layer permits these malignant cells to escape destruction by killer immune cells, which are unable to detect the cancer cell antigens. The systemic enzymes are able to detect and remove this fibrin coating, permitting the immune cells to again kill the tumor cells. Additionally, immune cells become stimulated by enzymes to increase production of *"tumor necrosis factor"* which can attack and destroy tumor cells, as well as cells infected by viruses. Systemic immune therapy has prolonged the life for many patients, and in the case of cancer of the pancreas, one third of pancreatic cancer patients have been cured by using systemic enzyme therapy.

In Europe and Japan, orally administered enzymes have been clinically used for more than 40 years to treat and cure disease.

Enzyme therapy has become a valuable aid in the cure of many diseases, their effects range from:

- Providing a natural **anti-inflammatory effect**, as opposed to anti-inflammatory drugs which are harmful and toxic to the liver and kidneys. Enzymes are safe and assist the body in healing naturally and free from pain. And are now being used to treat inflammatory responses in Parkinson's, Alzheimer's, CFS, FMS, and Autism.
- Provides an **anti-fibrosis effect**, removes scar tissue from excessive surgeries effectively as if it was a meal. They can remove **fibrin deposits from tumors, uterine fibroids, endometriosis, fibrocystic breast disease, arterial sclerotic plaques, fibrosis of the lungs, renal kidney fibrosis, keloids, etc.**
- They have **Blood cleansing effects** – they can dispose of **(fibrin)** dead matter and waste products that affect cells and organs that can thicken the blood and cause clot formation. Normally **waste products** are cleaned up by the liver, but given to the toxic build up condition that the liver normally endures due to an unhealthy lifestyle, this process of removal is impaired. Systemic enzymes can help to take the strain off of the liver by ridding the blood of excess fibrin and reduce the stickiness of blood cells, which are two main factors in **strokes and heart attacks due to blood clots.**
- Can help **Auto-Immune illness** – auto-immune disorder can attack the body's own tissues, such as in **multiple sclerosis, rheumatoid arthritis, lupus, FM,CFS,** and enzymes can restore the body's equilibrium and tone down the immune function and "eat" inappropriate antibodies.
- **Viral, Bacterial, and Fungal Infections** -in vitro studies, enzymes have shown promising effects on viral, bacterial, and fungal organisms. Enzymes can recognize the proteins that are foreign in the blood and inhibit viral replication through their "lock and key" mechanism, thus rendering the viruses inert.

The use of enzymes have allowed science to research new field of studies of how enzymes can be used to treat diseases. In their search science has also discovered a new and potent enzyme called *"Serrapeptase"* that has powerful anti-inflammatory effects. *Serrapeptase* was originally found in the silk worm, where it is naturally found in the intestine. This enzyme melts a hole out of the cocoon enabling the moth to emerge out of its fibrin based cocoon. Now, science is producing this enzyme commercially through fermentation.

Serrapeptase is enteric coated to pass safely through the intestines, from where it is transported through the circulatory system to the cells and tissues throughout the body. It has the ability to dissolve avital (non-living) tissue without damaging living cells. It's inflammation-modulating effects have been found to be superior to those of other *proteolytic enzymes,* and among other conditions, it has been used to ease symptoms of chronic sinusitis, traumatic injuries, post operative inflammation, cystitis(bladder inflammation), epididymitis, and elimination of bronchopulmonary secretions.

Unlike other biological enzymes, serrapeptase affects only non living tissue such as old fibrous layers that narrow the lining of our arteries, restricting oxygen and blood flow to the brain. It became widely known after Dr. Hans Nieper, a famous German doctor and research scientist, used serrapeptase to address arterial blockage in his heart patients.

Dr. Nieper described the amazing effects of the enzyme and quick recovery without for bypass surgery for the two patients - "women scheduled to have her hand amputated and a man scheduled for by-pass surgery" - after being treated with serrapeptase. However, there are still some cautionary notes that should be adhered to when using enzyme therapy that require supervised medical supervision, and that's for those people who are currently:

- Individuals taking prescription *blood thinner*s such as *"Coumadin, Heparin, and Plavix"*.
- *Hemophiliacs*.
- Any who is *scheduled for surgery* in less than two weeks.
- Individuals with known *Ulcers* of the stomach.
- Individuals with *gastrointestinal reflux disease(GRD).*
- Pregnant or Lactating women.
- Individuals taking *anti-biotics*.
- Individuals who are allergic to reactions of pineapple and papaya (the sources of two common *"proteolytic enzymes"* - "*bromelian and papian*".

(Key Reference Sources – Dr. Hans Nieper:"Silk Worm Enzymes for Carotid Artery Blockage") see also writings and experimental work employing serrapeptase supplementation to promote cardiovascular health information from the Nieper Foundation archive at the Brewer Science Library in Wisconsin (www.mwt.net/drbrwer/cardio.htm)

- **["Enzymes & Enzyme Therapy: How To Jump Start Your Way To life Long Good Health"] by Antony J. Cichoke, D.C.**
- www.answers.com/topic/enzyme
- Dr. William Wong. "What Are Systemic Enzymes & What Do They Do?
- www.serrapeptase.info/
- www.staytuned.ws/systemic_enzymes.html
- http://en.wikipedia.org/wiki/Enzyme

FINAL NOTE: With FM and CFS, enzymes are a crucial and important step in resolving the cure and remission of FM and CFS. Used along a proper recommended diet for FM and CFS can speed the healing and relieve you of discomfort and pain from the associated symptoms. Below are the recommended supplements of high quality that you can use.

Recommended digestive enzyme choices are – *Life Extension Foundation Supplements- "Enhanced Super Digestive Enzymes with Probitics" or "Enhanced Super Digestive Enzymes"(same company), and Garden of Life "Omegazyme", or "Omegazyme Ultra". Serrapeptase can be bought from "Cardiovascular Research" (must be of the enteric coating kind for proper digestion). Dosage – Follow label recommendations.*

Boosting Intercellular Glutathione Levels for FMS /CFS*** - In a study assessing anti-oxidant levels in patients with FMS in comparison to healthy controls, the study found that glutathione levels were significantly lower in the FM patients. Also the glutathione levels and morning stiffness was found to be significant. The conclusion: Increased free radical levels were considered responsible for the development of FM stating - "These findings may support the hypothesis of FM as an oxidative disorder." *(2005, Rheumatology International Journal- Volume 25, April).*

Bioactive Whey Protein Isolate** - (can supplemented/substituted as a meal) Is by far one of the best natural remedies for Fibromyalgia. It is also the one thing that has the most actual peer reviewed research and tens of thousands of related studies. Bioactive whey protein isolate is microfiltered and undenatured 90% protein isolate that contains immune system enhancing properties that are present in human breast milk that include – Alpha-lactalbumin, Serum albumin, and Lactoferrin which are all called bioactive proteins. These proteins contain exceptional amounts of Cysteine, the all-important molecular precursor of "Glutathione". Cysteine is an amino acid and when it is combined with glutamate and glycine, it forms Glutathione. Glutathione is arguably the most important water soluble anti-oxidant ffound in the body, and without adequate supplies other important anti-oxidants such as vitamins C and E cannot properly protect the body. Glutathione is known to be essential to immunity, oxidative stress, and over all well being, and reduced levels are associated with a host of diseases. Therefore Glutathione is essential for everyone.

Bioactive whey proteins has been clinically proven to increase glutathione levels in the body. Research studies have proved that it enhances both healthy and deficient immune systems, and is safe for those with auto-immune diseases, celiac disease, chronic fatigue syndrome, fibroblast, graves' disease, lupus, etc, and is validated as an effective nutritional and biological supplement by the medical community FDA and Health Canada. *(Ref- Bounous G, Molson J.: Med Hypotheses. 1999 Oct;53(4):347-9 – Glutathione Precursors, the Immune System and Chronic Fatigue).* Bioactive whey protein isolates can be found and purchased online, It is highly recommended for FMS and CFS.

There is also evidence to support that the use of **N-acteylcysteine (NAC)** as a natural remedy for FMS, (N-A-C) N-Acetylcysteine – is a precursor to Glutathione, as well as **Alpha Lipoic Acid and the amino acid Cysteine. Note:** When taking N-A-C, it is recommended to take 500 to 1,000mgs of vitamin C a long with it.

Essential Fatty Acids (Fish Oils)* - Definitely one of the important requirements in treating and healing FMS and CFS. (see section on Essential Fatty Acids and FMS/CFS and managing Cytokine Inflammation) for more information. Recommended supplements are _Udo's Oil Blend by UDO's Choice (provides a perfect blend of omega 3's, omega 6, and omega 9 fatty acids in a ratio considered ideal). Spectrum Naturals "Organic Flax Borage Oil". Second choice "Enzymatic Therapy" Eskimo-3 Fish Oil._

Liver Therapy* – Fatigue is one of the most common complaints in patients with liver problems. Everything that we eat and drink has to go through the liver, such as foods, drugs, supplements, etc. The build up and the accumulation of waste materials that have been stored deep down in liver tissues tend to create toxins, and harmful acids that have been produced by the consumption of animal proteins that aggravate muscle inflammation and spasms in FM and CFS.

The liver, the main organ of detoxification is involved in the elimination of these toxic substances from the blood and their conversion into less harmful substances that can be safely excreted into bile (and eventually the feces) and urine. Researchers have linked several chronic disorders including that of FM and CFS to impaired hepatic detoxification (sluggish liver), the symptoms of which are depression, general malaise, headaches, digestive disturbances, allergies, and chemical sensitivities, pms, and constipation.

This resulting toxic overload on the body means that physiologically the unwanted waste materials have to go somewhere, after all we don't have the mechanisms to make them disappear, like taking out the garbage out to the street on the appropriate day of the week!
Depending on the inherited constitution of the individual, the most likely place for these toxins to re-accumulate is in the weakest organ system of the body. Where the joints and bone structure are inherently weak, this scenario may result in toxic accumulation in these areas, which contributes towards an inherited disposition to Rheumatoid arthritis.

Where the lymphatic drainage system is not functioning properly, toxic waste accumulates in the tiny lymph nodes situated in the areas surrounding joints and following tracks of blood vessels and nerve pathways -i.e., below the surface of the skin at the pressure points where the pain felt in FM is often related to the swollen lymph nodes at these points where there is insufficient lymphatic circulation to move the waste products and insufficient capacity of the liver to deal with the waste products. Recent research has found a link in patients with FM with decreased metabolic energy levels and decreased levels of **_"Glutathione"_** and anti-oxidant nutrients both of which are extremely important for detoxification of xenobiotics (drugs and chemicals) and metabolic waste products, in the body.

The best approach to detoxification is to approach this slowly, gradually sliding into it over a period of a few weeks and continuing for several months until the medication can be reduced to a minimum (gradually and under supervision) and eventually exchanged for herbal and nutritional alternatives. It is also important to prevent the body from undergoing severe toxemia as waste material is finally dumped into the blood stream for disposal. This involves gradual changes and herbal/ nutritional support.

Also, a multi-clinic research study placed chronically ill patients suffering from CFS and FM and related disorders on a comprehensive detoxification program which included a hypoallergenic diet plus food supplements after 10 weeks. Symptom improvements was mirrored by normalization of heptatic detoxification. In a study conducted by Donaldson et al., Fibromyalgia patients were helped considerably in the relief of symptoms with mostly raw vegetarian diet. After 7 months 19 out of 30 participants had symptoms scores that were no different than those found in normal healthy women of the same age group. The recommendations for a slow slow detoxification are suggested below: For a complete fast detoxification see section on liver detox and whole body cleanse. Taking care of the liver is an important step towards recovery from FMS and CF. A clean and healthy liver will help you speed up the healing processes. *(Ref' Anja Morris-Paxton M.Dip.Herb BS (USA) M.Sc. (PAN) M.A.(UK)*

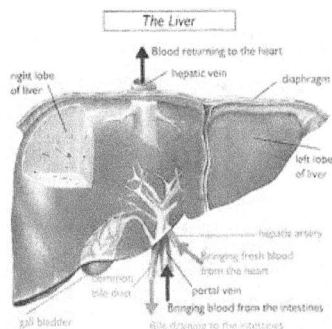

Slow Liver Detoxification

- Avoid *grapefruit*, as this contains **'Naringin'**, which prevents liver detoxification.
- Avoid **salts**, as this will contribute to the cellular imbalance that prevents detoxification
- Avoid **wheat and dairy products**, if possible, as it will slow the detoxification
- Avoid **coffee, tea, cola's, alcohol, sugary foods, and artificial sweeteners**
- Try to consume the following on a daily basis: a large raw mixed vegetable salad, two fresh fruits, lightly steamed vegetables, beans or lentils or any other vegetable proteins, large skinned potato, grilled fish, brown rice as much as you can eat, important to take in plenty of fluids (preferably distilled water), herbal teas are OK that include **milk thistle, dandelion,** will help with liver detoxification, take additional **buffered vitamin C, CoQ10** to increase energy levels, and **Ginkgo biloba** to increase circulation.
- Supplementing with **SAM-e (pronounced sammy)**that has pain relieving, anti-inflammatory, and anti-depressant effects has been found to help with liver

associated problems, and can reduce the number and severity of tender points in FMS. A New Zealand study concluded that SAM-e supplements helped restore normal liver function in people with chronic liver diseases! The study also concluded that SAM-e worked to protect and even reverse liver damage from drugs, alcohol, acetaminophen, steroids, and lead toxins.

- **Alpha Lipoic Acid** – 200 to 300mgs a day to support liver detoxification and Glutathione metabolism.
- **Glutathione** – For your liver to function properly it must have Glutathione. Glutathione is also synthesized from SAM-e, when a healthy liver produces SAM-e, it is then turned into glutathione which is your liver's natural anti-oxidant.

Adrenal /Thyroid Extracts*** – Supporting the adrenal glands and the thyroid is an important necessary step in healing FMS/CFS. See the section on adrenal and thyroid health for the required supplements of choice.

Vitamin D** – Vitamin D deficiency has become quite acceptable recently and it's also become a hot topic in the news as well, with many people being prescribed vitamin D supplementation by their perspective health care physicians. The importance of vitamin D in human nutrition cannot be over stated.

Considered a fat soluble vitamin slash-hormone, it's role in the human body has many important functions besides it being noted for bone strength and preventing osteoporosis, it also serves to modulate cell growth, insulin production, heart health, neuromuscular and immune function, and reduction of inflammation.

Obtaining sufficient vitamin D from sources alone is difficult and naturally present in very few foods. The flesh of fatty fish (such as salmon, tuna, and makerel) and fish liver oils are the best sources. Small amounts of vitamin D are also found in beef liver, cheese, and egg yolks. Vitamin D in these foods is primarily in the form of D3. Fortified foods provide most of the vitamin D in the American diet, as in milk. In 1930's, a milk program was implemented in the United States to combat rickets(bone disorder), then a major problem. Now their also fortified in ready to eat breakfast cereals, some brands of orange juice, yogurts, margarines, and other food products. And both the United States and Canada mandate the fortification of infant formula's with vitamin D.

Sun exposure of course is the other natural way to obtain sufficient amounts of vitamin D. And it is important that during the summer months we get as much sun exposure as we can, that is one the best ways to get vitamin D synthesis by spending at least 30 minutes of sun exposure between 10 am and 3 pm when the sun is at its strongest level at least 2 to 3 times a week. Dietary supplements are another logical choice in which sales and popularity of vitamin D has increased significantly. But in supplements vitamin D comes in two forms, D2 (ergocalciferol) and D3 (cholecalciferol). Both forms are also equally effective in raising serum vitamin D levels in the body.

Fibromyalgia and vitamin D deficiency very often have completely identical symptoms. And a large number of people have been misdiagnosed with Fibromyalgia when they simply have a vitamin D deficiency. A deficiency of vitamin D may result in some of the same symptoms that FM patients often experience, chronic pain,, muscle weakness, arthritis, and auto-immunity. It is also one of the most frequently recommended supplements for people with FM and CFS, and with good reason. Researchers found a significant association between moderate to severe vitamin D deficiency and newly diagnosed FM.

It was noted in one particular study in Glasgow, Scotland, that only 16% of FM patients in a small study had adequate levels of vitamin D, suggesting implications for treatment. Among 36 patients, 28% had levels of vitamin D that was considered deficient. 62% of the patients with FM had levels considered also insufficient. 90% of the patients were also women with the average age being 47. *(Source reference: Jan A, et al "Serum 25-hydroxy vitamin D levels in patients with Fibromyalgia" BSR 2012; Abstract 231.*

How Vitamin D Works With Pain & Inflammation

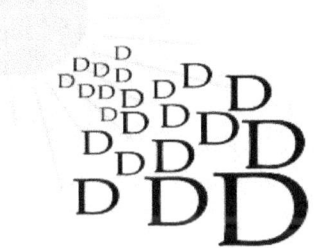

Some studies have reported that vitamin D may reduce the risk of pain and inflammation in those with FMS by lowering the production of **"cytokine"**, a protein that is responsible for inflammation. Vitamin D has also been used to treat FM in several studies and observations, and low levels have been known to cause muscle pain and weakness. Make sure you get ample amounts of vitamin D through your die and/or through supplementation. There are many studies and research that do show deficiencies, so it would be of best interest in those who suffer from FMS and CFS to include vitamin D in their diet. Some FM and CFS experts recommend between 1,000 iu's to 2,000 iu's of vitamin D.

(Resources- "The Vitamin D Solution: CFS/FM"; CFS pages 4,12,67; FMS pages 4, 6, 12, 65-68) -("The Vitamin D Cure: Chronic Pain & FM", page133-136) - ("T

St.John's Wort* – This herb can be an effective treatment for FM and CFS because it helps to relieve depression and promotes restful sleep. St. John's Wort does this by helping to restore serotonin balance back into the body, and serotonin is one of the most important neurotransmitters that FM and CFS patients have a deficiency in. St. John's Wort works on the same pathway as prescription drug (SSRI's) serotonin-reuptake-inhibitors do, and is considered equally effective, but safer with less side effects.

It is also not recommended to take St. John's Wort with any prescription anti-depressants, amphetamine drugs (Ritalin and Adder all), stimulants(coffee, caffeine), and any foods that contain "tyramine" which include aged cheese, aged or cured meat, sauerkraut, soy sauce, and other soy condiments, beer on tap, and wine.Other interactions include – tricyclic dugs, protease inhibitors, statin drugs, blood thinner medications(Warifin/Coumadin), sulfa drugs, and anti-inflammatory drugs. Make sure when taking St. John's Wort that you take it away several hours before taking any medications or foods containing tyramine.

St. John's Wort is considered a MAO inhibitor and can interact adversely with tyramine containing foods causing high blood pressure, rapid heart rate, and delirium.

St. John's Wort has been shown to be helpful in FM and CFS because of its ability to relieve depression and improve sleep quality which is a big issue in those who suffer from these symptoms. Make sure the St. John's Wort that you buy is standardized for 0.3% hypericin content and the standard dosage is 900 to 1,800mgs.

FMS and CFS Diet* – The Fibromyalgia diet is the most simple part of this healing protocol for FM and CFS.** After all "we are what we eat" if we eat foods that heal, such as quality protein, vegetables, vegetable juices, good fats (EFA's) that heal, distilled or filtered water, and unrefined sea salt, and understand and learn about food intolerance, you will then be on your way towards a fast recovery from FM/CFS. Nutritious wholesome food is where it all begins, its also rather simple to understand about healthy eating.

If we eat like crap and live a destructive lifestyle of junk food consumption, sugar, drugs, smoking, etc. What do you think happens? Our body starts to malfunction, organs become toxic and unable to function correctly, symptoms of illness start to arise, then throw in the stress factor and what do you think you get? Well, anything from high cholesterol, high blood pressure, heart disease, diabetes, IBS, leaky gut syndrome, arthritis, Crohns disease, Alzheimer's disease, CFS, FMS, and many others.

Adhering to a successful diet is one of your main goals in recovering from FM and CFS. And by eliminating and avoid the bad junk and processed foods you will be on your way to curing FM/CFS. *(See the recommended Diet for FM/CFS: The Road to Recovery)*

General Support Anti-Oxidant Protection

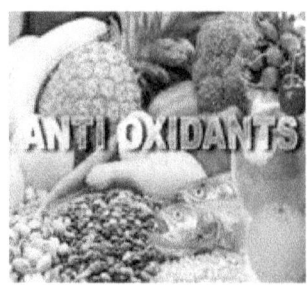

Anti-oxidants* – more and more studies are finding out that high levels of oxidative damage – reactive oxygen molecules that damage important cellular structure like

DNA – in people with fibromyalgia and related disorders like chronic fatigue syndrome. One of the key oxidants implicated in these disorders is called *peroxynitrite*. Researchers from Washington State University have hypothesized that anti-oxidants may help minimize damage from *peroxynitrite* and subsequently improve the severity of the symptoms. **Anti-oxidants like <u>blueberies</u> anthocyaninsitamins C & E, Selenium, pomegranate polyphenols, N-acetyl-cysteine, and Reduced Glutathione.** *(Pharmacotherapy. 2004 Nov;24(11): 16446-8).*

<u>**Easing Systemic Inflammation Naturally**</u> – High levels of systemic inflammation have also been reported in people with FMS and CFS. As a result, easing inflammation with specific nutrients can go along way in helping people with the disease feel better. Here are some suggestions that help relieve the inflammation quite substantially – **(1) Black tea theaflavins** can help turn off specific genes in your DNA that express inflammatory cytokines. **(2) Curcumin** is a compound found in *tumeric*. It has been shown to inhibit the effects of the master inflammatory molecule, called NF-kappaB. **(3) Omega-3 polyunsaturated fat**s have been shown to inhibit cyclooxygenase-2, an enzyme used to produce powerful pro-inflammatorys prostaglandins. *(J Rheumatol Suppl. 2005 Aug; 75:6-21)*

General Dosage Range For Supplements Concerning FMS and CFS

<u>**Multi-Vitamin/Mineral supplement:**</u> **can be purchased in powder formulas or in capsules. Take as directed per label use or instructed by health care physician.**

<u>**SAM-e**</u> **– 400-1200mgs daily in dived dosages**

<u>**Melatonin:**</u> **.03 - 3mgs**

<u>**D-Ribose**</u> **– 5 grams**

<u>**Chlorella**</u> **-1 to 3gms**

<u>**CoQ 10 w/ Shijalit**</u> **- 100-300mgs**

<u>**Acetyl-L-Carnitine**</u> **-1000 to 2000mgs**

<u>**Vitamin D**</u> **– 5000 to 8000 iu's daily, depending on blood test results**

<u>**Omega 3**</u> **–**

<u>**Probiotics**</u> **– per label instructions**

<u>**Super Dismutase (SOD)**</u> **– as per label instructions**

<u>**Vitamins A, C, E, and Zinc**</u> **– normally found in anti-oxidant formulas, take as per label instruction.**

<u>**B Complex Vitamins**</u> **– 50 -100mgs strength**

NADH – 5-20mg daily in dived dosages

DHEA -15 – 25 for women and 25 – 75 for men

5-HTP – 50 – 200mg

Fish Oils – 1400mg/day of EPA and 1000mg/day of DHA

Plant derived SOD blend – including SODzyme and GliSodin: 2,100mg daily
Creatine – 1.25 grams

Safety Concerns

Fish oils – If you are taking anti coagulating medication or aspirin, consult with your physician, as fish oils taken long term can thin your blood.

Melatonin – do not use if you have asthma or if you've been diagnosed with auto-immune disease.

D-Ribose – this product may lower blood glucose, consult your doctor or other health care practitioner if you are taking glucose lowering medication.

Curcumin – do not take this product if you have gallbladder or gallstones. If you are taking anti coagulants or anti platelet medications, or have a bleeding disorder, consult with your health care physician first.

Creatine – people with kidney dysfunction should avoid creating supplements

Vitamin D – do not exceed more than 10,000 iu's a day unless recommended by your phsician. Vitamin is also not recommended with people who have kidney disease, or hyperparathyroidism or sarcoidosis and those who use cardiac glycosides(digoxin) or thiazides diuretics should consult with their physician before using vitamin D.

Following Blood Tests That Provide Helpful Information

- Vitamin D (25-hydroxy) assesses vitamin D status
- Omega Score – assesses the blood fatty acid profile
- Red Blood Cell (RBC) magnesium: assesses blood magnesium levels
- Female Panel/Male Panel – for identifying hormonal insufficiencies
- DHEA – (available in male & female panels)

Additional Healing Methods To Explore in Healing FMS and CFS

Vitamin C Saturation* - Other areas to explore in the natural healing of FMS and CFS that has worked before that may seem a bit too easy for some is called "saturation therapy with vitamin C" used along with the use of calcium/magnesium supplements.

For some that have FMS/CFS it has been one of the most effective therapies for relieving the symptoms of FMS/CFS. The safety and the effectiveness of large amounts of vitamin C are well established. Large doses of vitamin C have exceptional pain relieving and even mood lifting properties.

Since the time mega-scorbate therapy was first introduced in the late 1940's by Dr. Fred R. Klenner, MD, and up to today as used by Robert Cathcart, MD, there is a surprising safe track record. Vitamin C is far more safer than any drug, period.

Magnesium Potassium Aspartate*** - with up to almost 10 million Americans that suffer from fibromyalgia and chronic fatigue syndrome, with the most common listed complaint in the doctors office being fatigue, lack of energy and pain. Magnesium potassium aspartate was first developed in 1957-1958 by Dr. Hans Neiper, a brilliant German physician and medical researcher that has cured thousands degenerative diseases worldwide. Recognized for his work at top cancer research centers, including the prestigous "Sloan-Kettering Institute for Cancer Research in New York,, and through his extensive clinical experiences, Dr. Nieper has both developed and established a line of alternative, non-toxic substances that are less stressful to the immune system. His motivation for developing this product was his revelation that cells of the female breasts on becoming cancerous lose magnesium.

Dr. Nieper thought why not conceive a mineral transport system to correct the magnesium deficiency in these cells and stimulate the immune system. His development of magnesium potassium aspartate became successful world wide as a substance for the protection of cardiac tissue destruction and arrest, enhancement of liver functions, and the detoxification of digitalis. And its been said that potassium magnesium aspartate also decreases the death rate from heart attacks.

It has been found to be effective for the relief of fatigue and lack of energy attributed to a variety of origins. In both uncontrolled and double-blind studies totaling nearly 3,000 patients, 75-91% experienced pronounced relief of fatigue with supplements of potassium and magnesium aspartate. By just using one gram(1,000mgs=1gram) of each, in divided dosages, a beneficial effect was usually noted after 4 to 5 days, but sometimes 10 days were required.. Usually patients continued treatment for 4-6 weeks and most patients continued to do well after supplementation was discontinued. *(Hicks, J. "Treatment of Fatigue in General Practice: A Double-Blind Study', Clin. Med., Jan., 1964. 85-90)*

In his book, "The Doctors' Vitamin and Mineral Encyclopedia," Dr. Sheldon Saul Hendler writes, "The primordial oceans on this planet were rich in magnesium and potassium. Sodium rules the seas today, but the waters within our cells remains true to the "primordial soup" from which all life arose, rich in magnesium and potassium. Optimal health depends upon the maintenance of this condition."

Magnesium is required for ATP synthesis and is a co-factor of more than 300 enzymatic reactions involving energy metabolism. A magnesium deficiency can result in muscle weakness, muscle fatigue, lack of coordination, loss of appetite and depression. Researchers at the University of Southamptom in the United kingdom recently reported that patients suffering from CFS have low blood levels of magnesium and supplementation improves their energy levels and moods.

Magnesium is not a trace mineral but a major entity in the body, and is absolutely essential for life. Most of it is in the bones and intracellular fluids. It is also necessary for every major biological process including the metabolism of glucose, production of cellular energy and the synthesis of nucleic acids (RNA) and proteins. It is also interesting to note that a magnesium deficiency are the same as those associated in CFS and FM. And it is no wonder that many people with FM and CFS do very well with magnesium supplementation.

Aspartic Acid and "ATP": Energy Production

Aspartic acid, a non essential amino acid, pays a vital role in in energy metabolism. It activates formation of specific enzymes that in turn increase ATP(adenosine triphosphate) production resulting in more energy and more oxygen in the blood. Increasing the formation of "ATP" is one of the *__most important factors in over coming muscular fatigue__*. As a potassium or magnesium salt, it is useful in physiological cellular function. Intracellulary, aspartic acid is converted into oxaloacetate, an important substrate in the Krebs Cycle where food is converted into energy. It is also a carrier molecule for the transport of potassium and magnesium into the cell, as well as an excitatory neurotransmitter in the central nervous system. CFS/FM may result from lowered cellular energy due to low levels of aspartic acid.

Protects and Detoxifies the Liver by Removing Ammonia

Dr. Neiper explains: "Chronic liver inflammation can also cause excessive production of ammonia which further damages the liver as well as intellectual capacity. Therefore, excessive ammonia must also be eliminated. This can be accomplished by supplying potassium-magnesium-aspartate, which causes more ammonia to used in urea synthesis and thus be eliminated via kidneys. This principle, by the way, was discovered by my friends Laborit and Weher in Paris in 1958. Fatigue is a common complaint with liver complaints.

Fatigue Syndromes

Fatigue syndromes of all kinds are particularly responsive to Potassium-Magnesium-Aspartate therapy. Magnesium levels have been reported to be low in all CFS suffers. Sevberal studies have shown that regardless of the cause of fatigue, Potassium-Magnesium-Aspartate provides substantial benefit in the prevention of fatigue with the additional benefit of being able to reverse it in 80% or more of cases. Usually one gram is taken twice per day. Additionally, a deficiency of **L-Carnitine** has been seen in some CFS sufferers. _One gram of L-Carnitine three times a day has led to improvement in CFS symptoms in recent investigations. Results have been reported within 1 to two weeks._ Dr. Nieper has often prescribed these two substances together. (*__References - F. Nagle and colleagues of the FAA Oficce of Aerospace Medicine 1963;63-12;1-10__*)

According to researcher and author Earl Mindell, aspartic acid increases stamina and endurance in athletes, and has become popular among endurance athletes. { **Gaby, A.R.,"Aspartic Acid salts and fatigue",** *Curr. Nutr. Thera.,* **Nov. 1982**}

Potassium and Energy

Magnesium also enhances the transport of potassium into cells. Malaise is properly the most common symptom off chronic potassium deficiency and muscular weakness is almost always noticed. Potassium is important for healthy nervous system and a regular heart rhythm. It aids in the proper muscle contraction and works with sodium to control the body's water balance. It is also important for chemical reactions within the cells and aids in transmitting electrochemical impulses. It also regulates the transfer of nutrients to the cells. {**Somer, Elizabeth, The Essential Guide To Vitamins and Minerals, Second edition, Harper-Collins, NY, NY 1990**}

NOTE: Potassium magnesium aspartate is also associated with improving the <u>adrenal stress tolerance</u>, lowering blood pressure, reversing arrhythmias, increasing muscular endurance, and encouraging sounder sleep.

FYI: Potassium-Magnesium-Aspartate -[**United States Patent Office; Patented Nov. 21, 1961:(3,009,859)** *Potassium Aspartate and Magnesium Aspartate Fatigue-Recovery Promoting Process and Composition*s]

<u>**Note: See also Magnesium and Malic Acid**</u>***

<u>**Calcium and Magnesium Supplementation**</u>* even around rather low RDA levels (about 1,000mgs of calcium and about 400mgs magnesium daily, in divided dosages) can make a big difference in muscle health and happiness. A deficiency in either mineral can cause tetany, or muscle spasm, among other symptoms. General to moderate exercise can help also, so start slowly and work your way up gradually. Yoga stretches and walking are also two good ways to begin as well. *(reference – "Doctor Yourself" A Natural Healing That Works" by Andrew Saul, Ph.D)*

The other effective way that has been employed by many with crippling diseases is *"Vegetable Juicing".* The effects one gets from fresh vegetable juice is often found to be very invigorating. Juicing with fresh vegetables and fruits are one of the fastest ways to optimal health and recovery from disease, period!

I would recommend to purchase the many books on juicing for simple recipes that you can enjoy the many health benefits. Live raw foods have wonderful healing affects and are a quick way to feel energized and healthy! *(Recommended reading - "Juice Fasting & Detoxification" by Steve Meyerowitz). Excellent manufacturers are Jarrow, Life Extension, Solgar, country Life, Twin Labs.*

<u>**Acetyl-L-Carnitine**</u> (ALC) -* One of the most <u>essential substances for the mitochondria cells</u> to produce energy and in the export of toxic waste materials from cells. It has also been found to be low in patients with CFS and FM. Because fatigue is a hallmark of FM and CFS, it seems logical to suppose that ALC supplementation, can improve cellular energy levels in those with CFS/FM. Based on all the current studies and ALC's important functions in the body with energy production and fat metabolism

(triglycerides), it can a vital and necessary step in healing the symptoms of CFS and FM.

(References - "Amantadine and L-Carnitine treatment of Chronic Fatigue Syndrome". Plioplys AV, Plioplys S., CFS Syndrome Center, Department of Research, Mercy Hospital, Chicago, Ill 60616, USA, Neuropsycholbiology, 1997;35(1):16-23)

- *"Carnitine is essential for the mitochondria energy production. Disturbances in the mitochondria function may contribute to cause fatigue seen in CFS patients. Previous investigations have reported decreased Carnitine levels in CFS. Orally administered L Carnitine is an effective medicine in treating the fatigue seen in a number of chronical neurological diseases. Amantadine is one of the most effective medicines for treating the fatigue seen in multiple sclerosis patients, isolated reports suggest that it may also be effective in treating CFS patients. Formal investigations of the use of L Carnitine and amantadine for treating CFS have not been previously reported.*

We treated 30 CFS patients in a crossover design comparing L Carnitine and amandatine. Each medicine for two months, with a two week wash out period between medicines. L Carnitine or amatadine was alternately assigned as first medicine. Amantadine was poorly tolerated by the CFS patients. Only 15 were able to complete 8 weeks of treatment, the others had to stop taking the medicine due to side effects. In those individuals who completed the 8 weeks of treatment, there was no statistically significant difference in any of the clinical parameters that were followed. However, with L Carnitine we found statistically significant clinical improvement in 12 of the 18 studied parameters after 8 weeks of treatment. None of the clinical parameter showed any deterioration. The greatest improvement took place between 4 and 8 weeks of L Carnitine treatment. Only 1 patient was unable to complete the 8 weeks of treatment due to diarrhea. L Carnitine is a safe and very well tolerated medicine which improves the clinical status of CFS patients,. In this study, we also analyzed clinical and laboratory correlates of CFS symptomatology and improvement parameters".

Dosage: 500mgs – 2 capsules twice a day equal 2 grams and take for 2 to 3 months, then drop down to 250mgs to 500mgs/day or stop it altogether. ALC is also important to take if you suffer from a Mitral Valve Prolapse and / or elevated triglycerides. L-Carnitine can also be substituted for ALC.

Anti-Inflammatory Agents For FM Pain

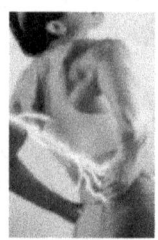

Inflammation is an immune response; a response from infections, irritations, or an injury. Immune cells are called to a localized site within the body through the blood stream. The blood vessels near the site become miraculously permeable and the site becomes very warm and red due to the increased blood flow(warm, hence the inflammation). Inflammation is part of the body's natural defense mechanism against injury and disease, and with FM its a constant state of chronic pain that never goes away called chronic inflammation.

Today modern medicine is starting to admit that chronic inflammation is the main contributing factor to all chronic degenerative diseases, and the root cause of the two greatest killers in America: Cancer and Heart disease. Depression, asthma, pancreatitis, Parkinson's, Lupus, anemnia, kidney failure, psoriasis, Fibromyalgia, and fibrosis, might just be the start suspected diseases that have a root cause of chronic inflammation. Beyond of what you eat, you should be careful about how you live: diet and lifestyle are two separate things. When the body is loaded with toxins, it can respond only in one way: chronic inflammation. Smoking, pesticides, cleaning chemicals, allergens, dust, contaminants, herbicides all contribute to toxic overload just as much as nutritional deficiencies do.

Pathogens, as we've already seen cause infections that lead to inflammation. We've already discussed stealth viruses, but there are many more pathogens (parasites, bacteria, and yeast) that are also contributing. If you don't get enough sleep, your IL-6 markers can go thru the roof. If you are on drugs, anti-biotics steroids, birth control pills, they are killing off the good bacteria in your body. Candida can flourish. And don't forget chlorinated water. Anything that kills off good bacteria allows candida to flourish. And finally there is stress, stress eventually leads to depression and depression has been linked to the inflammatory response.*[Licinio J. et al.* "The role of inflammatory mediators in the biology of major depression: central nervous system cytokines modulate the biological substrate of depressive symptoms, regulate stress-responsive systems, and contribute to neurotoxicity and neuroprotection." *Mol Psychiatry, 1999 Jul:4(4):317-27]*

Anthocyanins – are the water soluble flavonoid pigments in fruits and vegetables that help inhibit inflammatory COX-1 and COX-2 enzymes. [British Journal of Sports Medicine, 2006] Fruits such as – black currant, cherries, oranges, raspberries, red currant, acai berries, goji berries, blue berries, cranberries, red grapes, red wine, black berries, and egg plants.

Berries- are wonderful anti-oxidants – raspberries, acai berries, goji berries, blue berries, cran berries, and straw berries are all needed to fight chronic inflammation, and all anti-oxidants are natural anti inflammatory.

Boswellia - a rain forest herb that has shown in clinical studies improvements in patients with osteoarthritis, and rheumatoid arthritis, its active ingredients help to block the production of inflammatory prostaglandin hormones and other inflammatory chemicals.

Butterbar - A plant from the UK and Europe, that has amazing anti inflammatory and anti spasmodic abilities(prevents cramps). Butterbar has shown to treat allergies(hay fever) just as well as prescription medications and may be far superior to traditional allergy medications currently given. An extract of butterbar called "Buterbur Ze339", was just as effective as as Claritin and Tavist with no drowsiness; dosage 50mgs daily with meals. **["Treating intermittent allergic rhinitis: a prospective, randomized, placebo and anti histamine controlled study of Butterbar extract Ze 339."** *Phytotherapy Research Vol. 19, Issue 6.]*

<u>Vitamin C</u> – works best when taken as a vitamin C complex(bioflavonoids, quercitin, rutin, hesperdin), along with vitamin E to reduce inflammation. Daily dosages 1,000 to 2,000mgs to protect cells from inflammation induced damage. (see vitamin C saturation therapy in FM/CFS healing protocol).

<u>Carnosine</u> – can inhibit pathological glycation(the boding of sugars to proteins) reactions in the body which are known to contribute to inflammation. Dosage at least 1,000mgs a day in dived doses, or 300mgs of the European drug aminoguanidine.

<u>Cat's Claw</u> – a potent herb with a long history as a remedy for inflammatory arthritis. Recent cell culture experiment at the Albany Medical College, New york, Studies show that cat's claw inhibits inflammation by blocking the activity of NF-kB.

<u>Curcumin*</u> – found in Tumeric, a spice from India, is also a powerful anti oxidant that is active against a range of bacteria and fungal infections. It is also a powerful liver tonic that can help reduce cholesterol levels and thin the blood as well. It was found in a study at Cornell University that curcumin blocked the activity of Cox-2 effectively. Curcumin is also being used as an anti cancer remedy. Curcumin should not be taken if one is taken blood thinners, or suffers from gallstones or obstructive gallbladder disorder. Daily dosage is 2.8mgs a day.

<u>Ecklonia Cava Extract</u> **(ECE)*****– an important food derived from a specific brown algae found off the coast of Japan and Korea, and is one of the most powerful anti oxidants known, and a powerful anti inflammatory that repairs arteries, lowers blood pressure, removes plaque, and normalizes blood sugar. ECE could very well be the most powerful anti oxidant known in nature, approximately 10 to 100 times more powerful than other polyphenols. Its ORAC score is more than 8,300.

Martin Pall, Ph.D performed some ground breaking research on multiple chemical sensitivity, CFS, FM, PTSD, Gulf War syndrome, and a host of other conditions. Dr. Pall discovered that ECE was immensely potent in reducing the radical scavenging activities of peroxynitrate, the DPPH radical (another potent oxidant), and even reversed oxidized LDL levels. ECE has also extraordinary anti inflammatory properties, and inhibits Angiotensin-converting enzyme (ACE) responsible for high blood presure (Angien leads to constriction of the smooth muscles and arteries, which reduces blood flow and raises blood pressure).

In controlled studies lasting 8 weeks, ECE reduced the time it took FM patients to fall asleep by 47 minutes, increased total night time sleep by 1.6 hrs., improved sound sleep by 80%, boosted energy levels by 71%, reduced pain 31%, reported better days, and general conditions improved by 39%, better brain function and blood flow(brain fog). The results of the study have shown Ecklonia Cava Extract to be an important part of recovery in healing FM/CFS. It was also interesting to note that ECE was effective in helping men recover from erectile dysfunction(ED) and in a 6 month study of 31 men with ED, ECE performed better than Viagra in all parameters (orgasmic function, intercourse satisfaction, overall satisfaction) except for erectile function, which showed ECE equal to Viagra. With side effects reported!

It also bares to note that ECE does not work as quickly as Viagra does, and to get these benefits, ECE must be taken daily for a period of time, however the results are gratifying and worthwhile in the long haul. ECE attributes its effects by improving peripheral blood circulation around muscles and nerves that are involved in sexual function as well as the penile artery. It does this by rejuvenating damaged endothelial cells to produce nitric oxide, increasing dilation of the blood vessels by 50%.

A recent Harvard study at the "Joslin Sachool of Diabetes" directly implicated that ECE compounds have been found to also be potent aldose reductase inhibitors, which may be of benefit for patients with metabolic syndrome, syndrome X, or diabetes. ECE has shown to drop blood sugar levels quickly, and even if you cheat on your diet, blood sugar quickly normalizes.

To date there have been no known toxicities reported with using ECE, it is manufactured from an edible algae, and is considered a food. There are also no known drug interactions with using ECE. One serving of ECE is equivilant to 10 servings of fruits and vegetables
 ECE will be my one of my personal favorite's in battling FM and CFS, the health benefits are just too amazing to not pass up! ECE is normally sold under the name "Seanol". And can be purchased online and also under "Swanson's Vitamins".

Algoran-FS - this is a new formulation using *Ecklonia Bicyclis*, and like all their products , its 98% pure; standardized 25 to 1 extract. To potentiate the product Cordyceps Sinensis (medicinal mushroom) has been added and used for over 2,000 years, and Gynostemma Pentaphylum (or Jiaogulan), another Chinese herb and Huperzine. This formula can help cover and relieve many of the associated symptoms that plague FM/CFS sufferers. From an anti-fatigue, anti-inflammatory effect, increases libido and sexual function, regulates blood lipids, potent anti-oxidant, improves sleep quality by 89 to 95%, fights hypertension, anti-tumor, improves healthy blood sugar levels and insulin response, and increases cellular immunity which is very important in healing and re-establishing a healthy immune system. For purchasing see www.eckloniacava.com or www.mnwp.org/ece/. For further research and information on these extraordinary products please see www.mnwelldir.org/docs/nutrition/ece.htm.

Ecklonia Bicyclis*** does everything listed above that Ecklonia Cava does with one exception; it's actions are targeted, meaning it seems to go where it is needed to do good. Ecklonia Cava has a general effect, while Ecklonia Bicyclis has a targeted effects.

Guaifenesin*** – is a popular expectorant drug usually taken orally either in liquid (syrup) form or in capsules and tablets to assist the bringing up (expectoration) of phlegm from the airways in acute respiratory tract infections. Guaifensin is also sold under many brand names such as – Guai-Aid, GuaiLife, Ethex 208, Humibid, Mucinex, and Robitussin. It is usually included in many other over the counter cough and cold remedy combinations in conjunction with "dextromethorphan" and/or "phenylephrine" and/or "acetaminophen."

Because of its uricosuric (*gout drugs*) effect, guaifenesin was chosen in the 1990's for the experimental Guaifenesin Protocol for Fibromyalgia. Researched heavily by Dr. St. Amand, who claimed that guaifenesin could treat fibromyalgia symptoms by removing excess phosphates from the body, which he believes to be the cause of fibromalgia. According to Dr. St. Amand, he strongly believed that the removal of phosphates would supposedly lead to a reversal of all fibromyalgia symptoms, which would essentially be close to a cure as possible. Dr. St. Amand also claimed that he has successfully reversed all fibroblast symptoms in 90% of his patients.

Additionally, Dr. Amand himself claimed to have had fibromyalgia at one time in his life and has been pain free for decades since his use of Guaifenesin. Given these claims, many people on the mailing list decided to try it.

While some people experienced positive effects from it, and others did not no matter how carefully the treatment plan was followed. This involved avoiding products containing salicylates.

During the 1990's, Dr. Robert Bennet, a recognized expert in the field of fibroblast, decided to do a study on Guaifenesin with the aid of Dr. St. Amand as the technical advisor to the study. The results of the long term study showed that Guaifenesin had no effect on Fibromyalgia. The results of the study revealed Guaifenesin had no effect on fibroblast. It was also determined by Dr. St. Armand that patients included in the study must have unknowingly been exposed to sal, which he believed can block the effects of Guaifenesin. Dr. Bennet countered, by saying that if there were sufficient quantities of low levels of salicylates to block Guaifenesin, then this should have caused a decrease in urinary uric acid. Low levels of salicylates are known to have this effect. But unfortunately the lab tests did not show that this occurred. Thus it was determined by Dr. bennet that there were no such exposure to salicylates, to which later Dr. Bennet went on to say that the Dr. Armands success was due to a placebo effect.

However, contrary to what many doctors and skeptics may say about placebo effects. Additional studies have been done about Guaifenesin since then, and in 1996, medical literature has stated that Guaifenesin can have beneficial effects on skeletal muscle relaxant properties. This was a fact that many people in the fibroblast community were not aware of. It is also listed in the Merck Index, a drug handbook, which lists Guaifenesin as having a muscle relaxant effect. Guaifensin has been also known to have a neurological effect that most doctors in the medical community are unaware of, because it is no longer used in humans for this effect.

However, it is used for this effect in veterinary medicine. And a slightly different form of Guaifenesin called *"Guaifenesin Carbamate"*, is used in humans as a muscle relaxant, and is sold under the name of **"Robaxin."** This may have also been the reason why it helped some people in the study conducted by Dr. St. Armand. Guaifenesin also has pain relieving capabilities and has the ability to act as an anti-coagulant as well. All in all, I believe that Guaifenesin should be mentioned and used as a Fibromyalgia/CFS treatment protocol. The research and medical studies are out there for your information and benefit to be hold, so I do feel that no matter what conflicting studies that may be out there in medical literature. Results are results, and most people that have had Fibromyalgia do swear to its healing effect, and I do believe it warrants mention in this treatment protocol for Fibromyalgia and chronic fatigue. Its worth a try, and if it can help you well then its a go, why miss out on it!

Dosage used: 600mg to 3600mg per day divided into two dosages which was commonly used in case studies. However, dosage may depend on your response and can vary from person to person, hence the wide difference 600mgs to 3600mgs. Your progress of treatment concerning guaifenesin is measured by symptomatic improvement, which involves scanning the body for tender points or spasms in muscles and ligaments. The size and severity of these are then noted and regularly checked till they decrease and disappear altogether.

References & Resources - *("The Truths & Myths of the use of Guaifenesin for Fibromyalgia/ Guaifenesin: One Medicine, Several Effects," by Mark London; 12/05/2010-09:47:42) "excellent article very well worth reading"*

("What Your Doctor may not tell You About Fibromyalgia: The Revolutionary treatment That Can Reverse the Disease" by Dr. St. Armand) (Excellent book & reviews)

("A Randomized, Prospective, 12 Month Study to Compare the Efficacy of Guaifenesin Versus Placebo in the Management of Fibromyalgia"; Robert M. Bennet,MD, Professor of Medicine & Chairman Division of Arthritis & Rheumatic Diseases; Oregon Health Sciences University, Portland, Oregon; Sharon R. Clark, Ph.D., Pual St. Armand, MD.) see www.myalgia.com/guaif2.htm

("The Guaifenesin Guide: For Treating Chronic FATIGUE, Fibromyalgia, & IBS" by Gregory K. Penniston)

Chapter 24

Traditional Medical Treatment For FMS & CFS

"Our way of life is related to our way of death."
Framingham study, Harvard University"

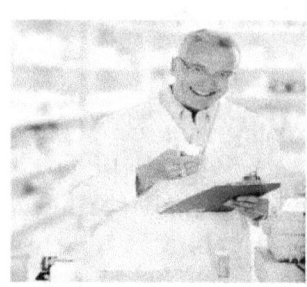

Traditional medical treatments for FMS and CFS have not been very effective, unfortunately. Most of these medicines prescribed have sort of a hit and miss situation, with side effects galore. And with a syndrome or disease that basically affects the entire body and mind, the prescriptions given have creating a whole new set of symptoms for these poor souls that suffer from FMS and CFS. Conventional medical treatment therapies have been ineffective for most FMS patients and no better than taking a sugar pill.

<u>The traditional drugs of choice include a wide range of medicines that include:</u>

- **<u>Anti-Anxiety medications -</u> (benzdiazepines) – Klonopin, Xanax, Ativan, Busbar,Valium, tranene, Serax, Librium, Tegretol, Trileptal, Symbax, Risperdal.**

These are a class of drugs know as benzodiazepines, used for anxiety medication and their usually addicting that patients normally build up a tolerance so that the drug eventually loses it's effectiveness. These medications are loaded with side effects that cause further health problems – depression, fatigue, memory loss, brain fog,, sleep disturbance, mania, agitation, nausea, tinnitus, low blood pressure, edema, ataxia, tremors, sexual dysfunction, asthenia, pro-longed drowsiness, trance like condition that may continue for a number of days, and headaches.

- **<u>Anti-Depressants</u> - (selective serotonin re-uptake inhibitors: SSRIs)** such as **Prozac, Celexia, Paxil, Luvox, Cymbalta, Lyrica,** and **Trazadone, Elavil.**

These type of drugs are of course given for depression as well as help to induce sleep. Anti-depressants help to increase a person's ability to hang on to serotonin, by increasing the brains use of serotonin, which is one of the neurotransmitters in FM patients that have been noted to be deficient in. serotonin deficiency is linked to depression and mood disorders, lowered pain threshold, poor sleep, excessive carbohydrate consumption(cravings) and mental fatigue. Some of these med's do seem to help and the results and improvements vary from person to person. It is also best to avoid prescription tranquilizers, as they often make FMS symptoms worse. **<u>Note:</u>** <u>All SSRI's are partially broken down in the liver and can create liver malfunction in some patients depending on long term use.</u> Those who are using SSRI's should be cautious of taking these types of medication.

According to Dr. Joseph Glenmullen, of Harvard Medical School, recently reported on the many dreadful side effects associated with anti-depressant medications, which include neurological disorders, sexual dysfunction in up to 60% of users, debilitating withdrawal symptoms including (halucinations, dizziness, electric shock-like sensations, nausea, and anxiety) and decreased effectiveness in about 35% of long term users.

(Side effects) such as dry mouth, daytime drowsiness, increased appetite, constipation, withdrawal problems, muscle pain, weakness, changes in sex drive, impotence, low thyroid, low blood sugar, tremors, itching, rash, diarrhea, loss of appetite, dry skin, heart beat irregularities, irritated stomach problems, increased aggression, suicide (prozac) sluggish liver function, and addiction. And many more.

- **<u>Pain medicine</u> - opiods, nonopiod analgesics, Oxycotin, Vicodin, Percosets, Darvocet or Traumadol (Ultram)These medications can be very addictive and impair mental and physical abilities.**

(Side effects) – The most troublesome side effects of pain meds (opiods) is constipation, other side effects are drowsiness, effect on breathing, confusion or delirium, nausea, muscle twitching, serious withdrawal problems, and addiction problem, light headiness, sedation, vomiting, itchiness, and skin rashes.

- **<u>Muscle Relaxants</u> such as Flexeril (cyclobenzaprine), Baclofen, and Zanaflex.** Muscle relaxants can be quite sedating and cause drowsiness, and sometimes used as a sleep aid. However, the side effects include gastritis, fatigue, low blood pressure, can give you that out of touch feeling as well and cause liver damage & failure, nausea, vomiting, blurred vision, speech disorder, constipation, and basically poison!

- **<u>Anti-Convulsants</u> – Lyrica, Gabitril (tiagabine), Neurontin (gabapentin), Topamax.**
These drugs were originally designed to help control seizures. They are now being used to block nerve associated pain (neuralgia) caused by herpes zoster, chronic headaches, and have not been helpful for FMS and CFS. But often cause the same related symptoms that are associated with FMS and CFS. **The side effects** are many that might sound the same as if I were describing the symptoms of FMS and CFS – weakness, fatigue, fluid retention, thought disorder, weight gain, itching, brain fog, back pain, involuntary muscle twitching, tremors, depression, etc.

- **<u>Sleeping medicines</u> – Seraquel, Ambein, Sonata, Restoril.**
Sleep medications are short acting drugs that promote sleep that usually last for 4 to 6 hrs. the problem is that, yes, they can put you to sleep, but eventually your body builds up a tolerance to the drug and you usually wind up either taking more of the drug or continuing on a different stronger kind and/or another type of drug like anti-depressants which help boost the body's serotonin levels to induce sleep, and muscle relaxants (Flexeril) will usually be prescribed along with it as well. Not all are basically bad, there are some effective ones like ambein.

But they have their side effects as well, such as – withdrawal symptoms, fatigue, short term memory loss, hangovers, mood disorders, anxieties, muscle aches and joint pains (you already have-FMS), flu like symptoms, sluggish liver function, dizziness, lack of concentration, dependency problem (addiction), depression, constipation, urinary tract infections, heart palpatations, and upset stomach.

- **Corticoidsterones – Betamethasone(Eelestone), Budesonide(Entocort EC), Cortisone(Cortone), Dexametasone(Decadrone),Medrol dose packs (Melthylprednisone), and Prednisone(Prelone).**

- These drugs have powerful effects and understanding how they work and how they can be safely taken is very important in their use. They are excellent in reducing pain, but do have serious side effects that can be classified as dangerous. Long term use can eventually cause health problems, such as thinning of bones, impairment of wound healing, hypertension, depression of the immune system, and have been noted to cause mental disturbances.

Corticoidsteroids can also create problems with nutritional deficiencies in the rate of enhancing excretion of vitamin C, potassium, and zinc. They can pose a serious threat to the absorption of vitamin D, and cause water retention. One one would be wise if under going cortisone therapy to increase their supply of vitamins and minerals. There are also better and safer natural alternatives which you will discover later by reading this book.

- **Stimulants** – (amphetamines) **Adderall, Conerta, Cylert, Focalin, Ritalin, Metadate.** These drugs are all used to increase adrenalin. They can also be very helpful in increasing a persons energy, but do you remember the saying "speed kills". These drugs are all incredibly hard on the adrenal glands (your stress coping glands), with the exception of "Provigil", And long term use can cause adrenal fatigue or at least and full blown "Addison's disease (adrenal failure at its worst). Provigil – a narcolepsy drug is also being recommended for fatigue in FMS and CFS.

This medication is designed to keep you from falling asleep, and yes, it can wake you up in the morning and make you more alert. However, this drug will interfere with your normal circadian rhythm (sleep wake cycle). That is also the worst thing that you can do is to take a medication that interferes with normal sleep and wake cycles. Anything that will disrupt your normal ability to fall into a deep restful sleep, should be avoided. **(Side Effects from Amphetamines)** - include insomnia(big problem), anxiety, depression, aggression, nervousness, irritability, rapid heart beat, high blood pressure, tourette's syndrome, tics(abnormal muscle movements), headaches, seizures, aplastic anemia, visual disturbances, liver dysfunction,

- **Nonsteroidal Ant-inflammatory drugs (NSAIDs) - Bextra, Mobic, Ibuprofen, Celebrex, Naprosyn, Vioxx (is now banned)**

Long term use of these drugs have been known to cause unwanted side effects – accelerated joint destruction, high blood pressure, intestinal permeability which can lead to more inflammation. These drugs cover up symptoms and don not address the cause, and are not meant for long term use. Memos from the FDA over a study by one of their own scientists, Dr. Graham, who estimated **"Vioxx"** had been associated with more than 27,000 heart attacks or deaths linked to cardiac problems.

Furthermore, NSAIDs have caused 10,000- 20,000 Deaths a year. And a person taken NSAIDs is 7 times more likely to be hospitalized for gastrointestinal adverse effects. The FDA also estimates that 200,000 cases of gastric bleeding occur annually which leads to 10,000 to 20,000 deaths each year!

Some of the anti-depressants like *Cymbalta* may allow fibromyalgia patients to avoid pain med's altogether. Cymbalta acts by increasing brain levels of serotonin along with secondary neurotransmitters, norepinephrine. Clinical studies have also noted that this dual effect reduces chronic muscle pain and although not yet clinically approved by the FDA, it does seem to be very promising though.

IMPORTANT: If you are currently on any medications and don't think you need to be anymore, never stop taking them abruptly; always work with your doctor to taper off. You could face serious reactions if you stop suddenly.

Conclusion:

As you can see from the traditional recommended treatments above that there are many different types of medications used in treating FMS and CFS. Physicians try and make the best choice possible in dealing with the associated symptoms of FMS, and it can become very difficult for them to prescribe the proper medication and the right dose for the right reason. Now physicians are required to prescribe a limited number of drugs, even if another one may be better suited for your particular needs.

Also, you should be well informed and educated of any potential side effects if contemplating medication use of these drugs currently being used for FMS and CFS. As the typical treatment for FMS and CFS does not cure or completely eliminate this dreaded disease/syndrome, and long term use of these medications can cause alternate health problems and conditions on top of suffering from FM and CFS.

Prescription medications offer little little hope, and a study conducted by the Mayo Foundation for Medical Education and Research demonstrated the need for FMS and CFS treatment beyond drug therapy. The studies revealed that medications currently prescribed for FMS and CFS still suffer from the same persistent symptoms as they did years before from the start of the disease and showed little or no change from many of the surveys that were given. In conclusion many of the recommended medications weren't making any significant impact.

I believe that an integrative approach which combines a judicious and limited use of prescription drugs along with nutritional therapy by combining other alternative means, such as a proper nutritional diet, detoxification therapy, lifestyle change, and a supplement protocol offers the best hope in beating and curing FMS and CFS, as laid out in this book.

"Treating the symptoms of disease resolves nothing but treating symptoms itself, when you treat the root cause of the disease", it no longer exists! And that is what we are aiming to do here.

When approached correctively and diligently, a natural and alternative treatment will achieve complete relief from FMS and CFS symptoms. By laying out a well approached plan in getting to the cause of the problem, hence when it all started, and by eliminating certain dietary foods and adapting to a healthy lifestyle of living and proper diet. You can be self assured that fibromyalgia will be a memory of the past and you will be fibro' free once and for all. Below you will see the basic crucial steps that you need to follow and adhere to.

Chapter 25

"Crucial Steps" in Creating Balance and Healing in Reversing FMS & CFS

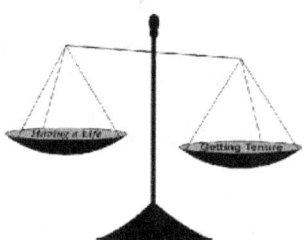

1. **Encourage a Healthy Diet***** – Your master eating plan for your bio-chemistry. Eliminate food allergies, employ a specific dietary protocol and add supplemental *"vitamins/minerals"*, *"enzymes"* and *"probiotics"* for proper absorption and health to prevent malabsorption syndrome. Make it a habit of including therapeutic raw foods at least twice a week, whether through juicing or iin its natural state. Avoid or eliminate junk foods, processed foods, alcohol, smoking, etc. Encourage yourself to lead a balanced and healthy life style!

2. **Do a Whole Body Cleanse & Detoxification Program***** – for chronic viral, myocoplasma, and or bacterial infects (candida albicans/yeast over growths), detox heavy metals, toxins and yeast over growth. Required in assuring complete recovery from FMS and CFS and general health status. (See section on whole body detox program.)

3. **Balance Neurotransmitters***** - restore your neurotransmitters, low serotonin states.

NOTE: SEROTONIN – one of the most important neurotransmitters in healing FMS and CFS helps regulate sleep, digestion, pain, mood, and mental clarity. Serotonin also helps by:

- *Raising the pain threshold* (having less pain), **and by blocking substance-P.**
- Lets you fall asleep fast and stay asleep throughout the night.
- Regulates your moods. "The Happy Hormone" reduces anxiety, carbohydrate cravings, and depression.
- Reduces cravings and over-eating syndrome.
- Increases a person's mental abilities.
- Regulates normal stomach motility (transportation of food-eaten) and reverses

(IBS) irritable bowel syndrome. Surveys also show that as many as 73% of FMS patients have irritable bowel syndrome. There are more serotonin receptors in your intestinal tract than in your brain. And emotional stressful situations can cause the body to release adrenaline, cortisol, and insulin. These stress hormones stimulate the brain to secrete serotonin. Long-term stress and poor dietary habits can deplete the body's serotonin stores.

4. **Balance Hormones (Endocrine)** *** – balancing the hypothalamus, pituitary, thyroid, adrenal, estrogen-progesterone, and testosterone are all vital in restoring the proper hormonal balance back to your body. Your hormones are a direct reflexion of your personality.

5. **Restore Deep Restful Sleeping Patterns***** – *are extremely important* to the complete health of your well being in reversing FMS and CFS. Healthy sleeping patterns is the most opportune time of self healing and revitilization.

NOTE: Studies and surveys have also shown that individuals who were prevented from going into deep sleep for a period of a week develop the same symptoms associated with FMS and CFS; fatigue, diffuse pain, depression, anxiety, irritability, stomach distress, and headaches. Sleep deprivation will also markedly increase inflammatory cytokines (pain causing chemicals) – by a whopping 40%. ***Therefore restoring deep restorative sleep is one one the most important steps in beating/curing FMS/CFS, if not the most important step of all!*** (see sections on sleep/serotonin/substance-P, cytokines and GH).

6. **Stress Management***** – *(One of the main possible causes of FM/CFS)* A big must and necessity in keeping calmness and balance within your delicate hormonal system and your immune system.

NOTE: Over 65% of Fibromygic and Chronic Fatigue people *reported physical and emotional stress as being the major cause or initiating factor in acquiring Fibromyalgia and CFS*. My belief and experience as a Holistic Health Practitioner is that chronic stress and trauma are the underlying "catalyst" for the onset of (HPA) dysfunction in FMS/CFS. As well as Auto-Immune Disorders too. Several studies have many times demonstrated how chronic stress undermines the normal hypothalamic-pituitary-adrenal axis (HPTA) function.

7. **Specific Nutritional Supplement Program***** - by utilizing special and a specific supplement protocol for your required needs in eliminating disease and restoring health is an essential requirement in creating the proper balance in your recovery from FMS and CFS.

8. **Boost Your Immune System***** – Boosting your immune system through high anti-oxidant foods, supplements, and sufficient sleeping patterns, are very important requirements to ward off disease and to keep your immune system functioning in a normal and healthy way.

9. **A Change in Lifestyle***** – Is a necessary essential requirement in playing a

vital part in healthy living. <u>Weekly "**Exercising**" helps to reduce stress levels, boost the immune system, balances hormone levels and helps slow down age related diseases</u>. Including stress mangement techniques like Yoga, Meditation, Tai-Chi, or any other technique that you may like to find relaxing. A Lifestyle change is like setting a healthy course of action in your journey of life, living life as healthy and clean as possible by eating correctly and by avoiding unhealthy substances that destroy and weaken your health. (This is a must concept)

Conclusion

The beauty of the human body of God's great creation, is that God gave us the ability within to heal virtually all diseases known to man. Once you realize that the human body always strives to heal itself through the wonderful laws of Nature and the Universe. We all have the ability to heal whatsoever afflicts us, given the proper mind set and diet. The body will do the rest.

Man created drugs and chemicals, nature created raw healing foods that nourish us to live and be fruitful. It is a concept that we as humans have lost sight of. Everything that grows in nature is meant for our capability to survive. In the beginning, God created the heavens and all that exists on earth, pristine land, vegetation, oxygen giving trees, plants, humans, and animals. Everything we need to live, survive, eat and flourish is provided for us, and that includes food as our medicine to cure illness and disease.

We just have to revert back to our natural ways by eliminating un-natural elements from our diet and well being. Disease will dissipate and eventually run its course as the body will always strives to heal itself, given of course the proper rest, foods, and mind set.

RESOURCES & REFERENCES

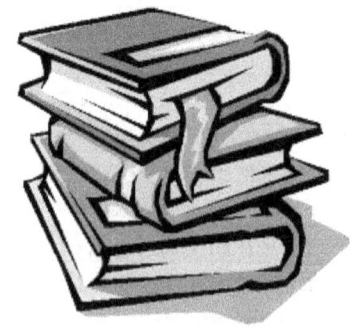

RECOMENDED BOOKS FOR READING

"Bee Pollen, Royal Jelly, Propolis, and Honey", by Rita Elkins, M.A.
"The Longevity Solution: Stabilized Royal Jelly" by Dr. Cass Ingram, DO
"The pH Miracle: Balance Your Diet, Reclaim Your Health" by Robert O. Young
"The Diet Cure" by Julia Ross, M.A.
"Barry Sears, Ph. D., "The Zone Diet"

"The Anti-Aging Manual: The Encyclopedia of Natural Health" by Joseph B. Marion

"Renewal: The Revolutionary AntiAging Manual" by Timothy J. Smith

"The Right Dose: How To Take Vitamins & Minerals Safely" Patricia Hausman

"The Omega-3 Miracle" Gary Gordan, M.D.

***_"The Colostrum: Life's First Food" " Daniel G. Clark, M.D._

***_"The Colostrum miracle: The Anti-Aging Super Food that Can Boost Immunity & prevent Premature Aging" by the editors of the doctors' living magazine._

"The New Truth About Vitamins & Minerals" Bill Sardi

"What Your Doctor May Not tell You About Fibromyalgia Fatigue" R. Paul St. Amand, M.D.

"From fatigued To Fantastic" Jacob Teitelbaum

***_"Super foods: The Food & Medicine" David Wolfe._

*** _"Natural Healing Foods" by Pamela Young._

"The Official Anti-Aging Revolution: Stop The Clock, Time Is On your Side" Ronald klatz

"Brain Boosters" Potter & Orfali

"Breakthrough Cures: revolutionary Answers to the deadlist Diseases" richard deandrea & John Wood

Susan Somers, "Bombshell: Explosive medical Secrets"

"From Hormone Hell To Hormone Well" Genie James & Randolph, Jr.

"The Miracle of Bio-identical Hormones" Michael Platt

"Anti-Aging Cures: Life Changing Secrets To Reverse the Effects of Aging" Dr. James Forsythe

"Foods that help Win the Battle Against Fibromylagia" Deirdre Rawlings

"Eat to treat Fibromyalgia" Kristie Leong

"Auto-Immune The Cause & The Cure" Annesse Brockley

The Phytogenic Hormone Solution" Saundra Koke

"Cure Your Auto-Immune & Inflammation" Gregory Barton

Dr. John Lee's "Hormone Balance Made Simple" John R. Lee

"Balance Your Hormones Balance Your Life" Claudia Welch

"Solved The Riddle of Illness" Stephen E. Langer

"Permanently Beat Hypothyroid Naturally" Caroline D. Greene

"Alternative Cures" Bill Gottlieb

"Glutathionine" Carl Rowe

"Tired of Being Sick & Tired" Michael Berglund

"Are You tired & Wired?" Marcelle Pick

"The 25-Hour Pharmacist" Suzy Cohen

"Super Immunity: The Essential Nutritional Guide for Boosting Your Body's Defenses to Live Longer, Stronger, and Disease Free" Joel Fuhrman.

"Feeling fat, Fuzzy, or Frazzled?" richard shames

"Everything You Need to Know About Enzymes" Tom Bohagar

"The Inflammation Syndrome" Jack Challem

"The Anti Inflammation Zone" Barry Sears

"The Auto-Immune Epidemic" Donna Jackson

"Living Well With Auto-Immune Disease" Mary J. Shomon

"The Real Cause The Real Cure" Bill Gottlieb

"Natural remedies For Chronic Fatigue" Michael Massie

"Fibromyalgia Basics" Pati Chandler

***"Could It Be B12?: An Epidemic of Misdiagnosis" -the underground classic that has saved lives, by Sally M. Pacholok, R.N., B.S.N. - Jeffrey J. Stuart, D.O.

"The Candida Cure" Ann Boroch

"Real Food: What To eat & Why" Nina Pianck

"Pain free 1-2-3: A Proven Program for Eliminating Chronic Pain Now" Jacob Teitelbaum

"Thyroid Power" Richard Shames

"Living Well With hypothyroidism" Mary J. Shomon

***"Adrenal Fatigue: The 21st Century Stress Syndrome" James L. Wilson

"The Endocrine System Overview" Susan Hiller-Sturhofel

"I'm Not In The Mood" Judith Reichman, M.D.

"Adaptogens: Herbs for Strength, Stamina & Stress Relief" David Winston

"15 Chronic Illnesses & Their Treatments" James M. Lowrance

"Healthy Sex drive, Healthy You" Diana Hoppe

"Aphrodisiacs: Proven Sex Boosters" Tony Xhudo, M.sc., H.N./B.C.

"Sex Drive solution For Women" Jennifer M.D. Landa

"The Ultimate Guide To Enhancing Your Sex Life For Men & Women" Tony Xhudo M.Sc., H.N./B.C.

"Incredible Sex (52 Brilliant Ideas)" Marcelle Perks

"The Sexy Years: Discover the Hormone Connection: The Secret to Fabulous Sex, Great Health, and Vitality, for Women & Men" Suzanne Somers

"Diagnosing and Treating Common nutritional Deficiencies" James Lowrance

"Pregnenolone: The Super Hormone" Billie J. Sahley

"Thyroid Diseases, Conditions, Auto-immunity and Cancers" James L. Lowrance

"Thyroid Disorders and Treatments: Underactive and Overactive Glands" James L. Lowrance

"Figuring Out Fibromyalgia: Current Science and The Most Effective Treatments" Ginerva Liptan.

"Yoga For Fibromylagia" Shoosh Lettick Crotzer

"Reversing Fibromyalgia : The Whole Health Approach to Overcoming Fibromyalgia Through Nutrition, Exercise, Supplements and Other Lifestyle Factors" Dr. Joe M. Elrod.

"Leaky Gut Syndrome" Elizabeth Lipski

"One Cause Many Ailments: Leaky Gut Syndrome: What it is & how it may be Affecting Your Health" John O. A. Pagano. D.C.

"Increased Intestinal Permeability aka Leaky Gut Syndrome: The Science of Achieving Digestive Health" Case Adams.

"Digestive Wellness: Strengthen the Immune System & Prevent Disease Through Healthy Digestion" Elizabeth Lipski.

***"I Was poisoned By My Body: The Odyessy of a Doctor Who Reversed Fibromyalgia, Leaky Gut Syndrome, and Multiple Chemical Sensitivity – Naturally!" Gloria Gilbere.

"Toxic Overload: A Doctor's Plan for Combating the Illnesses Caused by Chemicals in Our Foods, Our Homes, and Our Medicine Cabinets" Paula Baillie-Hamilton.

"The Blood Sugar Solution: The Ultra healthy program for Losing Weight, Preventing Disease, and Feeling Great Now" Mark Hyman.

"Clean: The Revolutionary Program to Restore the Body's Natural Ability to Heal Itself" Alejandro Junger.

"Toxic Relief: Restore health & energy through fasting & detoxification' by Don Colbert.
"Stress management for Dummies" Allen Elkin.
"The Ultimate Stress Relief Plan for Women" Stephanie McClellan, M. D.
"Time Alternative Medicine: Your Guide to Stress relief, Healing, Nutrition and More" Jeff Kluger.
***"The Relaxation and Stress Reduction Workbook (New harbinger Self-help Workbook) " Martha Davis.
***"Handbook of Stress Medicine and Health" Cary Cooper.\

REFERENCES & SELECTED STUDIES

(Endocrine Abstracts, 2011- 26 P225). GH supplementation remains a valuable option in those who suffer from fibromyalgia and chronic fatigue.

(Endocrine Abstracts, 2011- 26 P225)

(Kremer JM, Lawrence DA, Petrillow GF, et al. Effects of high dose fish oil on rheumatoid arthritis after stopping nonsteroidal anti-inflammatory drugs. Arthritis Rheum 1995;38:1107-14)

References – (Faigin, Rob. Natural Hormonal Enhancement. Extique Publishing: Cedar Mountain, NC. 2000.)

(Jamieson, James and Dr. L.E. Dorman. Growth Hormone: Reversing Human Aging Naturally. Published by J. Jamieson: St. Louis, MO, 1997)
(Brand-Miller, Jennie, et al. The New Glucose Revolution. Marlowe & Company: New York, 2003)

(HGH Magazine). www.hghmagazine.com. "Fiber helps manage HGH, Insulin, and Cholesterol." "Potassium and HGH – What your doctor does Not tell you." "Whey protein Supercharges HGH Supplements."

References & Sources - (A randomized, double-blind, placebo-controlled study of growth hormone in the treatment of Fibromyalgia; AM J Med. 1998 Mar.;104(3):227-31; Bennet RM, Clark SC, Walczyk J. department of Medicine, Oregon Health University, Portland 97201, USA

"Superfoods: The Food & Medicine of the Future" by David Wolfe.

"Grow Young with HGH: The Amazing Medically Proven Plan to Reverse Aging" & "The Official Anti-Aging Revolution" by Dr. Ronald Klatz.

"BombShell" by Suzanne Somers

Anti-Aging Cures: Life Changing Secrets To Reverse The Effects of Aging" by Dr. James Forsythe

"Younger Sexier You" by Dr. Eric Baverman

"Your Secret to the Fountain of Youth: What They Don't Want You To know About HGH: Human Growth Hormone" by Dr. James W Forsythe

"Growth Hormone: The Methusalah Factor" By James Jamieson

Chinese traditional herbal Medicine Vol II. "by Michael tierra, L. Ac., O.M.D., AHG and Lesley Tierra, AHG (Lotus Press, 1998), www.tibetgojiberry.com

"Chinese Tonic Herbs" by Ron Teeguarden (Japan Publications, 1984)

[Ceda GP, Ceresini G, Dentil L, Marazini G, Piovani E, Banchini A, Tarditi E, Valenti G. alpha-Glycerylphosphorylcholine administration increases GH response to GHRH of young and elderly subjects Horm Metab Res. 1992 March;24(3):119-21. Chair of Gerontology and Geriatrics, University of Parma, Italy.]

[Choline Info.org]

[L-Dopa Stimulates Release of Hypothalamic Growth Hormone-Releasing Hormone in Humans; KAZUO CHIHARA, YOICHI KASHIO, TETSUYA KITA, YASUHIKO OKIMURA, HIDESUKE KAJI, HIROMI ABE AND TAKUO FUJITA]

References – (Faigin, Rob. Natural Hormonal Enhancement. Extique Publishing: Cedar Mountain, NC. 2000.)

(Jamieson, James and Dr. L.E. Dorman. Growth Hormone: Reversing Human Aging Naturally. Published by J. Jamieson: St. Louis, MO, 1997)
(Brand-Miller, Jennie, et al. The New Glucose Revolution. Marlowe & Company: New York, 2003)

(HGH Magazine). www.hghmagazine.com. "Fiber helps manage HGH, Insulin, and Cholesterol." "Potassium and HGH – What your doctor does Not tell you." "Whey protein Supercharges HGH Supplements."

[References – Natural products inhibitors of the enzyme acetylcholinesterase;Brazilian Journal of Pharmacology;10/26/05;16(2):258-285, Abr./jun. 2006 ; Revisao Jose M] - (PMID: 8206111, PMID:3093909, PMID: 1677361)

References & Resources - Goji Berries – *Yu MS, Leung SK, Lai SW, et al (2005). Neuroprotective effects of anti-aging oriental medicine Lycium barbarum against beta-amyloid peptide neurotoxicity. Exp. Gerontol. 40 (8-9): 716-727.*

Gan L, Hua Zhang S Laing Yang X, Bi Xu H (April 2004). "Immunomodulation and anti-tumor activity by a polysaccaride-protein complex from Lycium barbarum". Int. Immunopharmacol. 4 (4): 563-569.

Department of Pathophysiological, Beijing Medical university, Beijing China; Sheng Li Xue Bao. 1998 June; 5093): 309-14.

Cancer Instiute, Ningxia Medical College, Yinchuan, China;Zhong Xi Yi Jie. 1991 Oct. 11,(10):611-2, 582.

Laboratory of Neurodegenerative Diseases, Department of Anatomy, The University of Hong Kong, Hong kong.Exp gerontal. 2005 August-Sept; 40(8-9): 716-27.

Antioxidant Research Group, Faculty of Health and Social Sciences, The Hong Kong Polytechnic University, Kowloon, Hong Kong SAR, China. Br J Nutr. 2005 Jan; 93(1) 123-30.
[References – Life Extension Foundation/Heath Article; Fibromyalgia and Obesity Link; Ursini 2011]

(Reference – Akiko Okifuji, Gary W. Donaldson, Lynn Barack, Perry G. Fine. Relationship Between Fibromyalgia and Obesity in Pain, Function, Mood and Sleep. *The Journal of Pain*, 2010; 11 (12): 1329 DOI: 10.1016/ j.jipain.2010.03.006)

[References – Life Extension Foundation/Heath Article; Fibromyalgia and Obesity Link;Ursini 2011]

- References – (Regleson, W., et al. 1994, DHEA –"The Mother Steroid")
- (Baschetti, R. 1995, chronic fatigue and licorice (letter)

(References -*Liberman, J., et al; Mood, performance & pain sensitivity: changes induced by food constituents. J. Psychiat. Res., 17(2): 135-145, 11982-83), (Braverman, E., R, Pfeiffer, C., C. :Suicide and biochemistry. Biol. Psych., 20: 123124, 1985.) (American Journal of Medicine, Nov.20, 1987, Vol. 83, supp.5A.)*

(Clinical rheumatol. 2009 Apr;28(4):365-9. Doi: 10.1007/s 10067-009-1093. Epub 2009 Jan 23.)

(Chronic fatigue syndrome, Fibromyalgia, Lupus, Rheumatoid Arthritis, Scleroderma, MCS: the mercury connection. B. Windham, (ED.) 2009).

(ATSDR MMGs and ToxFAQs; Anon 1993;Who 1998; CIS 1999; Roberts 1999; Dupler 2001;Ferner 2001)

[Acupuncture Electro res. 1996 Apr-jun, 21(2):133-60, Omura Y, Shimotsuura Y, Fukuoka A, Fkuoka H, Nomoto T]

The Food Pharmacy by Jean Carper 1997 ISBN 0-671-71502-X Simon & Schuster Australia)

(Reference -Fluoride: The Aging factor, Dr. John Yiamoyuiannis, Ph.D)

(Dr. Larry Clapp, Ph.D. In "Prostate Health in 90 Days")

[Ref' – Artical; Fish Oil For Fibromyalgia and Chronic Fatigue Syndrome; Dr. Roger Murphee, Feb. 24, 2012]

[Lancet 341:49:1993, American Journal of Physiology, 258; 603: 1990, and the Annals of Allergy, 1990],

(Additional Resources "Indican Test"- "Pizzorno, J., Murray, M. textbook of Natural Medicine. 2nd ed. New York, Churchhill. 1999; p 245-246) -(Todd J. Clinical diagnosis and management by laboratory methods. Philadelphia, PA: WB Saunders. 1979: p 592-593)

(References- "Worls Review of Nutrition and Dietetics"; Cereal Grains: Humanity's Double Edged Sword; Loren Cordain;199(PDF) (Vitamin Research Product: Lectins; Carolyn Pierini)
(Weston A. Price Foundation: Be Kind To Your Grains; Sally Fallon and Mary G. Enig; Jan. 2000)

(References and Resources)
(Leaky Gut Syndrome, Professor Keith Scott Murphy)
(Leaky Gut Syndrome: A Modern Epidemic Part I & II, Jake Paul Fratkin, OMD)
(Leaky Gut Syndrome: The Internal Terrorist – Gloria Gilbere)
(Leaky Gut Syndrome: Breaking The Vicious Cycle – Dr. Leo Gallard)

(Sources & References – CNR, Center for Nutritional Research; Colostrum & Auto-Immune Disorders; John Balmier, MS; www.icnr.org)

("The Colostrum Miracle" and "Colostrum Life's First Food" by Daniel G. Clark, M.D.)

(Henderson D. (2000) Colostrum: Nature's Healing Miracle. CNR Publications, Sedona, Arizona)

[References – Henderson D., Mitchell D., Colostrum – Nature's Healing Miracle, CNR Publications, Salt Lake City, UT. 1999.]
[Walker M, "The Benefits of Bovine Colostrum", Health Products Business, April, 1999.]

[Rona Z., "Bovine Colostrum emerges as immunity modulator". Alternative Health Directory, Vancouver, BC.,Canada.]

[Burke E, "Athletes; Have You Heard About Colostrum?", health Journal, Vol. II,

No. 13: July 21,1999]

[Klatz R., Kahn C., Grow Young with HGH, Harper Collins, New york, NY, 1997.]

(References- Jacobsen S, Danneskiold-Samsoe B, Anderson RB. Oral SAM-e (S-adenosylmethionine) in primary fibromyalgia. Double blind clinical evaluation. Scand J Rheumatol. 20.4 (1991): 294-302 – Tavoni A, Vitali C, Bombardi S, Pasero G. Evaluation of S-adenosylmethionine in primary fibroblast. A double-blind cross-over study. Am J med. 83.5A (1987)(: 107-110)

(References -Liberman, J., et al; Mood, performance & pain sensitivity: changes induced by food constituents. J. Psychiat. Res., 17(2): 135-145, 11982-83), (Braverman, E., R, Pfeiffer, C., C. :Suicide and biochemistry. Biol. Psych., 20: 123124, 1985.)

(The Journal of International Medical Research;1992; 20:182 – 1189)

(Ref- Dr. Ralph Heinicke, Xeronine and Cell Regeneration; Noni Juice, Xeronine, Damnacanthal & Scientific Studies), (Fairchild, Diana, Noni:Aspirin of The Ancients, Hawaii: Flyana Rhyme, 1998)

Recommended reading - "Superfoods: The Food and Medicine of The Future" by David Wolfe and "A Physician's Guide To Natural Health Products That Work" by James A. Howenstine.

(Ref - "A Physician's Guide to Natural Health Products That Work"- 2009, Dr.Ralph Heineke)
(References, Oz, M, MD & Roizen, M, MD, Authors of You: Being Beautiful, "Call Ribose One of the Decade's 'real Nutritional Heroes'. "PR Newswire. 2009. HighBeam research.(Dec. 14, 2009)
(Teitelbaum JE, Johnson C, St Cyr J. The use of D-Ribose in chronic fatigue syndrome and Fibromyalgia: a pilot study, J Altern Complementary Med. 2006 Nov. 12 (9):857-62).

(Teitelbaum JE, Johnson C, St Cyr J. The use of D-Ribose in chronic fatigue syndrome and Fibromyalgia: a pilot study, J Altern Complementary Med. 2006 Nov. 12 (9):857-62).

(Suraj P Agarwal, Phytotherapy Research, Volume 21, Issue 5, pages 401-405, May 2007)

(Key Reference Sources – Dr. Hans Nieper:"Silk Worm Enzymes for Carotid Artery Blockage") see also writings and experimental work employing serrapeptase supplementation to promote cardiovascular health information from the Nieper Foundation archive at the Brewer Science Library in Wisconsin (www.mwt.net/drbrwer/cardio.htm)

- ["Enzymes & Enzyme Therapy: How To Jump Start Your Way To life Long Good Health"] by Antony J. Cichoke, D.C.

- www.answers.com/topic/enzyme
- Dr. William Wong. "What Are Systemic Enzymes & What Do They Do?
- www.serrapeptase.info/
- www.staytuned.ws/systemic_enzymes.html
- http://en.wikipedia.org/wiki/Enzyme

(Ref- Bounous G, Molson J.: Med Hypotheses. 1999 Oct;53(4):347-9 – Glutathione Precursors, the Immune System and Chronic Fatigue)

(Ref' Anja Morris-Paxton M.Dip.Herb BS (USA) M.Sc. (PAN) M.A.(UK)

(Source reference: Jan A, et al "Serum 25-hydroxy vitamin D levels in patients with Fibromyalgia" BSR 2012; Abstract 231.

(Source reference: Jan A, et al "Serum 25-hydroxy vitamin D levels in patients with Fibromyalgia" BSR 2012; Abstract 231.

(Resources- "The Vitamin D Solution: CFS/FM"; CFS pages 4,12,67; FMS pages 4, 6, 12, 65-68) -("The Vitamin D Cure: Chronic Pain & FM", page133-136) - ("The Power of Vitamin D", page 25-34) – ("Vitamin D Prescription":FM on pages 4, 20, 23,80-84, 171, 185, 198-199) and see also www.vitamindwiki.com – the most vitamin D information on the web!

(Pharmacotherapy. 2004 Nov;24(11): 16446-8).

(J Rheumatol Suppl. 2005 Aug; 75:6-21)

(Hicks, J. "Treatment of Fatigue in General Practice: A Double-Blind Study', Clin. Med., Jan., 1964. 85-90)
(References - F. Nagle and colleagues of the FAA Oficce of Aerospace Medicine 1963;63-12;1-10)
{ Gaby, A.R.,"Aspartic Acid salts and fatigue", *Curr. Nutr. Thera.*, Nov. 1982}

{Somer, Elizabeth, The Essential Guide To Vitamins and Minerals, Second edition, Harper-Collins, NY, NY 1990}

<u>FYI</u>: *Potassium-Magnesium-Aspartate -[United States Patent Office; Patented Nov. 21, 1961:(3,009,859) Potassium Aspartate and Magnesium Aspartate Fatigue-Recovery Promoting Process and Compositions]*

(Source – "Doctor Yourself" A Natural Healing That Works" by Andrew Saul, Ph.D)

(Recommended reading - "Juice Fasting & Detoxification" by Steve Meyerowitz). Excellent manufacturers are Jarrow, Life Extension, Solgar, country Life, Twin Labs.

(References - "Amantadine and L-Carnitine treatment of Chronic Fatigue Syndrome." Plioplys AV, Plioplys S., CFS Syndrome Center, Department of Research, Mercy Hospital, Chicago, Ill 60616, USA, Neuropsycholbiology, 1997;35(1):16-23)

Mol Psychiatry, 1999 Jul:4(4):317-27]

["Treating intermittent allergic rhinitis: a prospective, randomized, placebo and anti histamine controlled study of Butterbar extract Ze 339." Phytotherapy Research Vol. 19, Issue 6.]

(References & Resources – Anon: Foods interacting with MAOI inhibitors. Med Lett. Drug Ther. 1989; 31:11-12)

(Brown CS & Bryant SG: Monoamine oxidase inhibitors: safety and efficiacy issues. Drug Intell. Clinical Pharmacy 1988; 22:232-235)

(Da prada M, Zurcher G, Wuthrich I et al: On tyramine, food, bevarges and the reversable MAO inhibitor moclobemide. J. Neural Transm. 1988; 26(Suppl):31-56)

Drs. Staroscik et al., Molecular Immunology; Bovine Colostrum's PRPs ability to regulate activity of the immune system, and hormones of the thymus gland; Allergies & Auto-Immune disease.

Playford RJ. (1999) Bovine colostrum is a health food supplement which prevents NSAIDs induced gut damage. Gut 44(5): 653-8.

Henderson D. (2000) Colostrum: Nature's Healing Miracle, CNR publications, Sedona, AZ.

"Colostrum: Life's First Food – The Ultimate Anti-aging Weight-Loss and Immune Supplement": Daniel G. Clark, MD., Kaye Wyatt.

"The Colostrum Miracle: The Anti-aging S Immunity & prevent Premature Aging": The Editors of The Doctors' prescription for Healthy Living magazine.

Goronzy JJ, Weyand CM. The innate and adaptive immune systems. In: Goldman L, Ausiello D, eds. Cecil Medicine. 23Rd ed. Philadelphia, Pa: Saunders Elsevier; 2007: chap 42.

Ghosh S, Vestrgaard, M, Pedersen, O, Serjrsen, K. (2007) Biological activity of bovine milk on proliferation of human intestinal cells. Journal of Dairy research 74(1):58-65. Bovine milk contains a number of biological that affect growth development of human intestinal tissue. The degree of activity depended on the stage of lactation.

Drs. Tortora, Funke & Cast; Microbiology "Clinical studies show that IgE (Immunoglobulin), found in bovine colostrum, may be responsible for regulating *allergic response."*

Ebina, T., et al., "Treatment of multiple sclerosis with anti-measles cow colostrum. "Med Microbiol Immunol (Berl), 1984; 173(2):87-93.

Lamoureux, G. et al., Transfer Factor of Proline-rich Polypeptides from Bovine Colostrum: A clinical and immunological study of the effects of transfer factor on multiple sclerosis. Clin Exp Immunol. 1981 March; 43(3): 667-564.

Also please read for further interesting information concerning diet and auto-immune diseases the book by Dr. Fuhrman titled "Eat To Live."

Ransberger K: Enzyme treatment in comparison with immune complex diseases. Arthritis Rheuma 1986; 8: 16-9.

Ransberger K., Van Scaik W: Enzyme therapy in multiple sclerosis. Der Kassenarzt 1986;41: 42-5

Murray, MT, Pizzorno J: Encyclopedia of Natural Medicine 2nd ed. Prime Publishing, Rocklin, CA; 1998.

Biochemistry, Mary Campell, Ph.D., and Shawn Farrel, Ph.D.; Jan 23, 2011 National institute of Health: Proteolytic Enzymes

"Enzymes – A Drug of The Future", Prof. Heinrich Wrba MD and Otto Pecher MD.

"Enzyme Nutrition: The Food Enzyme Concept" by Dr. Edward Howell

FIBROMYLAGIA/CFS RESOURCES

AFSA-"The American Fibromyalgia Syndrome Association, Inc." - www.afsafund.org/resource.htm

NFA -"National Fibromyalgia Association" www.fmaware.org

"Fibro Pharmacy" - www.fibropharmacy.com

Directory of Fibromyalgia Health Care Professionals -

Fibromyalgia Protocols

Fibromyalgia Resources on WebMD

Fibromyalgia Treatment Center
Mededia

"Fibromyalgia Solutions – www.fibromylagia-solutions.com/resources.html

Fibromyalgia Support - "World's Largest Fibromyalgia Site" - www.fibromyalgiasupport.com

National Institute of Health – www.nih.gov

National Sleep Foundation – www.sleepfoundation.org

Institute of Functional Medicine (IFM) – www.functionalmedicine.org *800-854-3402*

The American Association of Naturopthic Physicians (AANP) – *www.naturopathic.org* *(This organization can help you find a naturopathic physician in your area.)*

The American Chiropratic Association (ACA) – *www.acatoday.com* *(Many chripractors have a strong nutritional background on herbs carry physician-only formulas as well as other certified supplements. Chiropractors will also know which physicians practice alternative medicine)*

The Broda O. Barnes, MD Research Foundation Inc. - *www.brodabarnes.org* *(great resource for thyroid information)*

Clinical Pharmacology – *www.clinicalpharmacology.com (a great reference for clinicians on medications and herbals)*

The American Holistic Health Association (AHHA) – *www.ahha.org*

The American Holistic Medical Association (AHMA) – *www.holisticmedicine.org*

Professional Referral Network – *www.healthreferral.com*

Council for Responsible Nutrition (CRN) – *www.crnusa.org*

Alternative Medicine Network – *www.altmednetwork.net*

Health resource – *www.thehealthresource.com*

OTHER HELPFUL WEB SITES

www.antiagingdoctor.com***
www.drrodgermurphee.com
www.curezone.com***
www.prohealth.com
www.homeopathyandmore.com
www.herbdoctor.com ***
www.preventdisease.com
www.co-cure.com***
www.diagnose-me.com***
www.icnr.org/home-page/colostrum-a-autoimmune-disorder.html

www.lef.org
www.life-enthusiast.com
www.chineseherbacademy.org

LABS & TESTING

ZRT Laboratory -www.zrtlab.com (Comprehensive Hormone Profile Tests for at home saliva & blood-spot tests that you can order yourself without a doctor. Measures your dhea, cortisol, testosterone, estrogen, and thyroid, among others. Easy reports to follow and read which can be submitted to your doctor. 866-600-1636

Life Extension Foundation -www.lef.org/goodhealth 888-884-3666

Aeron LifeCycles – www.eron.com 800-631-7900

EnteroLab.com – 972-686-6869 – Specializing in stool testing for gluten and other food sensitivities, and gastrointestinal disorders.

ARL – Analytical Research Labs, inc. - (Hair Analysis Test) www.arltma.com 602-995-1580

TESTING FOR NUTRITIONAL DEFICIENCIES

Cristiana Paul, MS (Nutritionist) -www.cristianapaul.com

ARL – Analytical Research Labs, inc. - (Hair Analysis Test) www.arltma.com 602-995-1580.

Nutritional Test Descriptions – www.nutritionaltest.com
(a good site that covers testing for nutrition, digestive, hormones, and toxic metals and minerals)

The Right Diagnoses From Health Grades. (www.rightdiagnosis.com)

PRODUCTS & SUPPLEMENTS

Redmond Realsalt – ww.realsalt.com
Gourmet Salts -www.seasalt.com

Allergy Research Group -www.allergyresearchgroup.com (quality supplements)
Country Life – www.countrylife.com *(quality supplements)*
Enzymedica – www.enzymedica.com *(very good line of supplements catered to specific health illnesses)*
Enzymatic Therapy – www.enzymatictherapy.com
Garden of Life – www.gardenoflife.com
Jarrow – www.jarrow.com
Life Enhancement – www.lifeenhancement.com

Life Extension Foundation – www.lifeextension.com
Natural Factors – www.naturalfactors.com
Nature's Made – www.naturemade.com
Nature's Way – www.naturesway.com
Solgar – www.solgar.com
Solary – www.solary.com
Physician Formulas – www.physicianformulas.com
Swanson Health Products – www.swansonvitamins.com *(huge selection of quality products at a great price)*
Thompson Research, Inc. - www.thompsons.com

www.ingramcontent.com/pod-product-compliance
Lightning Source LLC
Chambersburg PA
CBHW080243290526
45790CB00005B/1684